HOME TREATMENT *for* ACUTE MENTAL DISORDERS

HOME TREATMENT *for* ACUTE MENTAL DISORDERS

An Alternative to Hospitalization

David S. Heath, MB, ChB, FRCPC

MT

Published in 2005 by
Routledge
270 Madison Avenue
New York, NY 10016
www.routledge-ny.com

Published in Great Britain by
Routledge
2 Park Square
Milton Park, Abington
Oxon OX14 4RN
www.routledge.co.uk

Copyright © 2005 by Taylor & Francis Group, a Division of T&F Informa.
Routledge is an imprint of the Taylor & Francis Group.

Printed in the United States of America on acid-free paper.

10 9 8 7 6 5 4 3 2

Library of Congress Cataloging-in-Publication Data
  Heath, David S.
    Home treatment for acute mental disorders : an alternative to hospitalization /
David S. Heath.
      p. cm.
    Includes bibliographical references and index.
    ISBN 0-415-93408-7 (hardback : alk. paper)
    1. Mobile emergency mental health services. 2. Crisis intervention (Mental health
services) 3. Home-based mental health services. 4. Mentally ill—Home care.
[DNLM: 1. Home Care Services. 2. Mental Disorders—therapy. 3. Crisis
Intervention—methods. 4. Mobile Health Units. WM 35 H438p 2004] I. Title.

  RC480.6.H438 2005
  362.2'4—dc22   2005006595

6/15/09

Contents

v

Acknowledgments

I want to begin by thanking three people who got me started in mobile crisis home treatment. First is Canadian psychiatrist Dr. Fred Fenton, whose book on his landmark Montreal Study first gave me the idea. Second is ex-Director of Psychiatric Services at Grand River Hospital, Kitchener, Ontario, psychiatrist Dr. David Barnes, who certainly created "an environment that tolerates risk taking." Third is social worker James Holland, the first manager of the Hazelglen Program, the first mobile crisis home treatment service in Canada, who ably translated our ideas into practice and provided strong leadership.

This book would never have gotten past the first two chapters if Brunner-Routledge editors Toby Wahl and Bernadette Cappelle had not recognized the need for a book on an uncommon subject. They were able to take my original idea and mould it into a much more interesting form. Paula Hendsbee edited my first two chapters for the proposal.

Much of what I know about treating patients in Mobil Crisis Home Treatment I have learned from the Hazelglen staff. For many evenings we met in a book group summarizing their experience, skills, and knowledge into a format suitable for a book. For that I thank Cathy Beebe, Maura Campbell, Colleen Cranch, Subaida Hanifa, Pauline Potzold, Glennis Yantzi, and psychiatrist Jim O'Doherty.

The current manager of Hazelglen, social worker Fred Wagner, has shared his experience and knowledge of community treatment and has given his time generously to review the manuscript.

Homewood Health Centre librarian Joyce Pharoah and her staff have provided invaluable help obtaining articles. For computer help I thank Joyce Effinger, Alan Stones, Alex Heath, and Diane Shelton; Janice Kutasinski provided secretarial help.

I thank Trish Stiles, Dr. George Awad, and Dr. Anysia Rusak for help with editing.

Many people have been very hospitable and did their best to make my site visits worthwhile. They have been refreshingly frank and open in our discussions. I thank:

In the USA:

Edgar Wiggins and the staff of Baltimore Crisis Response, Inc.

In Canada:

Liz Howey and Dennis Rodrigue of the Acute Home Treatment Program, Victoria, B.C.

Dr. Guinhawa, Fyfe Bahrey, and the staff of the Acute Adult Psychiatric Home Support Team, Edmonton, Alberta.

In Britain, my entry into British home treatment was through psychologist Bruce Cohen's website. Bruce is now a Marie Curie Research Fellow at the Humboldt Universitat in Berlin, but was conducting research at the Bradford Home Treatment Service when I met him. He introduced me to Neil Brimblecombe—author of *Acute Mental Health Care in the Community: Intensive Home Treatment* and to Sarah Orme, who was a Research Fellow in the Psychology Division of the University of Wolverhampton (who, with Bruce Cohen, has contributed to Neil's book). Neil is now Nurse Advisor/Clinical Governance Coordinator for the West Herts Community NHS Trust. These people have been extremely generous, providing me with material I would never have been able to get on my own, and helping me to find my way about home treatment services in Britain.

I thank manager Fiona Winstanley of the Manchester Home Option Service and her staff; Professor Sashidharan and his Ladywood Home Treatment Team in North Birmingham; psychiatrist Geraldine O'Sullivan, and manager Sue Smith and staff at the St. Albans Community Treatment Team, and manager Kirt Hunte and his staff at the South Camden Crisis Response and Resolution Team.

I had very useful meetings with psychiatrist Marcellino Smyth in North Birmingham and psychiatrist John Hoult at South Camden. Dr. Hoult has been very influential in developing MCHT programs in Australia and Britain and generously shared his material with me.

I thank Professor Lorenzo Burti and Dr. Lasalvia for my stimulating and informative visit to the South Verona Community Psychiatric Service in Italy.

Finally, I thank my sister Susan Haine and her husband, John, for their hospitality during my British visit and, for her patience, my wife Frances.

Foreword

"There's no place like home . . ." Dorothy chants as she clicks together the red ruby slippers and hopes for magic transportation back to her home. In this 1939 movie classic, based on L. Frank Baum's novel, *The Wizard of Oz,* Dorothy desperately seeks the peace, comfort, and safety of the Midwestern farm home from which she came. The story begins as the young Dorothy character becomes frustrated with the conventions of the farm and seeks adventure through running away. Not unlike the course of an unstable mental illness as it unravels, she encounters many unconventional thrills, risks, and perils along the way. In Oz she makes new friends, many are actually existing companions from Kansas, but experienced in distorted ways.

Although these bizarre experiences are later explained away as a disturbing dream, and not a psychotic state, her experiences are perhaps not unlike the experience of unstable mental illness. She experiences distortions in reality not unlike hallucinations. A further similarity is the chemically induced sedation from the poppy fields that surround Emerald City. These have the unwelcome effect of slowing down her journey. Despite this and other obstacles encountered along her journey, she remains persistent in her intent to get to the wizard who she believes can help her return to the safety and comfort of her home.

Ultimately, Dorothy finds the wizard, and he does have the knowledge, skills, and ability to take her home. The wizard character is not unlike the mental health professional who helps to facilitate a journey from psychosis to stability. The wizard, who is initially on a bit of a grandiose and distant pedestal, only becomes helpful to Dorothy once he is brought down from the pedestal (by Toto, the little dog) and is able to interact with her more directly and honestly.

There are many reasons for choosing and emphasizing *Home* as we consider and put into contemporary context this significant work of David Heath. *Home Treatment for Acute Mental Disorders* is published at a time of acute psychiatric care crisis in the United States and elsewhere. The high and increasing cost of institutional and in-patient care has been the focus of attention and rationale for decreased access to in-patient care as well as decreased length of stay. Our historic paradigm which considers asylums to be the bedrock of security for the safe management of acute psychiatric illness continues to be challenged, yet providers, professionals, and bureaucracies have been reluctant to broadly accept alternatives to in-patient care.

My goal in presenting this preface is twofold. First I hope to frame *Home Treatment for Acute Mental Disorders* in the contemporary mental health service delivery era in which is it published. My second goal is to create an anticipation and excitement so that the reader jumps into the book ready to absorb, reckon with, and then make some positive action steps in the transformation of his/her own local mental health service system.

Through *Home Treatment for Acute Mental Disorders,* Dr. Heath helps to promote a shift toward a more contemporary and humane model of in-home or community treatment that is influenced but not necessarily driven by cost. Psychiatric home care is presented as a service that is supported by science and positive outcomes and is a preferred service by many in need of acute psychiatric care. This work combines international research on home care and mobile crisis units with the real experience of several comparable home or mobile crisis services to produce what is virtually a complete tool kit for Mobile Crisis Home Treatment (MCHT).

Never before in history have we known more about the management of acute mental illness. Our professional forefathers could only imagine the contemporary medications we now use. We have access to a host of evidence-based services, including MCHT, which have been demonstrated to humanely promote opportunities for successful recovery in the lives of those with mental illness.

Living in Charlottesville, Virginia, for the last 18 years and within the shadows of the homes of four early American presidents and thought leaders for over 18 years has resulted in the development of a personal appreciation for history. Albemarle County in central Virginia is the home of Thomas Jefferson as well as James Monroe. A bit north of Albemarle County is the home of James Madison, and further north, toward Washington D.C., is Mount Vernon, the home of George Washington. A bit toward the east, Williamsburg, Virginia, is the site of America's oldest public asylum, which was opened in 1773. While the American timeframe is short compared with the long and rich histories of most other countries, this 200-year timeframe encompasses a period that is relevant to the development of mental health services as we know them today.

Imagine having a family member with a mental illness in 1804. You are married to a sea merchant and this ill family member is your 18-year-old eldest son, who has a significant role in your family's sustenance through maintaining the family garden and tending to the livestock while your husband is at sea. Although he has always been a bit unusual and standoffish with outsiders, he has been a consistent, dedicated son, and also a provider for you and his three younger sisters while your husband is away. Your son develops the idea that the village constable has been possessed by a demon and has a plot to hire certain villagers to kill the members of your family. Furthermore, the only way to stop this constable is to communicate directly with the Queen. Initially, he only periodically talks of this; however, progressively over the last several days he has become irritable and preoccupied with scheduling an audience with the Queen. Eventually he assaults a villager who he believes is studying his movements to plan his murder. You know there are rumors that your son himself might be doing the devil's work. Residence in an asylum is suggested; however, this is out of the question financially for your family and he remains in a local jail for over a year, eventually dying of untreated tuberculosis.

The actual treatment options for the same clinical situation 100 years later in 1904 would not likely be considerably different. One area of significant advance by 1904 would be greater thought and attention to the idea that some mental defects represented patterns of disease, some of which could be treated. By this time in the U.S. there was a fairly clearly defined responsibility for state government in the funding and provision of institutional care for persons with mental illness and mental retardation. Good institutional care was clearly seen as state of the art.

A principal advocate for state operated asylums in the U.S. was Dorethea Dix. Her advocacy for a strong role for state government was based on her numerous visits to locally operated alms houses, jails, and other institutions throughout the East Coast. She was generally appalled by the state of most of these institutions. The unsanitary conditions not infrequently included poorly or unclothed individuals in cages or cells with unclean straw and dirt floors. She spared no detail in describing these wretched conditions in her written published accountings of these institutional tours. Locally operated institutions, she concluded, generally did not have consistent capacity either to fund or manage these institutions. She advocated for larger, more central government entities to assume this responsibility. Dix also spent time as a nurse working in military hospitals in the American Civil War and grew to value the benefits of military structure, order, and discipline as a part of the treatment of mental illness. She maintained that many mental cases could be cured through exposure to a stable clean environment. This early 20ᵗʰ century military influence shaped the design and structure of large asylums throughout much of the 20ᵗʰ century.

Another 50 years forward, 1954, puts us squarely into the era of peak institutionalization. At this time, your son in the original case scenario depicted above would have been much more likely to have been referred to an asylum as his paranoid delusions progressed. In an institution, ideally, he would have received counseling, structure, and a clean environment designed to promote sanity. This generally would have resulted in long stays in a large institution. Medications were used, but the medications of this era were generally non-specific and primarily served to sedate and tranquilize behavior. Many dramatic interventions were attempted, including insulin shock, cold wraps, straight jackets, and others.

The institutions of this era had a treatment and public safety mission. They were what today we might call a center of excellence. They contained experienced if not expert staff and offered management economies of scale that could not be achieved in local or smaller settings. There was still great professional debate regarding the ability of proper psychotherapy to cure or at least mitigate many of the symptoms of most mental illnesses. There was no clear consensus as to the cause of the most severe mental illnesses, but with the development and hope proffered by psychoanalysis at this time there was increased attention to families of origin, early circumstances, and traumas as causal in the development of major mental illnesses.

The next 20 years included the development of new medications and the accompanying hope that biological interventions could address at least some of the symptoms of our most severe mental illnesses. Many of the medications developed in this era had side effects that are extremely difficult to live with over time; however, they were effective in the control of many features of psychosis and depression and did enable many, for the first time, to realistically plan for life outside an institution. Over time, there became a progressive need for individuals to receive treatment in their own communities, if only as a temporizing measure until re-admission to an institution could occur. As the need for community mental health services continued to grow, services including case management, crisis intervention, and psychosocial support programs were developed. Gradually, there was increasing experience with the management of unstable illnesses in community settings. Institutional length of stay for some was reduced from years and decades to months and weeks. Still, institutions for the most part were the benchmark against which no care or community care was compared.

It is not uncommon to hear reference to this institutional-based era of the mid-20th century almost as if it were the good old days. For professionals, and probably particularly psychiatrists, there is a kind of familiarity and comfort with the vision of the orderly and controlled environment that is theoretically offered by an ideally funded and managed institution. By comparison, the often chaotic realities of community life can seem unwieldy and unmanageable. (That is, a controlled environment vs. an uncontrolled one.) Most contemporary mental health stakeholders know that the day-to-day realities of many institutions were often far from their originally idealized vision. Clearly there is a place for longer-term and intensive hospitalizations for some individuals with very treatment resistant illnesses who cannot live safely in a community.

A host of developments have occurred within the last quarter century that have had a dramatic impact on the lives of persons with mental illness. Never before in history have we known more about mental illnesses and never before have we had the tools that we now have to facilitate treatment and recovery. These new tools have enabled thousands of individuals to live safely in community settings.

While 20 years ago there was considerable debate regarding the cause of many mental disorders, we now know that many of the most seriously disabling illnesses have a clear biologic and genetic basis. We have new medications that offer significant advances in terms of long-term tolerability and physical safety compared with medications that were available 25 years ago. We have an array of services that are supported by science and are designed to provide support and to promote independence and self reliance in community settings.

In 2002, President George W. Bush appointed a commission to conduct a thorough review of mental health services and to make recommendations for the enhancement of mental health service delivery in the U.S. Presidential mental health commissions are not common occurrences in the U.S., the last one having been a quarter of a century earlier and appointed by then-President Jimmy Carter. Roslyn Carter, the wife of President Carter, was the chairman of the Carter Commission. One of her remarks to the recent Bush New Freedom Commission was that a central difference between the commissions was that in 2002 there now exists a genuine hope and real potential for recovery, enabled by these new tools, that was not present even 25 years ago.

The two greatest challenges that lie before us as we begin this new century of mental health services include translating what we know so that all persons with mental illnesses have access to quality services that promote safe and productive lives and maintaining a focused research agenda that finds better ways to promote resilience, recovery, and even cure. The capacity to translate what is known in contemporary literature into practical, applied services is increasingly referred to as shortening the science-to-service gap.

In 2004, we know a great deal about what mental illnesses are and what it takes to provide a person with opportunities and tools to pursue a safe and productive life in their community. With *Home Treatment for Acute Mental Disorders,* Dr. Heath provides a wonderful compendium of the international science and the practical application of a level of care that many have been fortunate enough to participate in. Indeed, for most of us, there is no place like home; home is where the heart is and where we want to be, with properly trained natural and professional supports, as needed. Dr. Heath has made a wonderful contribution to our field with the writing of this book, and it is my hope that you will be inspired, motivated, and stimulated to look at your local services for opportunities to positively transform them such that more individuals have greater access to quality evidence-based services and tools that facilitate safe and productive lives. Psychiatric home treatment presents a level of service that resonates with the contemporary vision of the federal Substance Abuse and Mental Health Services Administration (SAMHSA): A life in the Community for Everyone.

Anita S. Everett, M.D.
Senior Medical Advisor
SAMHSA
Community Psychiatrist
Johns Hopkins University
Baltimore MD

Preface

In the 1980s I was the medical director of a general hospital psychiatric unit serving two medium, sized cities and the surrounding rural area, in south western Ontario. It was clearly too small for the size of the steadily growing population. Insufficient beds meant that acutely ill patients had to wait a dangerously long time to be admitted; our waiting list just kept getting longer and longer.

The provincial Ministry of Health policy was clear: no more funding for hospital beds—only funding for community programs. There was no clear solution in sight.

It was with great interest therefore, that in 1982 I read a review of "Home and Hospital Psychiatric Treatment" by psychiatrist Fred Fenton and his home treatment team at the Montreal General Hospital (Coates, 1982): "*The results are clear and consistent. Home treatment emerges as a safe, acceptable, effective, economic alternative to hospital care for all three diagnostic groups* [schizophrenia, affective psychosis, depressive neurosis]." Fenton's study (Fenton, Tessier, & Struening, 1982) is one of the five most respected studies comparing home treatment to hospital treatment.

Apart from reducing pressure on beds, Fenton's home treatment model appeared to have other advantages for our clinical population. Many patients balked at the prospect of admission to a psychiatric ward and would plaintively ask "Can't I just come in during the day?" We have a large population of recent immigrants from many different countries, for which hospital treatment was sometimes not a good fit. Many speak little or no English and a psychiatric ward could seem a rather alien place for them— unable to communicate, away from their customary food and families, which were often large and supportive.

We also have a large rural Anabaptist population: Amish and Old Order Mennonites, who eschew modern life—sometimes even government health insurance; they travel by horse and buggy, have very conservative attitudes, and don't want their family members exposed to such things as television and radio. Treatment at home would seem ideal for some of them; they have large close-knit families and a strong belief in mutual community support.

Based on Fenton's research, our home treatment program, called the Hazelglen Program, eventually opened in 1989. The results have been consistent with the research findings in Fenton's and others' studies; in other words, we have been able to treat many acutely ill patients at home, who would otherwise have needed admission, and almost all patients and families have preferred it to hospital.

Today, the same factors that spurred us to develop home treatment continue to fuel interest in community-based alternatives to hospital, and they fall into three broad categories. One is the lack of access to adequate in-patient treatment. In this era of managed care, reduction of hospital beds, and liberal mental health laws, patients cannot always get admitted to hospital when they need it; in-patient treatment they receive is sometimes inadequate, and they may be discharged prematurely without sufficient supports. "*This trend* [of in-patient beds closing], *might not be so troubling if we had a more viable system of care in the community. . . . However, the system in most places in the U.S. is not really there,*" stated Ronald Manderscheid, chief of the Survey and Analysis Branch of the Division of State and Community Systems in the federal government's Centre for Mental Health Services. (Lipton, 2001)

Another is the demand for out-of-hospital care from patients, families, advocacy groups, and legislators, (Wood & Carr, 1998), (Bazelon Centre for Mental Health Law, 2003).

A third factor is the recognition by mental health professionals that community-based treatment can have advantages beyond saving beds and cutting costs, especially for particular clinical populations—two other examples illustrate: patients with first episode psychosis (Fitzgerald & Kulkarni, 1998), and Black and south Asian consumers in Britain (Department of Health, 2000).

But which out-of-hospital alternative should be developed—and how should it be implemented?

In this book, I argue that short-term, mobile, intensive treatment in the patient's home with staff available 24 hours a day is emerging as the most versatile and effective alternative to hospital and is applicable to a broad range of patients with acute mental disorders who would otherwise need admission.

More than a dozen terms exist for this treatment model, presenting an author with a quandary: which one to use? In the U.S., the name for this model can be any of "mobile crisis treatment" (Zealberg & Santos, 1996)," mobile outreach service" (Gillig, 1995), "mobile psychiatric crisis intervention" (Reding & Raphelson, 1995) "mobile response" (Allen, 1999), "intensive outpatient treatment," or hospital diversion."

In Australia, "community treatment" (Hoult, 1986) is the usual term. In Britain, instead of the word mobile, "home" is used—as in "intensive home treatment" (Brimblecombe, 2001), "home-based acute psychiatric service" (Burns, Beadsmoore, Bhat, Oliver, & Mathers, 1993), and "home based care" (Marks, Connolly, Audini, & Muijen, 1994); other British terms are "crisis resolution service" (Department of Health, 2001), "early intervention service" (Merson, et al., 1992), and "out-of–hours service." Canadian programs are called "psychiatric home support," "acute home treatment" (Hibbard, Bahrey, Guinhawa, & Stevenson, 1998), or "mobile outreach."

I have exhaustively listed these synonyms to ensure readers will find a term that they recognize. In the absence of a current universally accepted terminology to describe mental health services, I have arbitrarily coined a combination term—mobile crisis home treatment (MCHT), the meaning of which I hope will be clear to readers on both sides of the Atlantic and will capture the essence of the book.

After seeing the benefits of MCHT for patients and their families firsthand since 1989, and reading about the increasing evidence for its effectiveness, it is gratifying to see that it is finally coming to the attention of national health policy makers. Almost simultaneously, between 1999 and 2002, the governments of the U.S.A., Canada, and Britain issued reports calling for the development and expansion of this type of community-based treatment model. The U.S. Surgeon General's report Mental Health: A Report of the Surgeon General stated: *"Mobile crisis services have developed in many urban areas to prevent hospitalization. . . . This new conceptualiztion of inpatient care and crisis intervention services minimizes the use of hospital resources; however, well-coordinated teams, sufficient community programs, and ready linkages are not widely available"* (Surgeon General, 1999). The Canadian Federal Government's Commission on the Future of Health Care in Canada recommended: *". . .home intervention to assist and support clients when they have an occasional period of disruptive behaviour that poses a threat to themselves or to others and could trigger unnecessary hospitalization"* Romanow, 2002). The Department of Health (2000) has very specific plans for this model: *"By 2004, all people in contact with specialist mental health services will be able to access crisis resolution services at any time. The teams will treat around 100,000 people a year who would otherwise have to be admitted to hospital. . . . Pressure on acute in-patient units will be reduced by 30%.*" The Australian government issued a similar report a decade ago (Commonwealth of Australia, 1992): ". . . *services for those experiencing acute episodes would include. . . community and home-based care.*" MCHT has since become well established in many parts of Australia.

Mobile crisis home treatment can provide an alternative to in-patient treatment for up to two thirds of patients destined for hospital admission and can reduce the length of stay for many others, according to studies reviewed in Chapter 1. All but one of these studies in five countries (and four continents) over the past 40 years have shown it to be less expensive and as effective as hospital treatment for selected patients. Studies find that most patients and their families prefer it to hospital admission.

Despite the widespread international interest in this treatment model, there is no comprehensive guide to establishing such a service. This book aims to fill this gap in the literature. The material in this book derives from four sources: what I have learned as a psychiatrist for 14 years in the Hazelglen MCHT service (which also included setting up a second service in a nearby town); a review of the literature on MCHT; and material developed for workshops on this model presented at Canadian and U.S. psychiatric conferences. Also, between 2001 and 2003, I visited six MCHT services, to learn firsthand how the model actually works in different settings and different countries, and to speak with local experts. Sites included Baltimore in U.S.A., Victoria and Edmonton in Canada, and Birmingham, Manchester, and St. Albans in Britan in Britain. To obtain a different perspective, I also visited the South Verona Community Mental Health Service in Italy.

This model is not wedded to any specific mental health system, and I have endeavoured to adopt an international perspective.

The book is both a review of MCHT and a practical guide to setting up and operating a service. It is divided into two sections. In the first section, the evidence base for MCHT is examined with historical and contemporary analysis. This has practical applications: clinical "pearls" derived from the research are highlighted and, also, knowledge of this research is useful in inducting new staff into the model and philosophy of this approach (McGlynn & Smyth, 1998). This section also describes how MCHT fits into mental health systems, with specific comparison to other hospital alternatives. The 20 components of in-patient treatment are described, followed by a discussion of how MCHT can serve as a substitute for hospital in particular cases. The second section builds on the first by providing principles and instructions to guide the development of an MCHT service. Profiles of seven MCHT services in the U.S., Canada, and Britain illustrate how this model actually works in practice. Its applicability to the treatment of patients with major depression, bipolar affective disorder, first episode psychosis, schizophrenia, postpartum disorders, and borderline personality disorder is demonstrated using case histories.

It is written for anyone who is planning, starting, operating, or working in such a service. It provides sufficiently detailed information to understand the evidence and rationale for MCHT and how it would fit in with the reader's local mental health system, and would enable them to set up a service from scratch. It will help administrators and mental health policy makers and planners to decide whether and how to create and fund such a service. It will be useful for orienting and training new staff, and will be a source for continuing education of current staff. It will therefore be of interest to psychiatrists, psychologists, nurses, social workers, occupational therapists, administrators, and mental health policy makers and planners. It will also be suitable for students of these disciplines with an interest in alternatives to hospital admission. Like most psychiatrists who spend most of their careers working in and around hospitals, I am more comfortable using the term "patient" than "client" so that is the term I use when I write.

Even though this book is about alternatives to hospital, it goes without saying that in-patient treatment is an essential part of any mental health system. At the same time, in a well-functioning system, patients should receive treatment that is not too much and not too little, whose intensity varies responsively according to their fluctuating needs, and is the least disruptive to their lives.

Introduction

'When I use a word, Humpty Dumpty said in a rather scornful tone, it means just what I choose it to mean—neither more nor less.'

—Lewis Carroll, *Through the Looking Glass*

Writing about community-based services is bedevilled with a Babel of labels, often sounding similar. This creates confusion: is the label synonymous for one clearly defined service model, or does it denote discrete sets of service components? (Catty, Burns, & Knapp, 2001).

Because of this, I chose to arbitrarily coin the term "Mobile Crisis Home Treatment." Mobile Crisis Home Treatment is defined as: *An alternative service to in-patient hospital treatment for individuals with acute mental disorders, who would otherwise need admission, offering short-term, intensive home-based treatment, with staff available 24-hours a day, seven days a week.*

CORE CHARACTERISTICS OF MOBILE CRISIS HOME TREATMENT (MODIFIED FROM SMYTH & HOULT, 2000)

- Is available 24 hours a day, 7 days a week
- Allows home visiting
- Allows rapid response
- Is able to spend time flexibly with the patient and their social network, including several visits daily if required
- Addresses the social issues surrounding the crisis from the beginning
- Allows medical staff can see patients in their homes and are available round the clock
- Allows medication to be administered and supervised
- Can provide practical problem solving help

- Is able to provide explanation, advice and support to families and caregivers
- Provides counselling
- Allows service to act as gatekeeper to acute in-patient care
- Allows involvement until the crisis is resolved
- Ensures that patients are linked up to further, continuing care

The confused etymology of community care models makes it difficult to write about them clearly. For example, Breslow (2001), writing about "mobile teams," and, in particular, a service in Britain (Merson, et al. 1992), mentions the terms "mobile crisis teams," "community outreach care," and "community based early intervention team" all in the same breath. Tyrer, a co-author, writes about the same service in a chapter entitled "Maintaining an Emergency Service" in a book on emergency mental health services in the community (Tyrer, 1995). It may seem picayune to pinpoint this use of four terms in a way that implies they are all synonymous, but as Catty, et al. (2001) have pointed out, the lack of an agreed terminology makes comparisons of services in different countries difficult. This has practical relevance when one examines why some studies of "mobile crisis teams" in the U.S. show no evidence of saving beds, whereas, studies of "home treatment" or "crisis resolution teams" in Britain do. Much depends on describing *exactly* what these services do, where and when they do it, for how long, and to whom. This is discussed further in Chapter 1.

To reduce such misunderstanding, and to ensure this book is as clear as it can be, the following is a set of definitions and a description of the anatomy of a typical psychiatric emergency, or crisis, its evolution, temporal course, and the different stages of intervention.

The words "care" and "treatment" are often used synonymously in this book, as in the rest of the mental health literature. "Care" tends to be used when describing the broad range of activities with patients, such as educating and supporting the family, and providing practical help with problems, whereas "treatment" is used more when describing specific therapeutic activities such as psychotherapy and giving medicine.

"Consumer" is meant to indicate a person who is a recipient of psychiatric treatment at times; in the U.K., the term is "user."

"Caregiver" means a family member, or friend who takes some responsibility for helping a patient; in the U.K., the term is "carer."

"Community-based treatment" means treatment provided outside of a hospital.

WHAT IS THE DIFFERENCE BETWEEN MOBILE CRISIS HOME TREATMENT AND ASSERTIVE COMMUNITY TREATMENT ACT?

One term not mentioned so far is assertive community treatment (ACT), with which MCHT is often confused but also shares some characteristics. MCHT is both more than ACT, and less than. More in that MCHT is aimed at a much broader range of psychiatric patients—anybody, in fact, who may end up admitted to a psychiatric ward. ACT, on the other hand, is usually limited to those with the most serious chronic mental illness. Less than, because it is short term, with the limited goal of stabilizing the patient's condition and referring them on. ACT is long term and has broad goals, such as obtaining employment and enhancing quality of life.

The differences between the two are summarized in Table 1 (Sainsbury Centre for Mental Health, 2001).

Table 1

	MCHT	ACT
Length of involvement	Short term, usually 2–4 weeks	Longer term, frequently several years
Patients	Anyone ill enough to be admitted to a psychiatric ward; may have no previous contact with psychiatric services	Have serious chronic mental illness
Referrals	Accepted from ERs, primary care physicians, and patients themselves	Usually require referral from mental health service
Hours of operation	May be 24 hour, or at least provides for some degree of care for patients round the clock	Usually more limited
Service delivery	Rapid response—may be within one hour	Longer response time, especially for patients not previously known to the service
Other	May act as gatekeeper to in-patient beds. Aims to stabilize patient's acute condition	Usually no gatekeeper role Broader goal—e.g., to enhance quality of life, obtain employment

---

SIDEBAR

MCHT and ACT Share the Same Roots

MCHT and ACT share the same roots. In Stein and Test's study (1980) of hospital vs. community-based treatment of patients in an emergency and in need of admission, the subjects entered the study at the same time that they presented at the Mendota Mental Health Institute seeking admission; they were randomly assigned by the admission office staff to hospital treatment or community treatment, and the community treatment team took over their care there and then. The only criteria were that they were residents of Dane County, aged 18–62, and had any psychiatric diagnosis other than severe organic brain syndrome or primary alcoholism. This description of operations sounds similar to MCHT: they were accepted into treatment immediately, and the patients were a broadly defined group—not necessarily limited to those with the most severe and chronic conditions. However, since 1980, the two models of service have evolved differently. Currently, according to recent guides to ACT operation (Stein & Santos, 1998; Allness & Knoedler 1998), ACT is recommended for the seriously and persistently mentally ill "patients in greatest need," not just with any psychiatric diagnosis. Furthermore, the intake process as described is elective and lengthier than an MCHT service accepting a patient in an emergency. Stein and Santos (1998) recommend patients be "taken in at a slow rate," (no more than five to six a month for a new team) because they require a great deal of time and the assessment and treatment planning activities are very time consuming. The issue is further confused by the fact that research studies of MCHT, such as Fenton, Tessier and Struening (1982) and Hoult (1986) were an attempt to replicate Stein and Test's work. But since these studies, ACT has developed into a more specialized service with a narrower focus.

Because Stein and Test's original treatment model can be subsumed under the definition of MCHT, their research study is included in Chapter 1.

WHAT IS A CRISIS?

The "c" word is the cause of much of the confusion in terminology. Tufnell, Bouras, Watson, and Brough (1985), in a paper on a British Crisis Intervention Team wrote, "The term crisis intervention has now become an umbrella covering a range of approaches to psychiatric patients in a wide variety of settings and consequently suffers from a lack of definition." They go on to say, "We describe here the first three years of the work of the Crisis Intervention Team, preferring to discuss the service it provides more in term of *home assessment and treatment* than *crisis intervention,* because of the difficulties of definition already noted in relation to the latter term. We define *an emergency* as an urgent demand for psychiatric intervention in the community." A senior psychiatrist in Britain, very involved with MCHT, implied crisis had become a buzz word: "we have to use the word crisis, in order to get the funding."

Crisis originally referred to a person's reaction to an external stress that overwhelmed him, and the concept was so broad that it likely was intended to embrace far more than the serious acute psychopathology that constitutes today's psychiatric emergency. Caplan (1961) defined crisis as occurring "when a person faces an obstacle to important life goals that is, for a time, insurmountable through the utilization of customary methods of problem solving." However, many psychiatric emergencies can arise in situations where stress may play only a minor role as a precipitant or perhaps none at all. Others include stopping medication, substance abuse, and disturbed brain biology.

Many practitioners likely no longer find the term useful, but accept it as part of the mental health/psychiatric lexicon. It is often used synonymously with psychiatric emergency. The American Psychiatric Association Task Force on Psychiatric Emergency Services produced a report entitled "Report and Recommendations Regarding Psychiatric Emergency and Crisis Services" (Allen, Forster, Zealberg, & Currier, 2002). In this report, they cheerfully use the word crisis numerous times—as in crisis hospitalization, crisis beds, and crisis respite, but understandably avoid defining it. Extensive definitions of psychiatric emergency are provided. We will likely continue to use the word crisis through habit; also, it goes easily with other words—crisis intervention rolls off the tongue easier than psychiatric emergency intervention. In this book, the term crisis is intended to be synonymous with psychiatric emergency, but I suggest narrowing the definition of crisis *intervention.* I think it is important to distinguish this from psychiatric emergency service because it is usually, but not always, a separate step that precedes specialist psychiatric emergency intervention.

WHAT IS A PSYCHIATRIC EMERGENCY?

The first American Psychiatric Association Task Force on psychiatric emergency services (as cited in Allen, et al., 2002) defined an emergency as, "an acute disturbance of thought, mood, behavior or social relationship that requires an immediate intervention as defined by the patient, family, or community." The second Task Force (Allen, et al., 2002) emphasize that *this service domain includes two levels of care; urgent* and *emergency.* They define an emergency as "a set of circumstances in which 1) The behaviour or condition of an individual *is perceived by someone,* often not the defined individual, as having the potential to rapidly eventuate in a catastrophic outcome, and 2) *The resources available to understand and deal with the situation are not available at the time and place of the occurrence.* Thus emergencies frequently involve a *mismatch of needs and resources for which the emergency service must compensate.*

"Central to the concept of an emergency is *the subjective quality,* the unscheduled nature, lack of prior assessment or adequate planning and resultant uncertainty, severity, urgency and conflict or failure of natural or professional supports, all of which contribute to the need for immediate access to a higher level of care."

"*Urgent problems, as opposed to emergencies, can be thought of as situations that have some or all of these features, but where the situation is evolving more slowly, the feared outcome is not imminent and attention can be delayed for a short time.*"

This definition hits the nail on the head. It will help us to understand why, for example, it is so difficult to compare and do research on different services in different locations. "The mismatch of needs and resources for which the emergency service must compensate" can help explain why MCHT appears to have a more positive effect in some settings than others, because the "usual" services, with which it is being compared, vary in quality; hence less "compensation" is required (Burns, et al., 2001).

WHAT DOES "MOBILE" MEAN?

The APA Task Force (Allen, et al., 2002) recognized two broad categories of service—hospital and community-based services; two approaches to providing service—residential and mobile; and two levels of access within each type of service—emergent or urgent (see Table 2). What is rarely clear in descriptions and discussions of emergency services is what "mobile" means. Three aspects of mobility are crucial in this context: *destination*—**where** the emergency service travels to—e.g., to the person's home, or, anywhere on the streets where a disturbed individual happens to be; *time*—at **what stage** in the temporal course of the evolving crisis does it kick into action; and *duration*—how **long** does it remain involved?

Failure to differentiate between these makes it difficult to compare services and draw any conclusions as to their usefulness.

WHAT DOES "OUTREACH" MEAN?

The word "outreach" is rather like the word crisis; the meaning has become so vague as to have lost its purpose. Frequently, it appears to simply mean any service provided where the patient is—in the street, or soup kitchen, or in their home—not in an office or an institution. My own MCHT service is called the Hazelglen *Outreach* Mental Health Service. The term originally had a more specific meaning describing services targeting such people as seriously ill patients who were difficult to engage and unreliable to follow with treatment, such as the homeless. *Collins English Dictionary* (1991) definition captures this more specific meaning "any systematic effort to provide unsolicited and predefined help to groups or individuals deemed to need it," and "propagating take-up of a service by seeking out appropriate people and persuading them to accept what is judged good for them." Engaging people on the fringes of society, such as homeless persons, and successfully providing psychiatric treatment to them takes specialized skills and knowledge, deserving of its own term: I would suggest confining its meaning to that activity.

To help myself understand the various community treatment models, I constructed a figure, "The Anatomy of a Crisis" to illustrate these models and the differences between them. Figure 1: "The Anatomy of a Crisis" illustrates the temporal course of a typical crisis or psychiatric emergency severe enough to warrant hospital admission. This diagram will be used throughout the book in order to illustrate and explain the different community treatment models.

Many clinical scenarios, of course, would appear different on this graphic representation. For example, some patients' crises may develop more acutely; the duration of time before they are admitted may be excessive; and the acuity may increase rapidly between Stages 2 and 5. The figure is simply a schematic representation to help the reader—and myself—understand the differences between community treatment models. The time between the different stages can vary greatly' from a few hours to days—or even weeks.

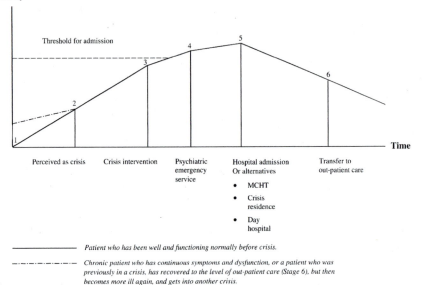

Figure 1 Anatomy of a crisis . . . or evolution and temporal course of a psychiatric emergency.

There are six stages in the typical psychiatric emergency severe enough to end up in a hospital admission.

Stage 1

The individual develops a psychiatric disorder, which gradually gets worse (solid line). In the case of a chronic patient (dotted line), this disorder is already present at a tolerable level and starts getting worse, or, they develop a second or third disorder; for example, a patient with schizophrenia becomes severely depressed or starts to abuse drugs. The dotted line may also represent a patient, not chronic, but one who has had a crisis, has gone through the stages to the out-patient Stage 6, and then, after a while, becomes more ill, and develops another crisis; for example, a depressed patient who partially recovers, but then becomes acutely suicidal again.

The time course of Stage 1 varies enormously: from hours to weeks or months. Much depends on the perception of the family and the community. The extent and quality of the person's social network is important. For example, a homeless, chronically psychotic man with hallucinations and delusions may be allowed to wander the streets of a large city for months without anyone batting an eyelid. However, if these same symptoms are noticed for the first time in a young man just home from college, the family are likely to whisk him off to the primary care physician or local emergency room within a day or two. The length of Stage 1 can be shortened for socially deprived individuals on the margins of society by "outreach" services, which can assertively intervene on their behalf.

Stage 2

At this stage, somebody, maybe the individual themselves, *perceives* the symptoms, behaviour, etc., as an emergency, and arranges for help; e.g., by calling 911, or by a visit to the ER or the primary care physician. Anyone in the social network may start the ball rolling: it can be family, employer, teacher, minister, or even a service provider such as a bus driver or store keeper—anyone the individual comes into contact with and reveals disturbing behavior to. The APA definition of emergency emphasizes the *subjective* element operating at this stage.

Stage 3

I refer to this stage as *crisis intervention*, which is defined in this book as *the first professional contacted; the service (often not mental health, but can be) to which the individual goes, or is taken, once the situation has been declared a crisis by someone.*

There are five crisis intervention services that are typically used in most settings, three of which are not specialized mental health services; the emergency room of a general hospital, police, primary care physician, and community crisis intervention service, including hot lines. Individuals already known to the mental health system may also be referred urgently to their psychiatrist or mental health worker. Any one of these may elect to send the person to the first mentioned service—the emergency room (dotted line). The individual may already be in treatment by a mental health professional at the time they become more acute. In this case their therapist will intervene at Stages 2, 3, and 4; perceiving the situation as a crisis, assessing it, and if necessary arranging in-patient treatment or a community alternative. See Figure 2.

It is at this stage, that a "mismatch of needs and resources" is perceived, as described in the APA definition; a similar concept to "insufficiency" (Christie, 1985) (see Chapter 2): it is then regarded as an emergency.

Stage 4

This is the psychiatric emergency service—a service specifically designed for psychiatric emergencies and manned by mental health professionals. Often,

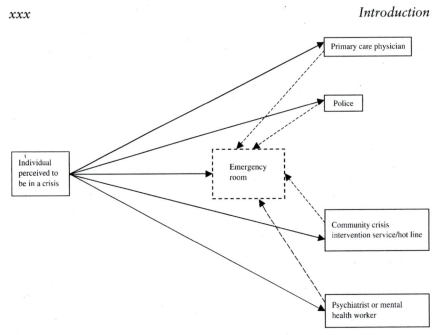

Figure 2 Stage 3, crisis intervention.

Stages 3 and 4 are combined, e.g., a patient walks into the ER and the triage nurse or the ER physician calls the psychiatric resident to see him. Or, they can be separate, a primary care physician, may send the patient to the emergency room to see the psychiatric resident on call, or the police take a person to the emergency room.

If the patient's condition is severe enough to be at or above the clinician's threshold for admission, the patient then goes on to Stage 5.

Stage 5

This stage is hospital admission, or its alternative, MCHT, crisis residence, or day hospital. This stage can consist of two parts: the hospital first, then early discharge to one of the alternatives. Or, the hospital treatment runs its conventional course, and the patient is discharged to out-patient care, Stage 6.

Stage 6

This stage is transfer to out-patient level of care e.g., a psychiatrist's office, mental health clinic, or primary care physician. The patient may then go on to complete remission or may have a bumpier course, with exacerbations reaching the level of a crisis again (Stage 2); for example, a depressed out-patient may become acutely suicidal again.

The essence of MCHT is that it provides an alternative to in-patient treatment; in research studies this is the outcome by which it is chiefly judged. Does it reduce bed usage? In the analysis of psychiatric emergencies in Figure 1, MCHT operates at Stage 5 and continues until Stage 6—transfer to out-patient care. However, in many actual clinical situations, its use is not restricted to Stages 5–6; as Joy, Adams, and Rice (2001) point out, the services they analyzed were not pure forms of a model: "they all used a form of home care for acutely ill people, which included *elements of crisis intervention* [italics added]." Because of their mobility and great flexibility, MCHT services often operate earlier in the course of a psychiatric emergency—at Stage 3 or 4—crisis intervention, or psychiatric emergency service. They also sometimes operate later in the course, extending into the early phase of Stage 6, thereby providing a more gradual transfer to out-patient care than may occur with in-patient care.

Because MCHT services sometimes don't just function exactly as an alternative to in-patient treatment—sitting passively, waiting to receive referrals from an emergency room—it can be difficult to examine how effective they are in replacing beds; *they have this other function added on—as a crisis intervention and/or a psychiatric emergency service.* The degree to which they engage in these functions gives rise to two broad types of MCHT. As Brimblecombe (2001) describes, there are two ways of structuring assessments in MCHT:

- Some also act as a crisis intervention/psychiatric emergency service in their own right, seeing the majority of urgent referrals or those potentially requiring hospital admission in their catchment area (Stage 3 or 4).
- Others only take referrals from other psychiatric services, after an initial psychiatric emergency assessment has already been carried out, for example, by a psychiatric resident (Stage 4). The MCHT then does a follow up assessment to check whether home treatment is practical as an alternative to admission. Therefore, they only commence their involvement with the patient at Stage 5.

The reader should keep these two structures in mind as they are discussed in later chapters. However, in real clinical life, most MCHT services are not pure versions: e.g., the Manchester Home Option team (in Chapter 3) takes referrals directly from ex-patients, (Stage 3). In the U.S., the crisis intervention/psychiatric emergency service function may be conducted by one mobile team, (Stages 3 and 4) who then transfer care immediately to another mobile team that does treatment only (Stage 5).

This book concentrates on MCHT as the primary (but not only) treatment with most of its activity confined to Stage 5. How much crisis intervention should be done by these teams, and the optimum combination of the two functions are very important issues for mental health policy. The implications for cost effectiveness and success at reduction of bed usage will be discussed further in Chapters 1, 2, 4, 5, and 6. MCHT services as described in this book would be classified as "mobile psychiatric *urgent* care services" (not emergency) within the American Psychiatric Association Task Force scheme (Allen, et al., 2002). See Table 2.

In this scheme, the Task Force's suggested standard for response time is within 4 hours for an urgent call, and availability at least 12 hours a day, 6 days a week, preferably with a schedule covering afternoons, evenings and weekend days, when other resources are hard to access. In contrast, the Task Force describes mobile crisis *emergency* services as having the capacity to manage patients at extreme risk of harm to themselves or others, extreme impairments in functioning, and with severe medical, psychiatric and substance abuse comorbidities. The standard for response time should be within 1 hour for emergency calls and availability 24 hours a day. Clearly, many of these patients could not be treated in the community and would need in-patient admission.

This preamble is necessary to enable the reader to appraise the research in Chapter 1 in the context of their own current mental health system and to be able to perceive clearly the role of MCHT in that system.

Table 2 Categorization of Psychiatric Emergency Services (Allen, et al., 2002)

	Hospital	Non-hospital residence	Mobile
Emergency	Psychiatric emergency service (in medical ER)		
	Psychiatric emergency service (specialty setting) • 23-hr beds • 72-hr beds	Psychiatric emergency residential facility (Acute Diversion Units)	Mobile psychiatric emergency service
Urgent	Psychiatric urgent care service	Psychiatric urgent care residential facility (Crisis Residential Facilities)	Mobile psychiatric urgent care service i.e., MCHT

Chapter One
Review of Research on Mobile Crisis Home Treatment

"In view of the consistently positive findings for this type of treatment, it is difficult to know why it has not been more universally adopted."

(Dean & Gadd, 1990)

"Community care alternatives are capable of reducing the need for in-patient treatment. The trouble is that we don't know to what degree. Current scientific knowledge is not sufficient to base a radical reduction of beds on."

(Kluiter, 1997)

Those with clinical experience of MCHT, who have seen admission to hospital averted many times, even for very sick individuals, and have witnessed the relief on the faces of the patients and their families, will share Dean and Gadd's enthusiasm and puzzlement. However, donning one's mental health services researcher hat, or one's mental health systems planner's hat, one has to agree with Kluiter; caution is required in adopting this model of care. All of the comparative studies are flawed to some degree; for example, questions have been raised about the degree to which their findings can be generalized to the general clinical population we deal with today, and we are often left in the dark regarding the conventional hospital-oriented treatment to which MCHT is compared.

The irony is that while we mull over these studies, and wrestle with whether MCHT can be an alternative to admission, we lose sight of the fact that what MCHT purports to replace—hospital treatment—has, itself, been poorly evaluated (Kluiter, 1997).

More and different kinds of research are clearly needed; in spite of this, however, critical reviewers have all come to positive conclusions in some

---

SIDEBAR

Common Flaws in Mobile Crisis Home Treatment Research

- Poorly defined target population: although severely mentally ill, it's unclear if they were in crisis and in need of immediate hospitalization
- Little information provided regarding the numbers and characteristics of patients excluded or dropped out
- Exclusions such as high suicide risk, or living alone, limit the generalizability to the average in-patient population
- Especially in older studies, the patients may be less ill than current patients admitted to hospital
- Control hospital-based services poorly described—it is hard to know what the experimental group is being compared to
- The control group treatment is far removed from today's superior conventional community-based out-patient treatment—so the comparison is not as relevant to today
- Family burden not measured
- The experimental treatment group is not a pure replacement of just hospital care; most of them engage in some form of crisis intervention (Stage 3) or psychiatric emergency evaluation (Stage 4), and many of them continue their involvement with the patient into the follow-up or out-patient phase (Stage 6 in the anatomy of a crisis diagram). See Figure 1.1
- There are limits to the general application of experimental programs because they employ special start up funds, enjoy the non-specific "Hawthorne effects" of being part of an experiment, and benefit from the contributions of charismatic individuals. (Thornicroft & Bebbington, 1989)
- Meta-analytic reviews may include research from countries with different health care infrastructures; the question of how well mental health care models travel is highly relevant

---

measure. Braun, et al. (1981) state "A qualified affirmative response to the question of the feasibility of deinstitutionalization can be given with regard to programs of community care that are alternatives to hospital admission . . . " Kluiter (1997) concludes that "community care arrangements are capable of reducing the need for in-patient treatment. The trouble is that we don't know to what degree." Joy, Adams, and Rice (2001) state "Overall, the review suggests that home care crisis treatment, coupled with an ongoing home care package, is a viable and acceptable way of treating people with serious mental illness . . . ." Burns, et al. (2001) declare "Our finding that in-patient control studies found a difference of nearly five days in hospital per patient per month in favor of home treatment (at one year) was open to question due to the difficulties of meta-analysis. . . . Nevertheless, if this finding is valid, it's magnitude is extremely significant clinically. Home treatment services achieved fewer days in hospital than services involving at least an initial period of in-patient treatment (in-patient control studies). We recommend that studies of home treatment compared with admission are no longer initiated, at least where hospitalization is used as an outcome measure."

Mobile Crisis Home Treatment (MCHT) has been the subject of at least 14 comparative studies, in five countries (and four continents), all but one of which have found it to reduce bed usage, to be less expensive, equally effective, and preferable to inpatient care.

Eight studies are randomized controlled trials in which patients presenting in an emergency are treated by MCHT or admitted to hospital; in three studies in one catchment area MCHT is compared to a conventional service (usually hospital based with traditional out-patient services) in a similar catchment area; and in three studies, there is a comparison of two different time periods in the same area: before and after the establishment of the MCHT service. All reported differences are statistically significant.

In each decade from the 1950s to the 2000s, research studies have shown MCHT to be less expensive, equally effective, and in some ways preferable to the contemporaneous hospital services. In the older studies, the hospital practices that are contrasted with MCHT are outdated; however, these studies are included in the review for two reasons. One is to show the historical evolution of this model, and, in particular, the consistent practical lessons that recur in each study—useful for understanding the key elements and principles described in Chapter 4. The other is the fact that some of these older studies were among the five that were of sufficient quality to be included in the 2001 Cochrane Library review of this model (Joy, Adams, & Rice, 2001). These five studies are Pasamanick, Scarpitti, and Dinitz (1967); Stein and Test (1978); Fenton, Tessier, and Struening (1982); Hoult and Reynolds (1984); and Muijen, Marks, Connolly, and Audini (1992).

COMPARATIVE STUDIES OF MOBILE CRISIS HOME TREATMENT

The Worthing Study: A Comparison of Two Time Periods, Before and After, 1958 (Carse, Panton, & Watt, 1958)

This, the first study of mobile crisis home treatment took place 40 years ago in the southeast of England in two towns, Worthing and Chichester. The

10-Month Period

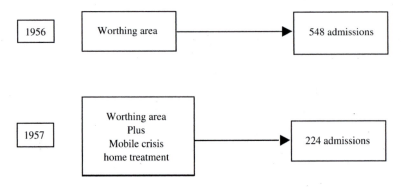

Figure 1.1 Worthing study.

Table 1.1

Practical Tips

Requirements for Success:
- Community acceptance of, and freedom from fear of, mental illness—achieved by talks and public hospital visits
- Cooperative patients
- Favorable home background
- Reasonable risk of suicide, danger to others
- Physically healthy patients

area, predominantly wealthy, high social class, with many retired persons, sounds an unlikely location to have a psychiatric bed shortage so severe as to force such an innovative approach. But that was the motivation: too many patients for too few beds. Then, as now, access to in-patient treatment had become limited. Admissions to mental hospitals in the U.K. had increased by 40% in five years in the 1950s, and the number of psychiatric beds peaked in 1954; but, there was a serious overcrowding problem. The only answer seemed to be to build more hospitals—until the regional hospital board decided to undertake a two-year pilot project to provide a mobile crisis home treatment service (termed "outpatient and domiciliary treatment service") to patients in the Worthing district, starting January 1, 1957. This district was deliberately chosen because it was 22 miles from the nearest mental hospital, Graylingwell, to show that it is possible to provide psychiatric treatment for large numbers of patients without the immediate availability of a modern mental hospital. It became known as the "Worthing Experiment."

All patients had to be referred by their primary care physician, and the service functioned as the only gatekeeper to the mental hospital. The area had a wide range of social classes, and, of particular interest, the highest proportions of elderly people of any town in Britain; how far it is possible to treat elderly psychiatric patients out of hospital was of urgent concern. Staff consisted of two and a half psychiatrists, at least four nurses, two orderlies, two social workers, and an occupational therapist.

Admissions to Graylingwell for the first ten months of the new service in 1957 were compared to those in the same months in 1956. The results were dramatic: 60% reduction in admissions from Worthing (from 548 to 224), compared to a 4% increase in admissions from other districts (Figure 1.1). The study is short on details; diagnoses are not described with the rigor and detail of today, clinical outcomes are not compared, and it is hard to compare the acuity of the patients with today's patients. Also, the program provided more community services in general beyond home treatment, making it difficult to separate out the specific role of home treatment in this result. Finally, there was no attempt to measure family burden.

The Worthing patients were mainly suffering from depression. ECT was used extensively, and modified insulin treatments were given. The main treatment was individual psychotherapy.

The Chichester Study: A Comparison of Two Areas, 1966 (Grad & Sainsbury, 1966)

A year later, Grad and Sainsbury (1966) replicated the Worthing Experiment in Chichester for the same reason: overcrowded mental hospitals. They compared two districts: Chichester, where community services were set up, including mobile crisis home treatment and a day hospital; and Salisbury, which had a hospital-centered service. The two areas were similar with respect to psychiatric population referred, except that the Chichester service received more elderly patients and organic disorders and fewer neurotics. Any bias, therefore, is toward more severe cases in Chichester.

Again, the results were dramatic: 14% of patients referred to the Chichester service were admitted to hospital, compared to 52% referred to Salisbury; 15% were treated in a day hospital and 16% treated at home, compared to 3% at home in Salisbury; and none in a day hospital (Salisbury, as in the rest of the U.K., already had an existing form of home treatment, but less extensive than the new service).

Such little consideration of community treatment appears to have been the norm in this era that in retrospect it would appear to have been comparatively easy to bring about such dramatic reductions in admissions. For

Table 1.2

Diagnoses—Chichester	
Organic psychoses	20%
Functional psychoses	40%
Neuroses	30%
Other	10%

Table 1.3

Diagnoses—Salisbury	
Organic psychoses	15%
Functional psychoses	40%
Neuroses	36%
Other	9%

example, many patients came into the mental hospital directly from their primary care physician, "this could occur without the hospital being aware that it was getting a new patient."

Family burden was measured, the overall result being no significant difference between the two services after one month (Grad & Sainsbury, 1968). However, there was a tendency for the hospital service to provide more relief in the less severe cases by way of more social work support to families, underscoring the need to provide more attention to families in home treatment.

Two-Year Follow-Up

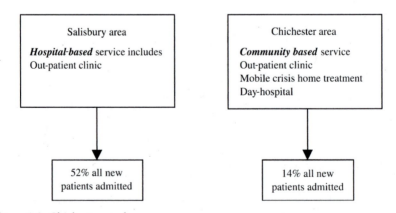

Figure 1.2 Chichester study.

Table 1.4

Practical Tips

- Adequate social support to family important

Most stressful to deal with:

- Body ailment preoccupation
- Importunate demanding behavior
- Suicidal concern
- Organic, bedfast patients

The Louisville Kentucky Study: A Randomized Controlled Trial, 1967 (Pasamanick, Scarpitti, & Dinitz, 1967)

A few years later, across the Atlantic, in Louisville, Kentucky, in the first American study of MCHT, Pasamanick, et al. (1967) focused on a different population of patients for home treatment: patients with schizophrenia. For the first time, the new neuroleptic drugs had opened up the possibility of treating these patients in the community instead of in the hospital. At that time, patients with schizophrenia were staying in hospital an average of 11 years, and, except for the drugs, were receiving only custodial treatment. Concern over this grim state of affairs seems to have been the driving force behind this landmark study.

The study was designed to determine:

1) whether home care for patients with schizophrenia was feasible.
2) whether drug therapy was effective in preventing their hospitalization.
3) whether home care was, in fact, a better or poorer method of treatment than hospitalization.

Viewing this study as a hospital vs. home care experiment, from the vantage point of today, is complicated by the incorporation of a drug vs. placebo experiment and by the fact that hospital care today bears little resemblance to hospital care at the time of the study. As described in the study, "In the hospital, between acute episodes, patients are mostly left alone to stare vacantly into space, to walk down the corridors and back again, to sit, rock and hallucinate, or to partake of inmate culture. In time, this lack of normal stimulation—intellectual, interpersonal, even physical—has usually resulted in deterioration and impairment of functioning which was wholly unnecessary."

The study compared 152 patients admitted over 25 months of intake, and followed for 6–12 months. They were assigned randomly to three groups:

1) Home on drugs
2) Home on placebo
3) Hospital

To qualify for home care, patients were required to:

1) Have schizophrenia, with psychosis severe enough to warrant hospital admission
2) Display no homicidal or suicidal tendencies
3) Fit within the age range of 18–60
4) Have family or family surrogate willing to accept and supervise them in the home and to report on their progress throughout the course of the study
5) Reside within 60 miles of Louisville

No criteria for diagnosing schizophrenia are given, and today the concept of this illness is much narrower. From the case descriptions, these patients certainly appeared psychotic, and would have warranted hospital admission; however, many of them would be diagnosed today as acute reactive psychosis and affective psychosis, by *DSM-IV* criteria.

All patients had been admitted to Central State Hospital because they were thought to need in-patient treatment. There, they were screened for inclusion in the study within one to four days. In the course of 25 months of patient intake, 163 patients were accepted for the study, and after 11 dropped out 57 were assigned to drug/home care, 41 to placebo/home care, and 54 to hospital controls.

To attempt to treat these acutely psychotic patients, for the first time ever in their homes, the study used public health nurses with no psychiatric experience whatsoever! This same feature, the use of public health nurses instead of psychiatric nurses, crops up again, 15 years later, in the Montreal study by Fenton, Tessier, and Struening (1982). The rationale for this choice was the high degree of public acceptance enjoyed by PHNs and their experience in caring for people at home (particularly with tuberculosis patients). Seemingly anachronistic now, the community treatment of a chronic disease like TB was thought to be a suitable model for home treatment of schizophrenia.

Training for the nurses consisted of a two-week orientation program and four weeks in the hospital observing and talking to staff and patients. By today's standards the treatment provided was astoundingly minimal. The nurse visited the patient once a week for the first three months, bimonthly during the second three months, and monthly thereafter. It is not made clear what attention patients received in between visits. Patients and family could phone and

6–30 Months Follow-Up

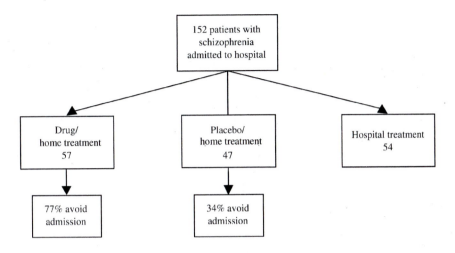

Figure 1.3 Louisville, Kentucky study.

talk to a nurse or psychiatrist, but in practice very few did. Dosages of neuroleptics were very low by contemporary standards e.g.; Trifluoperazine 2 mg three times daily, Thioridazine 100 mg three times daily.

The psychiatrist played an even smaller role. He devoted two days a week to the project and saw patients every three months. He assessed patients for research purposes and determined what progress had been made. He depended almost wholly on the report of the nurse in making treatment decisions. In practice, it became necessary for him to see patients more frequently.

The nurse was also responsible for the extensive research evaluation carried out on each patient, using a large number of rating scales. These included an in-patient multidimensional psychiatric scale; four psychological tests—WAIS, Bender Gestalt, reaction time, and Porteus Maze Test; and various nursing scales and checklists.

In spite of the therapeutic minimalism, the results were impressive. More than 77% of the drug/home care patients, but only 34% of the placebo/home care patients, remained at home throughout the course of the study (6–30 months). Home care patients functioned as well, or better than, hospital patients, whose initial hospitalization lasted, on average, 83 days, and almost half of whom had to be readmitted.

A major oversight in the study was the failure to compare family burden in the three groups, which must have been considerable judging from the case descriptions. (Family burden was measured, but it appears as though the results were not compared.) Costs were not analyzed, but home care was estimated to be less expensive than hospital care.

The Denver Colorado Study: A Randomized Controlled Trial, 1968 (Langsley, Pittman, & Machotka, 1968)

The next foray into MCHT took place in Denver, Colorado, in 1968 (Langsley, Pittman, & Machotka, 1968; Langsley, Flomenhaft, & Machotka, 1969; Langsley, Machotka, & Flomenhaft, 1971). Langsley's group, at the Family Treatment Unit of the Colorado State Hospital, were motivated not so much by concern over crowded mental hospitals, or lengths of stay, but more out of a belief that hospitalization was wrong and should be avoided if possible because it contravened the principals of family systems theory and family therapy. Hospitalization was seen as not only unnecessary, but also as harmful, disrupting individual and family life, fostering regression, causing significant social stigma and unnecessary expense. Also, as the Langley groups' research showed, hospitalization can lead to a greater risk of subsequent admission.

Although there is token recognition of the role of genetics and physiology, the authors' bias is clear, as shown by the use of quotation marks around "mental patient." Mental illness is seen as a result of inadequate coping with family problems and admission to hospital as "extruding and scapegoating" the patient, and avoiding the true problem—the family dysfunction. The study consisted of 300 patients, who were all assessed by a psychiatric resident on the admission unit as needing admission. They were assigned by random selection to one of two groups, hospital or family crisis treatment, which were systematically shown to be comparable in terms of demographics, diagnoses, previous admissions, and suicidality. Hospital treatment at the Colorado Psychiatric Hospital (a university teaching hospital) lasted 26 days on average, included individual and group therapy and drugs, and was considered "more than adequate when compared with that available in any mental health treatment setting."

This rather dated approach appears to have been extraordinarily successful. With only five office visits, one home visit, and a few telephone calls taking place over three and a half weeks, all experimental patients avoided admission over the acute treatment period.

Again, we see the theme of "therapeutic minimalism" as noted in the Pasamanick, et al. (1967) study: successful outcomes of what seems like inadequate treatment by today's standards.

It is impossible though, to determine objectively the acuity of these patients. There are major flaws in the study: it includes no diagnoses (presumably stemming from the family systems approach) and no descriptions of

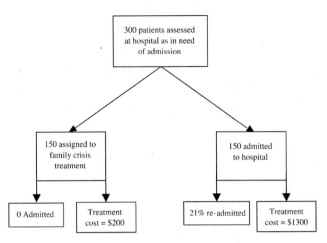

Figure 1.4 Denver-Colorado study.

typical cases. Patients were referred to as "psychotic." Was the threshold for admission to psychiatric hospital then similar to today (even before managed care)? One suspects not: no home care patient was hospitalized in the acute treatment phase, and no mention is made of exclusionary criteria, such as suicidal risk. Outcomes for the two groups were similar, and were determined by two scales that measured social functioning, and symptoms. During the six month follow-up period, none of the family crisis treatment patients were admitted. Twenty-one percent of the hospital cases had to be re-admitted. Six months after family crisis treatment had finished, 19% of the experimental group, were admitted—no greater than the rehospitalization rate of the controls, thereby demonstrating that admission had been truly avoided for most of the experimental group and not merely postponed. Lengths of stay for readmitted hospital treatment patients were almost three times that of family crisis treatment patients. Family burden was not measured; it was considered to be less for the experimental patients because of their rapid return to functioning thought presumably to offset any burden caused by psychopathology. Cost comparisons showed a huge difference: $1300 (U.S.) for hospital care compared to $200 for family crisis treatment, estimated from total salaries and overhead divided by an estimate of 350 patient per year.

The Madison, Wisconsin Study: A Randomized Controlled Trial, 1978 (Stein & Test, 1978)

The next study was a giant leap forward in mobile crisis home treatment. Stein and Test's research study and method of MCHT was more detailed and sophisticated than any previous studies and revealed a deep understanding of the many needs of chronically and severely ill patients (Stein & Test, 1978, 1980; Test & Stein, 1980; Weisbrod, Test, & Stein, 1980). They, too, were concerned about the harmful effects of hospitalization; the "institutional syndrome" described by Goffman, Wing, and others in the early 1960s; and the perseveration of the psychiatric system, repeatedly admitting patients whenever they were in a crisis. This observation is further evidence for the conclusion that "to hospitalize a patient is a major decision which forever after changes the attitude of both the patient and those who care for them" (Mendel & Rapport, 1969).

Stein and Test first tried out their ideas on 21 patients who had been in a state hospital for 3–18 months and who were considered not yet ready for discharge. These patients were all transferred to community treatment, and all but one avoided re-admission and attained a degree of autonomous living and functioning greater than the controls that stayed in hospital five months longer. Thus encouraged, Stein and Test developed an MCHT program called "Training in Community Living" (TCL), which addressed the five factors thought to be essential to keep patients out of hospital and give them quality of life. These were:

1) material resources—food, shelter, medical care, etc.
2) coping skills to meet the demands of community life—using public transportation, budgeting, meal preparation, etc.
3) motivation to persevere and remain involved with life through a readily available system of support.
4) freedom from pathological dependent relationships, defined as "one which inhibits personal growth, reinforces maladaptive behaviors and generates feelings of panic in its members when its loss is threatened." Hospital was thought to increase dependency, and, upon discharge, patients were usually returned to a highly conflictual family situation where another crisis was waiting to happen, resulting in the revolving door syndrome.
5) an "assertive support system" (dropping out is not allowed in Madison!). The program "goes to the patient" because the patient is frequently passive and interpersonally anxious which, combined with his severe symptoms, leads them to not show up for appointments.

Experimental subjects were all patients seeking admission to Mendota Mental Health Institute; they resided in Dane County (Madison) and district, were aged 18–62, and had any psychiatric diagnosis other than severe organic brain syndrome or primary alcoholism. Patients were quite ill; they had accumulated a mean of 14.5 months in psychiatric institutions spread over a mean of five hospitalizations. There were no exclusionary criteria, based on suicidal risk or risk of harm to others; experimental patients were admitted at the time of initial assessment only in rare instances. Patients were randomly assigned to two groups—65 TCL and 65 controls—who were admitted to a hospital that was regarded as "more than just custodial" with a high patient/staff ratio and, a wide variety of services, and where liberal use was made of aftercare services following discharge, which occurred after a mean of 17 days. The patients had a wide range of diagnoses, and approximately 50% had schizophrenia. The two groups were shown to be comparable.

Outcome was measured by the use of scales measuring social functioning, symptoms, self-esteem, quality of life, and family burden.

Treatment lasted 14 months; follow-up lasted 28 months. Of the 65 experimental patients, 12 were admitted in the first year, for a mean of nine days, compared to 58 (data not available on eight) controls, 21 of whom had to be re-admitted at least once.

The experimental group was less symptomatic, more satisfied with their lives, and spent more time in sheltered employment. There was one suicide in each group and no homicides. Family burden was less in the TCL group, some of that presumably due to the practice of removing the patient from dysfunctional families and setting them up in their own residences.

In contrast to the "therapeutic minimalism" in Pasamanick, et al. (1967) study, staff were all trained mental health professionals and treatment was very intense with daily contact, and two shifts (7 a.m.–11 p.m.) 7 days a week. Staff spent long periods of time with patients, accompanying them and participating in every facet of their lives. Cost comparisons between the two treatment modalities were the most exhaustive of all the studies and also showed the least difference. Cost included not only direct treatment

Table 1.5

Practical Tips
• "Can-do" philosophy; stress patient's assets, downplay symptoms
• Interventions are assertive, directive, flexible, and available 24 hours
• Support families and community as well as patients
• Prepare, and work with, the community at large
• Appropriate funding mechanism essential
• Attend to pathologically dependent family relationships

costs, but also indirect treatment costs, including social service agency use, law enforcement costs (e.g, overnight stays in jail) and maintenance costs such as social security and welfare. The experimental group treatment cost $797 more; however, patients in that group earned $1196 more—a monetary benefit of $400 more per patient per year over the added costs. An attempt was also made to quantify in non-monetary terms the added costs and benefits such as family burden, mortality, and days of employment/year. Based on the non-monetary analysis the home treatment group experienced added benefits. Social costs were also thoroughly measured using a family burden scale, number of arrests, suicidal gestures, and emergency room use; there were no differences except for a slightly greater use of emergency rooms for the control group patients.

12 Months Follow-Up Period

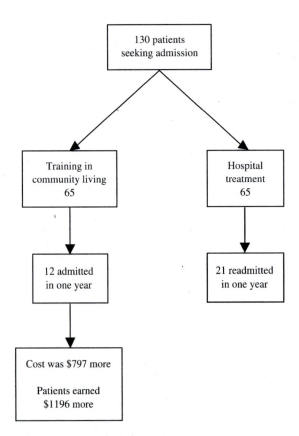

Figure 1.5 Madison, Wisconsin study.

The Montreal Study: A Randomized Controlled Study, 1982
(Fenton, Tessier, & Struening, 1982)

Fenton, et al. (1982) conducted a similarly detailed study in Montreal, Canada. The study was motivated by concern about maintaining clinically effective services, with shrinking budgets, with a goal of enhancing community treatment for the chronically disabled patient, mainly those with schizophrenia. The target group included not just patients with schizophrenia or other severe mental illnesses but any patient who would have required admission to the Montreal General Hospital. The experimental subjects were randomly selected from patients in the emergency room who required admission. Unlike Stein and Test's 1978 study, there were exclusionary criteria of immediate risk of suicide and dangerousness (15.7% thus excluded); also, patients had to have someone who could help with treatment (not necessarily family or cohabiting)—9% thus excluded. The other exclusions were similar to the Madison group; excluded patients had a primary diagnosis of substance abuse or organic brain syndrome, refused home care, or were under 18. A total of 46.5% of the patients were excluded on these grounds. Screening resulted in a cohort of 78 home care patients and 84 hospital patients. The two groups were analyzed as compatible; diagnoses (by ICD 8) were 40% schizophrenia, 30% manic depressive psychosis, 30% depressive neurosis. Clinical impairment was severe.

Staff consisted of a half-time psychiatrist, a Master's level social worker, and an RN. Continuing the curious tradition seen in Pasamanick et al.'s study (1967), neither the social worker nor the nurse had any clinical experience with psychiatric patients. The control hospital-based treatment was described in more detail than in other studies and consisted of a fairly active university general hospital psychiatric ward, with an average length of stay of 28 days. Outcome was measured independently using rating scales of mental status, role functioning, and family burden. Cost analysis was very extensive and included costs incurred by patients and their families for drugs, transportation, lost days from work, and extra care for housekeepers or nurses.

In summary, home treatment relieved signs and symptoms of psychiatric illness as effectively as hospital treatment, family burden was no greater—in fact, in one respect it was less; home treatment patients could continue to assume some of their responsibilities. Average cost of treating each control patient for a year was $3250, compared to $1980 for home treatment patients, which was 40% cheaper. Other costs, such as drugs, extra help, etc., were equal for both groups.

Table 1.6

Practical Tips

- The degree to which reality testing is impaired by delusions or hallucinations, or the degree to which patients can understand that their faculties are impaired, has an important influence on outcome
- Previous hospitalization predicts re-hospitalization
- Willingness of family or other individuals to support patients and participate in treatment is important
- Quality of relationships between family members and with the patient is important
- Home visiting is essential—builds rapport and teaches family members how to care for the patient and assume some of the tasks normally performed by experienced staff
- Telephone is used as a partial substitute for office visits; 24-hour answering service important

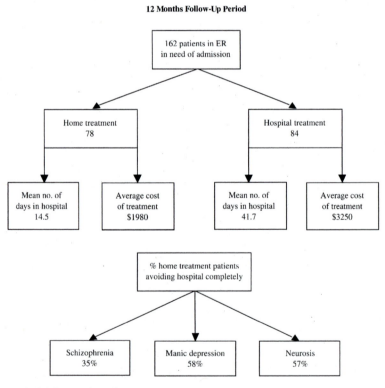

Figure 1.6 Montreal study.

The Vancouver Study: A Randomized Controlled Study, 1975
(Goodacre, Coles, MacCurdy, Coates, & Kendall, 1975)

In contrast to all the previous studies, and indeed all subsequent studies, this study conducted in Vancouver, Canada, in the early 1970s showed no advantage to MCHT. Subjects were 16–69, not primarily substance abusers, not referred under a magistrate's warrant or an Order in Council, or certified within the jail. The patients may have been more ill than those in other studies: "During the study period, staff shortages led to restricted admissions to the hospital, and consequently, the subjects of this study were drawn from a severely ill and highly prescreened psychiatric admission cohort." Diagnoses included: 48% schizophrenia, 14% psychosis, 29% neurosis and personality disorder, and 7% organic brain syndrome. Two hundred and twelve patients were randomly sampled from patients who had arrived at the Riverview mental hospital and had been accepted for admission. They were then randomly assigned to one of three groups—home treatment, hospitalization followed by home treatment, and hospital treatment followed by conventional services (physicians or hospital aftercare). Four hypotheses were tested: 1) some patients would avoid admission completely, 2) a shorter average length of first admission for those initially assigned to home treatment, 3) a smaller number of readmissions for both the home treatment and hospital plus home treatment groups, and 4) shorter hospitalization for patients who were followed up by home treatment. In contrast to the Madison study in which

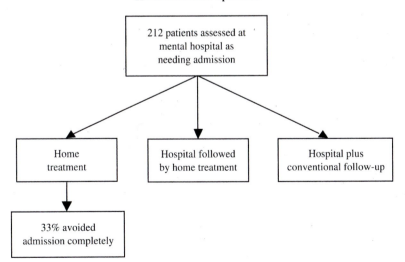

Figure 1.7 Vancouver study.

experimental patients were rarely initially admitted, 43% of these home treatment patients were admitted within the first week, usually because of suicidal or homicidal behavior or lack of support. The first hypothesis was supported; 33% of patients never went to hospital during the entire study year. The experimental patients who were hospitalized had lengths of stay no shorter than hospital treatment patients (hypothesis 2.). However, it's hard to know, what to make of this finding in light of some rather eccentric features of this study. In particular, in-patient hospital staff, who because of rivalry with home treatment staff, kept experimental patients longer in hospital than control patients, thus sabotaging the study. Hypothesis 3 was not supported; i.e., the readmission rate was similar for all groups—10 to 17%. The hypothesis that being assigned to home treatment reduced the total of hospital days was also not supported. Another unusual feature of this study was the idea that home treatment encourages admission: "The addition of home treatment seems to bring to light a number of acute family conflicts, suicide attempts, and disturbed and disturbing behavior in patients leading to arranged admissions in cases that otherwise would be overlooked." This phenomenon makes it difficult, therefore, to assess the finding of no difference in re-admission rates for the two groups. Possibly the control patients' out-patient follow-up was of such poor quality that relapses were overlooked. However, in spite of all these negative conclusions, the study did manage to treat 33% of seriously ill patients without any admission at all.

The Sydney Study, A Randomized Controlled Trial, 1984 (Hoult, Rosen, & Reynolds, 1984)

In 1979, the concept of mobile crisis home treatment spread to a third continent, Australia. There, Hoult (1986; Hoult & Reynolds, 1984), frustrated by the inadequacies of crisis-oriented hospital treatment, which ignored the underlying social causes of psychiatric illness, became interested in Stein and Test's work and decided to replicate it. One hundred and twenty patients presenting for admission, both voluntary and involuntary, to the state psychiatric hospital in Sydney, the Macquarrie Hospital, were randomly allocated to two groups: standard hospital and aftercare and "community treatment." Criteria were similar to Stein and Test: aged 15–65 and did not have a primary diagnosis of organic brain disorder or substance dependency. As in the Madison study, but unlike the Fenton study, suicidal or dangerous patients were not excluded. One difference from the Wisconsin study was in the use of certain previously identified boarding homes; if the situation between patient and family was intolerable, the patient was moved to a boarding home. Patients, who fell asleep when given their initial medication in the admission area,

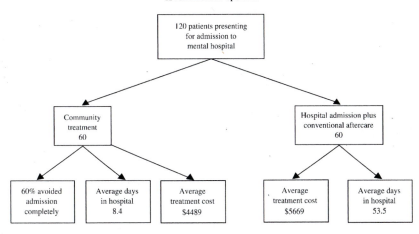

12 Months Follow-Up Period

120 patients presenting
for admission to
mental hospital

Community
treatment
60

Hospital admission plus
conventional aftercare
60

| 60% avoided admission completely | Average days in hospital 8.4 | Average treatment cost $4489 | Average treatment cost $5669 | Average days in hospital 53.5 |

Figure 1.8 Sydney study.

and those who refused to cooperate, were admitted to hospital first. Most were cooperative enough after two or three days of compulsory admission. Those who stayed in hospital were the responsibility of the team who cared for them after discharge. Both home and hospital treatment are well described. The hospital was modern, small, and provided treatment of a high standard followed by conventional out-patient care. Assessments were done independently at one, four, eight, and twelve months. Patients were quite ill; 60% presented as involuntary, 75% suffered from a functional psychosis, and 50% from schizophrenia. The results were positive: the study showed a marked decrease in bed usage—control: average 53.5 days; experimental: average 8.4 days—and a superior clinical outcome. Sixty percent of patients avoided admission altogether. Unlike the Madison study, the experimental group treatment was 21% cheaper, at $4489 (Australian) compared to $5669 for the control group.

Community treatment patients had a superior clinical outcome—(most studies show no difference): 71% of them, compared to 57% of control patients, had no psychotic symptoms at the end of the study year. Patients and relatives found community treatment more satisfactory and more helpful. One negative finding was that community treatment was not as effective in reducing the number of suicide threats and attempts as standard care, but unfortunately no data are provided. None of the community patients died; two of the controls did—one from a stroke, and one from drowning (possibly suicide).

Table 1.7

Practical Tips

- Accurately define presenting problem
- Threats of violence and suicide usually subside with supportive firmness and medication
- Community relocation can highlight role in interpersonal conflict in the crisis for the family
- Intensive help at the beginning forges important therapeutic bond with family and patient
- Involve patient and family in management program
- Personal, consistent case manager
- Assertively go to the patient and family
- Help with practical problems of living
- 24-hour access, rapid mobile response

The Bangalore India Study: A Randomized Controlled Trial, 1982 (Pai & Kapur, 1982)

In 1982, Pai and Kapur focused home treatment on a specific population—patients with first onset schizophrenia. The duration of illness prior to intake was from 4 days to 1 year, with an average of 149 days. The main aim of the study was different from other studies: to determine whether the family burden of this illness was directly proportional to the degree of the patients' psychopathology or their ability to function socially. Comparison of the two treatment modalities (hospital and home) seemed almost secondary and focused mainly on whether either had an effect on the three variables. Fifty-four patients were assigned alternately to home or hospital treatment after "they approached the psychiatric out-patient department." Details of the treatments were very scanty; home treatment is simply described as the nurse visiting regularly to assess the patient, dispense drugs, and counsel the family. The assessments were thorough, using rating scales administered by an independent researcher, and showed the superiority of home treatment. After six months, scores of psychopathology and family burden were less for home treatment patients, and their social functioning was better. Home treatment was also cheaper at 146 rupees, compared with 352 rupees for hospital treatment. Data on hospital admission rates for home treatment patients is not presented: "the home group remained in their own homes"—perhaps they weren't admitted at all. Average stay of the hospital group was 1½ months, ranging from 3 weeks to 6 months. A proportional relationship between the three variables was found and it was postulated that the

Six Months Follow-Up Period

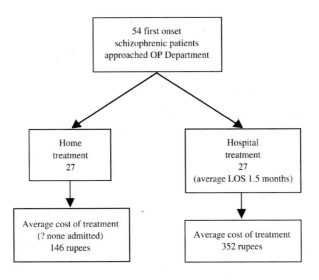

Figure 1.9 Bangalore study.

presence of an improving patient in the home, plus the visiting nurse's counseling and support of the family, were key factors in reducing family burden. Better followup in the home care group (in contrast to conventional out-patient followup) was thought to enhance compliance, and encouragement of usual activities at home was thought to improve social functioning.

The Birmingham Study I: A Comparison of Two Time Periods, Before and After, 1990 (Dean & Gadd, 1990)

In 1987, in Birmingham U.K., Dean and Gadd (1990) decided to investigate whether the mobile crisis home treatment findings established elsewhere could be generalized to Britain. Dean and Gadd's first study is different from the previous studies; it is more of a natural experiment in which MCHTs services' effect on bed utilization is measured over a 2½ year period—a comparison of two time periods: before and after MCHT started. There was no control group. The MCHT service was added to a multidisciplinary mental health team that had been previously set up at a resource centre, which provided a drop in service for patients with chronic mental illness and also groups for these and less seriously ill patients. Two community psychiatric nurses and two nursing assistants were added specifically for MCHT.

　　The catchment area, Sparkbrook, of 26,000, was a very poor inner-city district of Birmingham with many Asian immigrants, one of the 10 most

Two Year Follow-Up Period

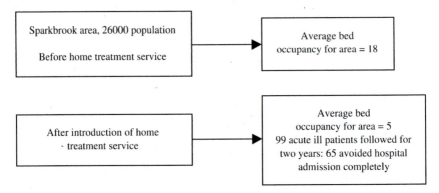

Figure 1.10 Birmingham study I.

socially deprived areas in Britain. Anybody could refer to the service, including patients themselves and their families. Subjects of the study were seriously ill, "who would normally have been treated in hospital"; they included those who were at suicidal risk, aggressive, non-compliant, or seriously psychotic. The study included 99 patients treated during a two-year period; 65 of them avoided admission altogether. Of these, 45% were depressed, 25% had schizophrenia, and 22% had some form of bipolar illness. Of those who had to be admitted, 21% were depressed, 23% had schizophrenia, and 35% had a form of bipolar illness.

Hospital admissions before the MCHT service averaged about 100 per year with a mean bed occupancy of 18; this fell to 5 over two years. There was no attempt to determine the effect of home treatment on clinical outcome, functioning, or family burden. Costs were not assessed. After one year, a 24-hour on call service was introduced, following which bed occupancy dropped from 10 to 5 days.

The authors point out that this type of study avoids any exclusions found in randomized controlled trials, such as organic brain disease and drug or alcohol dependence. It was the first British study since the Chichester study in 1966.

The Birmingham Study II: A Comparison of Two Areas, 1993 (Dean, Phillips, Gadd, Joseph, & England, 1993)

In 1990, Dean, et al. (1993) compared the Sparkbrook MCHT service with the hospital-based service in a demographically similar area, Small Heath. The Small Heath services consisted of 12–14 beds in a large psychiatric

12 Months Follow-Up

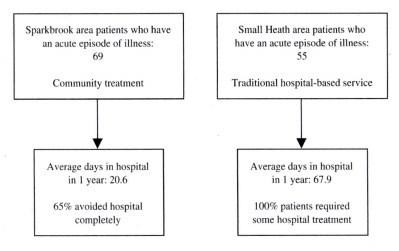

Figure 1.11 Birmingham study II.

hospital, day hospital, a rehab service with short- and long-term beds, and two community psychiatric nurses. All patients 16–65 having an acute episode severe enough to warrant hospital admission between January 1990 and February 1991 were followed, 69 in Sparkbrook, 55 in Small Heath. There were no significant differences between the two groups, and the initial severity of illness as measured by total score on the present state examination were the same. Thirty-five percent of the Sparkbrook group received some in-patient treatment during their acute episode, compared to 100% of the Small Heath group. Diagnoses in the home treatment and hospital-based group were schizophrenia, 42.38%; affective disorder, 28.25%; neurosis, 16.9%; paranoid state, 7.9%.

The Sparkbrook group had an average of 8 days in hospital at the first admission compared to 58.7 in Small Heath, and, on average, 20.6 days in one year, compared to 67.9. Clinical outcome was the same for both groups. Family burden measures showed less distress in the relatives of the Sparkbrook patients. Relatives and patients preferred MCHT.

The authors point out that this type of study avoids the exclusion of patients with organic brain disease and drug or alcohol dependency that occurs in randomized controlled trials. It is the first study since the Chichester study (Grad & Sainsbury, 1966) to examine MCHT in the context of a total psychiatric service in Britain.

Table 1.8

Practical Tips

Elements of the service considered responsible for reduced admissions:

- 24-hour on-call system
- Rapid response to referrals from any agency
- Proactive response to missed appointments and maintenance injections
- Patients disclose symptoms of their illness earlier, knowing they will not necessarily be admitted
- Existence of crisis resource centre—a comprehensive mental health and social service agency, which includes a "drop in" service. Focal point for referrals.

The Southwark, London Study: A Randomized Controlled Trial, 1992 (Muijen, Marks, Connolly, & Audini, 1992)

In the same year as the Birmingham study, also in Britain, the Maudsley group, embarked on a three year study to replicate the Madison and Sydney studies (Muijen, et al.,1992; Marks, Connolly, Audini, et al., 1994; Marks, Connolly, Muijen, et al., 1994; Knapp, et al., 1998). Unlike Madison and Sydney, but similar to Birmingham, the catchment area, Southwark, was a very poor inner-city district of London with a high proportion of immigrants.

The design was the usual one of random allocation of patients, independently assessed as needing admission from the Maudsley Hospital 24-hour walk-in emergency clinic. Generalizing from this study to real clinical practice is limited by the fact that the sample is limited to only 20% of those with previous admissions; the rest were first time admissions. The reason for this is not clear: the authors say, "The other 80% were excluded because the team would not have been able to care for this additional number of patients." The only other exclusions were patients with a primary diagnosis of addiction or organic brain damage; suicidal and dangerous patients were included, as well as patients on a section of the Mental Health Act. One hundred and eight-nine patients were randomized either to home-based care, called "daily living program" (92), or standard hospital care (97). Patients were followed up for a period of 18–20 months.

Diagnoses included 49% schizophrenia, 15–19% mania, and 23–25% depression in the experimental and control group, respectively. The control group treatment was well described and appeared of high quality.

The results were as expected from the two previous studies: an 80% drop in days in hospital (mean number of days in hospital: 18 in experimental group, 76 days control group). Clinical outcome and social outcome was comprehensively evaluated by independent researchers, at 4, 11, and 20 months, and favored the experimental group slightly.

Admission to hospital was used more often than in the Madison and Sydney studies: at entry, 29% avoided admission (a conservative estimate, as 12% of patients were admitted overnight before being allocated to the experimental group). At 18 months, only 12% of the experimental group had avoided admission. This difference in the three studies is not discussed.

Costs were significantly less for the experimental group, which is a curious difference to the Madison study, where the more expensive option of hospital admission was used much less (in that study, the treatment costs were more in the home care group). The difference in the two groups was 196 pounds mean weekly cost compared to 358 pounds; the experimental group was 45% cheaper. Unlike the Madison study, there was no evidence of any differential impact on employment on the 2 groups, so that was not factored in cost-benefit studies. Similarly, cost of family and informal care were no different.

One cannot finish the account of the Maudsley study without mentioning the very tragic occurrence that marred the study and had a demoralizing effect on the staff. Ten months into the study, and 7½ weeks after he had entered the study, a 45-year-old male patient killed a neighbor's baby. At first, publicity was minimal, but then, 14 months later, the incident was splashed over four newspapers and TV. A hospital audit exonerated the home treatment team, but the decision as to when to discharge experimental patients back to community home care was taken out of their hands and given to the ward staff. Following the audit, the average length of stay skyrocketed; for example, 17 patients who had admissions before and after had lengths of stay 300% greater.

Is there a lesson here? In the Vancouver study (Goodacre, et, al., 1975), one reason that lengths of stay of experimental patients was not less than controls was the feeling that ward staff were dragging their feet when it came to discharging

Table 1.9

Practical Tips

Important for survival of home treatment services:
- Enough staff trained in problem-oriented case management
- After-hours telephone rota
- Quick staff travel to patients' homes
- Systematic audit
- Access to quick specialist help and brief crisis admission
- Coordination of the team with other agencies
- Home treatment team to be responsible for any brief in-patient admissions
- Supportive funding and policies

18–20 Months Follow-Up Period

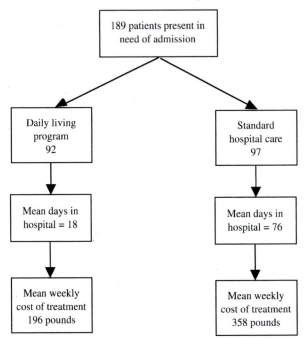

Figure 1.12 Southwark, London study.

home treatment patients. Perhaps for these services to achieve their full potential, control of discharge has to reside with home care staff, as is the case in many of the studies. This tragedy also raises another issue. Rather bitterly, the authors point out that when the patient committed his crime he would have likely been discharged, avoiding any responsibility accruing to the hospital. One "disadvantage" of home treatment of this long-term care type is that it prolongs the time that staff can be held responsible for patients' actions.

Another Birmingham Study—"Open All Hours": A Comparison of Two Areas, 1998 (Minghella, et al., 1998)

The MCHT service located in the Yardley/Hodge Hill area of North Birmingham in Britain is called the "Psychiatric Emergency Team" (PET), and its evaluation and description is of considerable interest for many reasons. Perhaps the most significant feature is that its development was specifically linked to psychiatric bed closures, and it is the first study to demonstrate exactly how, and to what degree, MCHT can replace inpatient care (Minghella, et al., 1998; Ford, et al., 2001; McGlynn & Smyth, 1998).

Furthermore, this model of MCHT has had an influence on development of the British national health service plan to develop 335 "crisis resolution teams" by 2004 with an expected reduction of 30% in demand for in-patient care (Department of Health, 1999). It is also used as a model for training purposes by the Sainsbury Centre for Mental Health. This is an organization affiliated with Kings College, London, that aims to influence national policy and encourage good practices in mental health services through research, training, and development. This study is the only one that was not first published in a peer reviewed journal; instead it was published as a book entitled *Open All Hours*, published by the Sainsbury Centre for Mental Health. This project benefited from the expertise of Dr. John Hoult, who imported his experience of MCHT from Sydney, Australia, and was the service's first psychiatric consultant.

The Sainsbury Mental Health Initiative awarded funding of 500,000 pounds to the Psychiatric Emergency Team in 1994 with three aims in mind:

- To support a home-based service that would offer an alternative to in-patient care
- To support a model that enables more people to receive acute treatment
- To reduce spending on in-patient beds and to free up money to develop longer term home-based care for those with the most severe needs—assertive community treatment.

The Sainsbury Initiative Award was used as bridging funds for the setting up of the new PET service over three years and enable a staged reduction of in-patient beds, which were halved from 41 to 20.

The study set out to compare two acute services in North Birmingham—Yardley/Hodge Hill and Erdington—both demographically similar inner-city areas with 90% White U.K. ethnicity and 14–15% unemployment.

The PET team and its work are described in great detail, but little information is given about services in the comparison area. The PET team comprised 9 mental health nurses, 2 social workers, 2 community support workers, 0.4 psychologist, and an administrator. Medical staff consisted of 1 consultant psychiatrist, plus 2 psychiatrists in training. Acute care in the comparison area was traditional hospital based, with a 23-bed in-patient unit and an after-hours on-call psychiatrist and social worker.

The design of the study was a comparison between consecutive patients admitted to hospital in Erdington and a series of matched patients in Yardley/Hodge Hill who had been admitted to hospital or accepted by PET.

All admissions to the Erdington in-patient ward over an eight-month period were assessed. Over the same period, a computer-generated random sample of one in three admissions to in-patient care or acceptance for PET were collected. The samples were then matched using the following criteria: gender, whether admitted in previous 18 months (yes or no), psychotic or neurotic illness, and age +/– 10 years. Previous studies have demonstrated that these factors are the best predictors of future in-patient bed usage (Marks, et al., 1994). This allowed 58 pairs to be matched (116 in all). The implementation sample consisted of 20 patients who were admitted upon referral and 38 who were accepted for PET. The target population is described as "those with a psychiatric disorder of such severity that they are at risk of hospital admission" and the commonest reasons for referral were onset or relapse of psychotic symptoms and risk of harm to self or others. Referrals, usually by phone, were accepted from primary care physicians, community mental health teams, and agencies such as social service departments and police. The team acted as a gatekeeper to the in-patient unit.

The pairs were not matched for severity of psychiatric illness at the time of the referral, and so it is not clear whether the 38 patients accepted for PET were as sick as the 58 who were admitted in Erdington—whether they would have required hospital level care. The BPRS was administered, but not immediately (within one week of entry into the study), but only 54% of implementation patients and 69% of comparison patients could be interviewed for this purpose. For those who were interviewed, there was no difference.

The patients were then tracked for six months. Service use and costs were measured. Untoward events, such as self-injury, violence, trouble with police, and suicide (there were none) were monitored and showed no difference.

BPRS was administered at six weeks, with a disappointing response rate (34%). The main diagnoses are shown in Table 1.10.

Table 1.10

	Implementation group	Comparison group
Schizophrenia	22%	24%
Affective disorder	24%	14%
Anxiety/depression	22%	16%
Other psychoses	10%	19%
Drug/alcohol	7%	16%

There were no differences found in clinical outcomes in the two groups. The BPRS response rate at 6 weeks though, was a disappointing 34.5%.

A detailed cost comparison was conducted by Ford, et al., (2001). Treatment of the hospital-oriented comparison group was 30% cheaper. In both follow-up periods, total costs were significantly lower for the implementation group. In the first six weeks the higher cost of community care for the implementation group was offset by the lower cost of in-patient care—a cost-benefit factor of 1.7:1. The cost-benefit factor rose to 5:1 in the 6–26 week follow-up period. In-patient care accounted on average for 50% of the total cost for the implementation group in the first 6 weeks and for 64% in the 6–26 week period. The respective figures for the comparison group were 99% and 85% (Figure 1.14).

Patient satisfaction as measured by the Client Satisfaction Questionnaire showed no difference. In both groups, over 70% were satisfied and 80% would recommend the service. This appears to be inconsistent with comments in the preamble to the study explaining its origins in the "clamoring" of consumers for a range of more sensitive services to be available 24 hours a day/7 days a week and including treatment in the home.

There were qualitative group differences in areas of dissatisfaction. The comparison group complained about the ward and hospital environment and wanted more choice of types of care, whereas the implementation group wanted more of the home treatment service: more time, more visits, easier access to the team.

Outcomes at Six Months

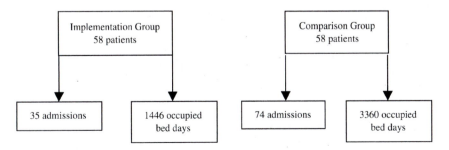

Figure 1.13 "Open All Hours" study.

6 Months Follow-Up Period

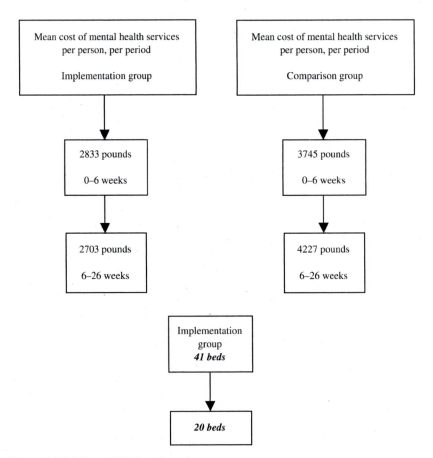

Figure 1.14 "Open All Hours" study.

Table 1.11

Practical Tips
• Service must be available after hours. This can be efficiently and effectively provided on an on-call basis overnight and by telephone
• It is absolutely crucial to prioritize those in high need
• Service should be multidisciplinary and include psychiatrists
• Service must be complementary to and integrated with other services
• Clear information about the service, how it operates, and how it can be contacted must be readily available to referring agents

- Teams must receive training in effective interventions, including those aimed at relapse prevention
- An acute community-oriented service costs less than an acute hospital-based service and bridging funds need only amount to an extra 1 pound per head over three years, but money must be recycled to sustain the system and a range of other support services must be in place
- An acute community service can work but there must be acute beds available—the service needs to be community-oriented, not exclusively community-based. Acute beds were needed both initially and in some cases after PET's involvement

---

South Islington Crisis Resolution Team: A Comparison of Two Time Periods, 2001 (Johnson, et al., 2001)

South Islington is an area of Inner London and is therefore of particular interest for MCHT research for two reasons. Questions have been raised as to whether MCHT can substitute for admission in an area where a) the threshold for admission is already high and b) many patients live alone, and homelessness and poor living situations are frequent, which makes home-based treatment less feasible. It will obviously be easier to reduce admissions in areas where clinicians have been relatively ready to admit, and patients relatively readily to go to hospital. This is not the case in Inner London where clinicians, managers, and patients are often eager to avoid it (Johnson, et al., 2001). There has been a bed crisis in London, often attributed to policies of bed closure and move to community being pursued too far, leading to a heated debate as to how far acute beds are replaceable.

The aim of this study was to compare outcomes and costs associated with management of crises before and after introduction of a "crisis resolution team" (CRT).

The primary hypothesis to be tested was that a) introduction of a CRT is associated with a fall in the proportion of patients in a crisis who are admitted to hospital and b) that patient satisfaction is greater, following introduction of a crisis resolution team. Unusually specific criteria are provided for "crisis":

1) Substantial deterioration in mental health and/or social functioning or significant disruption in support network/social circumstances of severely ill individual

2) Significant concerns re at least one of the following: Risk of harm to self or others, physically harmful self-neglect, risk of injury or harm from others because of a lack of caution or usual network

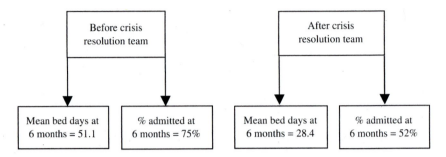

Figure 1.15 South Islington study.

Table 1.12

Presenting problem	Pre CRT	CRT
Psychotic symptoms	59%	75%
Depressive symptoms	53%	34%
Suicidal ideation	36%	26%
Anxiety	20%	17%

    no longer able to cope with caring role

3) Extent of deterioration such that professionals believe there is a need for an immediate change in management

Sample: all individuals aged 18–65 resident in South Islington and meeting criteria for crisis during six months pre-CRT (77) and ten months post-CRT (123).

    Socio-demographic characteristics of the two groups were similar: mean age was about 40, 51–53% lived alone, and 60% were single.

    Outcomes of this study in spite of the level of social deprivation were positive; less bed use, greater satisfaction and similar clinical outcomes—a replication of previous studies. However, the authors acknowledge the potential bias in such a design and plan on a randomized control study.

STUDIES OF HOME VISITING AND EARLY INTERVENTION

The following two studies are not really of Mobile Crisis Home Treatment as defined in this book—treatment for patients who are so acutely ill that they are candidates for admission. It is not clear how to categorize these studies: they are studies of "early intervention," home visiting, and other modifications of out-patient care. Admittedly, what the essential components of MCHT are has not been conclusively researched, but they are undoubtedly more than just home visiting. The subjects of these studies were simply not candidates for admission when the experimental intervention commenced.

The St. Georges Hospital, London, Study: A Randomized Controlled Comparison of Two Services, 1993 (Burns, Beadsmore, Bhat, Oliver, & Mathers, 1993; Burns, Raftery, Beadsmore, McGuigan, & Dickson, 1993)

In their introduction, the authors imply comparison of this study to those described above, in which patients at the point of requiring admission are instead diverted to an alternative community-based service. But, they then go on to say the study was designed to examine the effect of "adopting a more assertive community approach in a comprehensive psychiatric service." The services were not specially designed to provide MCHT and did not function like typical MCHT teams: they appear to be community mental health teams—described as " catchment area teams," which consist of medical staff, plus 1 full-time community psychiatric nurse, a half-time social worker and psychologist, and minimal occupational therapy. Acute bed provision was 0.2 per 1000. Most of the patients were not acutely ill: "many had minor time limited disorders." Only 12% of the experimental group and 20% of the control group are described as "urgent"; over 50% had no previous psychiatric history; and mean PSE scores were 40% lower than in the studies by Hoult and Muijen described previously. Even the psychotic patient's scores were only marginally higher than the non-psychotic.

The authors of the study had concerns about most of the previous studies of MCHT, in particular that one could not generalize the findings to routine clinical work for a variety of reasons. Some patient groups in a particular catchment area may not respond to MCHT or might suffer "relative neglect." Staffing levels and motivation are high in the teams of research studies. Both the Madison and the Wisconsin studies developed their services to meet large deficits in community mental health services, and the same positive results would not be found if MCHT were compared to a control group who had access to adequate community care and good primary care services.

With this in mind, Burns, et al. (1993) did a study that was more of a natural experiment. Of six clinical teams, three were to change their modus operandi to a "home-based" approach and they were each paired with a team carrying out conventional psychiatric care consisting of the usual out-patient clinic and in-patient unit, only using home visits for a few urgent

1 Year Follow-Up

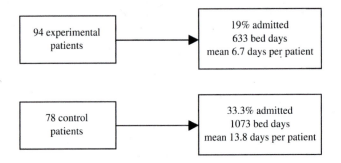

Figure 1.16 St. George's Hospital, London study.

cases. The experimental team underwent what sounds like very modest changes. These included the use of home visits, rather than clinic visits; the use of joint assessments by medical staff and another non-medical staff (in contrast to the usual assessment done by the psychiatrist); and earlier appointments with a maximum of two weeks' wait. All this was accomplished without any increase in the total number of visits, the mean number being 5.5–5.7. However, the experimental group spent an average of 5 hours and 23 minutes total treatment time including travel compared to 3 hours and 36 minutes for the control group, which the authors state is not statistically significant. None of the teams had a base in the community, and all but one lacked experience or training in home visiting.

The study randomly allocated patients to one of the 2 teams in each catchment area: a cohort of 94 experimental patients and 78 control patients was followed for one year. Over half were neurotic, mainly in states of depression and anxiety. Although allocation was random the groups were not completely comparable; 29% of the experimental group were psychotic, and 42% of the control group were psychotic. Statistically this is only adjusted for in the cost comparisons. Clinical outcomes and degree of satisfaction and family burden were the same for each group.

In spite of what appear to be minimal modifications to the method of care, differences in the two groups were substantial. The admission rate for the experimental group was 19% (633 bed days) compared to 33% (1073 bed days) for the controls—an overall mean of 6.7 days (experimental) and 13.8 days (control). Control patients incurred 57% higher costs.

These results came as a surprise to the authors, who had made no attempt to reduce hospital care. They attribute this outcome to the "experimental team's perception of which problems required hospital care and which could be dealt with out of hospital had changed," which is explained by the following factors:

1) More flexibility in work practices; i.e. if an initial assessment was inconclusive, the patient could be visited the next day to continue exploration: "they did not have to use admission for patients whose needs did not easily fit into a rigid clinic schedule."

2) An increase in conjoint working and consultation between medical and other staff (which meant less medical contacts—48% compared to 76% in the control group), and led to a "marked shift in a less medically dominated service, and an increase in psychosocial interventions."

3) "The study lends support to the value of a key-worker approach (patient assigned to non-medical staff person) even in relatively short-term treatments, and suggests that traditional patterns of working fail to fully utilize the potential of the multi-disciplinary team."

To put this study into context using the "anatomy of a crisis" Figure (Figure 1 in the Introduction), Figure 1.17 shows that these teams intervened chiefly at a point between Stage 1 and 2, before most patients' levels of clinical acuity reached a point where it was perceived as a psychiatric emergency severe enough to make them candidates for admission, which is likely why there was not greater patient or caregiver satisfaction in the experimental group.

Most of these patients were not facing hospital admission, avoidance of which is a large source of increased satisfaction. How did home visiting help to reduce hospital admission and bed usage? Details of clinical activity are scanty and one can only speculate. Most of these patients' problems did not reach the acuity of Stage 2, the crisis point. Crises are often the result of psychosocial stresses, interpersonal family tensions, difficulty in accessing conventional mental health services, poor compliance with treatment and caregiver's anxiety and helplessness. Possibly, home visiting mitigated these factors. It allows increased awareness of environmental and family problems; provides more opportunities to meet caregivers; and gives them support, reassurance, and tips on how to deal with the patient. Access to services was improved, and therefore likely prevented some patients' situations from becoming a crisis. The team operated without a waiting list, and outreach to the home sidestepped poor compliance and clinic no-shows; the proportion of patients who failed to attend their initial clinical assessments was significantly

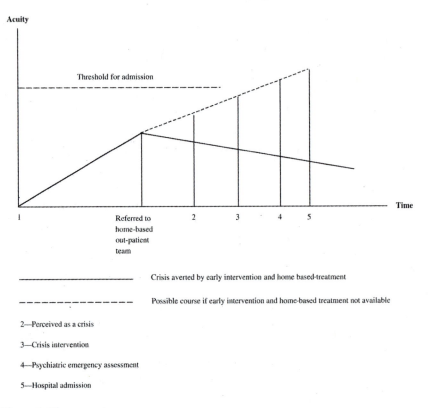

Acuity

Threshold for admission

Time

1

Referred to
home-based
out-patient
team

2   3   4   5

—————————————— Crisis averted by early intervention and home based-treatment

— — — — — — — — — — Possible course if early intervention and home-based treatment not available

2—Perceived as a crisis

3—Crisis intervention

4—Psychiatric emergency assessment

5—Hospital admission

Figure 1.17

lower in the experimental (7%) than in the control group (25%). When patients were encountered at Stage 4, psychiatric emergency assessment and the team's confidence and subjective perception about which problems required hospital care had changed as a result of their new way of providing care. In other words, the *clinical acuity threshold for admitting patients had been raised* (Figure 1.18). They were also able to respond more flexibly, and thus cope better with uncertainty and unpredictability. As Allen, et al. (2002) point out, in the discussion about what constitutes a psychiatric emergency in the introduction—"central to the concept of an emergency is the *subjective* quality, the unscheduled nature, lack of prior assessment or adequate planning and resultant uncertainty, severity, urgency, and conflict or failure of natural or professional supports, all of which contribute to the need for immediate access to a higher level of care."

In this study, home visiting probably reduced hospital bed usage for most of the patients by *prevention*; it helped to prevent the patient's acuity

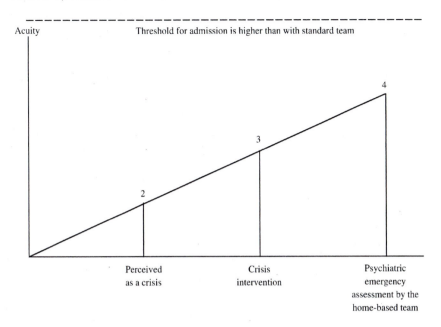

Figure 1.18

level from reaching the point where hospital admission is seriously considered. For some patients, it did actually provide an *alternative* to hospital— "the unscheduled nature and uncertainty" could be handled by the new, more flexible way of working; hence, as this was not perceived subjectively as an emergency, the team could still cope. It is an intriguing and important study, but for the most part should not be regarded as a study of MCHT providing an alternative to admission.

The St. Mary's Hospital, Paddington, London, Study, A Randomized Controlled Comparison of Two Services, 1992 (Merson, et al., 1992)

In the introduction to this study, Merson, et al. (1992) imply comparison with studies of MCHT aimed at acutely ill patients at the point of needing admission (Stein & Test, 1980; Hoult, 1986; Muijen, et al., 1992). They cast doubt on how valid generalizations may be from these studies because they were experimental and some of the gain may have stemmed from novelty and the enthusiastic commitment of research-oriented teams.

However, in this study, the patients were not acutely ill enough when enrolled to warrant hospital admission; therefore, it cannot be regarded as evaluating MCHT as an alternative to admission.

It is difficult to ascertain the clinical state of the target population. The subjects are described as "psychiatric emergencies," referred after visiting the ER of St. Charles Hospital or from the on-call psychiatrist or social worker of the hospital, which is located in Paddington, an inner-city district of London—one of the most socially deprived in Britain. But, when one examines how these patients were dealt with by the control "standard hospital" service, they don't appear to be emergent. They were referred to a psychiatric outpatient clinic, where they were seen for a mean of only 2.7 appointments, with "occasional domiciliary visits by senior psychiatrists"; none of them were admitted to hospital at the time of the referral.

One hundred patients were randomly allocated to a multi-disciplinary community based team (n = 48) or conventional hospital-based psychiatric services (n = 52) and assessed over a three-month period for psychopathology, social functioning, and treatments received. Criteria for inclusion in the study included: age 16–65, have a psychiatric disorder not primarily substance abuse, reside within Paddington, don't require mandatory admission, and not currently in contact with psychiatric services. Diagnoses were 40% schizophrenia, 25% mood disorder, and 27% neurotic and stress-related in the experimental group; 37% schizophrenia, 38% mood disorder, and 23% neurotic and stress-related in the control group.

The experimental service comprised 2 community mental health nurses, 2 social workers, a clinical psychologist, an occupational therapist and an administrator. They responded to referrals "within a few days" (which would suggest that they were not emergencies) and did not have 24-hour coverage. Most assessments were carried out in the patients' homes and close liaison was maintained with social agencies already in contact with patients. A case manager was assigned to each patient to coordinate all aspects of management.

The team did not appear to function like a typical MCHT service, given the low intensity of care; patients received a mean of only 5.2 visits. However, they were strikingly successful in reducing hospital bed usage, by 8-fold; the experimental group had a mean of 1.2 days, the hospital-based group, 9.3 days. Seven out of 48 patients from the experimental group (15%) and 16 out of 52 patients (31%) in the hospital-based group were admitted.

The authors are clear that this service did not provide an *alternative* to admission: "admission was not avoided in patients allocated to the experimental service and the difference in bed usage was accounted for largely by *early discharge,* rather than a *specific intervention at the time of presentation.* Use Figure 1.21 to understand this mechanism: early discharge to a home-based service, at Stage 5B shortens the time the patient spends at

3 Months Follow-Up

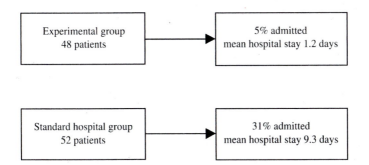

Figure 1.19 St. Mary's Hospital, Paddington study.

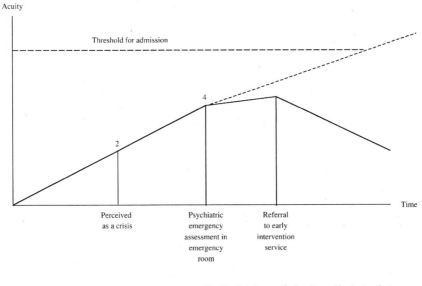

Figure 1.20

Stage 5, providing a more nuanced clinical response to the patients' psychosocial circumstances and clinical state. This study is similar to the Burns study in that home visiting, for most of the subjects, works by *preventing* hospital admission, rather than providing an *alternative*, likely by the same mechanisms as in that study. But, as shown in Figure 1.20, in this study, intervention was at Stage 3 and 4, crisis intervention or psychiatric emergency evaluation. These patients had gone first to the emergency room or had seen

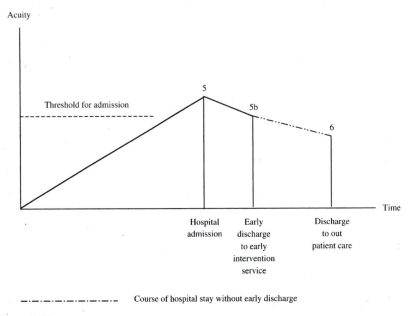

Figure 1.21

their primary care physician—likely perceived as in a crisis by themselves or those in their social network; but their clinical acuity was assessed as being below the threshold for admission.

One feature of the service contributing to its success in preventing admission was greater accessibility to mental health services—as in Burns' (1993) Study. Fifteen patients in the hospital-based service compared with one experimental patient did not receive a follow-up contact, reinforcing the greater take-up of the community service.

MOBILE CRISIS HOME TREATMENT IN U.S. MANAGED CARE; PATH, WEST HARTFORD, 1993 (PIGOTT & TROTT, 1993)

In the U.S., MCHT is used in managed care organizations. In West Hartford, Connecticut, Positive Alternatives to Hospitalization (PATH) has been developed (Pigott & Trott, 1993; Moy & Pigott, 1998). PATH is a 24-hour a day, in-home crisis intervention, triage, and treatment service founded by psychologists and is part of ConnectiCare (CCI), a 110,000 member health maintenance organization. HMO, PPO, and EAP managers refer psychiatric patients in acute crises presenting for hospitalization to PATH 24 hours a day, 7 days a week. A PATH provider (psychologist, psychiatric social worker, or clinical nurse specialist) meets with the patient and family wherever is most convenient, i.e., patient's home, emergency room etc., within one hour of referral. The referring case manager has to certify that without PATH's services the patient's condition warrants hospitalization. PATH's services were 100% reimbursed for the first three weeks of treatment when referred by CCI as an alternative to psychiatric hospitalization.

The majority of patients not referred to PATH were cases that were either hospitalized before CCI case managers were notified or hospitalized by a psychiatrist after refusing to allow PATH to assess the suitability of its services for the patient.

The first two years of PATH's operations with CCI were described by comparing in-patient utilization rates of patients who CCI case managers referred to PATH with those hospitalized without first being evaluated by PATH and managed by an out-of-state telephonic utilization review firm. It's difficult to compare the degree of psychopathology in the two groups, although to be referred to PATH in the first place the case manager has to certify that hospitalization is warranted. As shown in the following table, the patient group not assessed by PATH had a higher proportion of psychotic and bipolar diagnoses, and it is likely that in some cases more severe pathology was the reason why alternatives to hospital were not pursued. The authors admit that this is not a controlled study, describing their paper as a

Table 1.13 Diagnostic Comparability between PATH Referred and Not Referred Psychiatric Patients

Primary Diagnosis	ConnectiCare Cases Not Seen by PATH (%)	ConnectiCare Cases Treated by PATH (%)
Adult patients		
Depressive disorder	37.5	45.6
Psychotic disorders	19.7	10.7
Bipolar disorders	8.7	5.8
Personality disorders	16.6	19.4
Dual diagnosis (Psy/CD)	14.2	15.5
Other	3.4	2.9
Child and adolescent patients		
Depressive disorders	63.0	48.8
Disruptive behavior disorders	23.3	44.1
Psychotic disorders	9.6	3.6
Other	4.1	3.6

Table 1.14

Practical Tips
• Allow for lengthy initial visit; defuses tension and forges strong therapeutic alliance • Mobilize patient's support system • Single case manager • 24-hour care available • Flexible multimodal treatment approach

two-year "snapshot" of the impact of MCHT on hospital utilization in an HMO. Three hundred thirty-nine adult patients were hospitalized without first being evaluated by PATH, in contrast to 103 referred to PATH; we don't know what clinical factors determined the psychiatrists' decisions around hospitalization.

Of the 187 patients referred by CCI case managers, admission was averted in 151 cases (80.74%). During the two-year follow-up period, there were 45.9% hospital re-admissions of the non-PATH patients compared to 11.8% of PATH patients admitted or re-admitted. Average number of hospital days were 17.46 for non-PATH patients vs. 2.32 for PATH patients. Patients and their families were highly satisfied with PATH's services according to surveys submitted by CCI case managers.

MOBILE CRISIS TEAMS IN THE U.S.

MCHT services in the U.S. are often termed mobile crisis teams (MCT) and it is unclear whether they reduce hospital bed usage (Geller, Fisher, & McDermeit, 1995); much depends on what their goals are. Surveying these goals as stated in the literature provides a clue as to why reduction in hospitalization is not consistently demonstrated (Gillig, Dumaine, & Hillard, 1990; Alexander & Zealberg, 1999; Zealberg, Santos, & Fisher, 1993; Bengelsdorf & Alden, 1987; Gillig, 1995; Zealberg, Christie, Puckett, McAlhany, & Durban, 1992). Some of the goals of MCT, such as treating the crisis where it occurs and preserving the person's autonomy, are quite compatible with the aim of avoiding hospital admission; however, some are not, and may actually lead to increased use of hospitalization.

Goals that may conflict with avoiding hospital include:

- Providing service to difficult-to-reach persons
- Rapid response to police emergencies; these include someone threatening to jump off a ledge, hostage taker trapped by SWAT team, and intoxicated individual brandishing a weapon

- Case finding—related to next goal
- Reaching patients who lack insight, would not seek treatment on their own, and would refuse to come to hospital
- Reaching the homeless
- Initiating civil commitment
- Transporting disturbed individuals to the hospital instead of using the police
- Early intervention in a crisis

MCHT cannot provide an alternative to hospital treatment for all patients presenting in an emergency, especially those within the upper range of acuity, which likely includes many of those targeted in the above list of goals: those requiring civil commitment, transportation by police, or those involved in a police emergency. For an acutely ill patient to be treated at home, a minimum degree of cooperation and insight is required. This may exclude (but not necessarily) some of the patients described above; those who would not seek treatment on their own, need police transportation, or are difficult to reach. MCHT obviously requires the individual to be in a home, which excludes the homeless—although some of them can be treated by MCHT if they can be persuaded to go to a hostel or crisis shelter (see case history in Chapter 7). Case finding and early intervention may mean dealing with unscreened individuals at Stage 1 and 2 (Figure 1.1). As discussed in Chapters 4, 5, and 6, that may mean the team spends much of its time and resources on doing assessments on individuals who are not suitable for MCHT because their crisis is too mild or too severe, they have insufficient social support, they cannot cooperate, or their problem is more of a psychosocial one.

The study by Gillig, et al., (1990) of the mobile crisis team (MCT) at University of Cincinnati illustrates some of these points. The psychiatric emergency service associated with the university medical centre serves as the primary evaluation centre for psychiatric patients referred from a catchment area with a population of more than one million; it has both a mobile and a hospital-based component. The study compares the characteristics of patients who use each component. The MCT has round-the-clock capability and will evaluate in the field a person in a crisis who cannot, or will not, come to the hospital who has a probable mental illness or significant situational stress and will allow right of entry. The hospital-based service has an interdisciplinary staff and patients are seen around the clock on a walk-in basis. Data were collected on 100 consecutive contacts by MCT and a 100 randomly selected visits to the hospital-based emergency psychiatric service between February and June 1988.

Of patients seen by MCT, 39% refused to come to the ER and 37% did not realize they needed help. Even though the MCT was set up in response to a lobbying effort by friends and families of patients, or patients themselves, specifically to prevent hospital admission, 45% of MCT patients were admitted immediately or the next day, 14% involuntarily (40% of the hospital based emergency patients were admitted). The team saw a qualitatively different patient population than that seen by the hospital-based service. This group included elderly persons with organic illness, many of whom were referred by concerned family members who could not convince their loved ones to come to a hospital. The group also included shut-ins, physically disabled, and agoraphobic patients.

Although the Global Assessment Scale rating indicated both groups were equally impaired, it's not unreasonable to conjecture that some of these patients would never have been admitted were it not for the MCT; that they and their families would have quietly suffered at home, and never had contact with a mental health service. Or, perhaps, they would have had to deteriorate further before reaching the threshold of acuity for admission. In other words, the MCT may have served the entirely appropriate and laudable goals of treating the hard-to-reach patient and case finding, but that is not going to save beds.

Fisher, Geller, and Wirth-Cauchon (1990) raise similar issues. After their study failed to find an association between" mobile crisis capacity" and reduced rates of state hospitalization, they ask "What is the nature of linkages between mobile crisis teams, general hospitals, police departments, and other social agencies, and how do they affect the outcomes of mobile crisis intervention? Are there different 'styles' or approaches to mobile crisis intervention, and if so, are some more effective than others?"

Fisher's strategy was to compare Massachusetts state hospital admission rates across catchment areas with and without mobile crisis capacity, contrasting 20 catchment areas that had mobile capacity in 1986 with the group of 20 that did not. In each area, mobile crisis teams, hospital-based emergency services, and/or community-based clinics performed pre screening and crisis intervention functions. They controlled for social deprivation and stress, availability of community resources, and availability of general and private psychiatric beds. First and total admission rates were no different in areas with and without mobile crisis capacity. Fisher acknowledges that "having mobile capacity" is overly simplistic; how the services are structured, and how they are integrated into the rest of the mental health system and the existence of other key services for treatment and diversion are important variables and would be a profitable area of research.

Table 1.15

Practical Tips
• Therapeutic alliance strengthened by psychiatrist's presence on team, especially by ritual of physical examination
• Rapid alleviation of symptoms by medication including long-acting depot anti-psychotics and rapid tranquillization
• Leverage exerted on recalcitrant patients by threat of involuntary admission by psychiatrist
• Frequent home visits, often several a day; 24-hour telephone access; and periodic "check-ups" by telephone calls

Fisher conjectures that unnecessary hospitalizations prevented by mobile crisis intervention are "offset" by the admission of individuals needing inpatient care who are "discovered." It all boils down to what is meant by "mobile," what is the target group, and where and at what stage in the crisis the MCT intervenes Any MCT that meets its patients before Stage 4, psychiatric emergency assessment (Figure 1.1), runs the risk of netting so many unsuitable ones, that it defeats its purpose (of reducing hospital admission).

There are descriptions of mobile crisis services in the U.S. (Chiu & Primeau, 1991; Bengelsdorf & Alden, 1987; Zealberg, et al., 1992; Alexander & Zealberg, 1999), but very few studies are comparative: here are two—both comparisons of two time periods.

The Kalamazoo County, Michigan, Study: A Comparison of Two Time Periods, 1995 (Reding & Raphelson, 1995)

This study of "mobile crisis intervention" in Kalamazoo County, Michigan, did demonstrate reduced hospital admissions. Reding joined a pre-existing "mobile crisis intervention team," upgrading its function beyond triage for hospitalization to psychiatric treatment at the site of the crisis. Admission rates to the local state hospital one year prior to the new service, during the six months it operated and one year after it ended were compared. During the program period there was a 40% drop in admissions. After the psychiatrist, Reding, left, the rate of admission rebounded to the previous level.

There are lessons for the planning and administration of MCHT services in this study, which are elaborated on in Chapters 4, 5, and 6. Briefly, the psychiatrist's role was unsustainable—on-call 7 days a week, 24 hours a day—and the team met much resistance from the rest of the local mental health services with which it was poorly integrated. It ceased to function after six months.

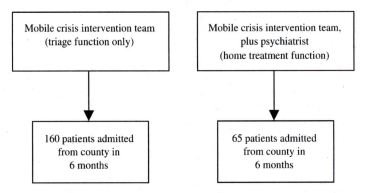

Figure 1.22 Kalamazoo County study.

30 Day Follow-Up Period

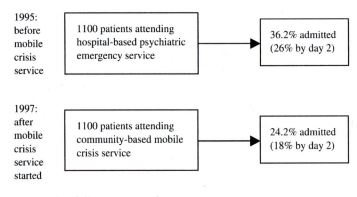

Figure 1.23 30-day follow-up period.

Table 1.16

Practical Tips

Features of program considered critical to reducing hospital admission:
- Active participation of a psychiatrist
- Ability to prescribe medication

Kluiter says that further research is needed to "look into what specific interventions (community or in-patient) are effective, neutral, or counter productive, and analyze treatment responses of well defined groups of patients." Szmukler and Holloway (2001) suggest that we need to become more deliberate and specific about in-patient treatment and its alternatives, reminding us that developments in community mental health services show how each of the functions of hospital (the 20 components of in-patient treatment described in Chapter 2) can be undertaken without automatic recourse to admission. This issue and just how MCHT and in-patient care fit together as components in today's complex system of mental health care are examined in Chapter 2.

A Comparison of a Hospital, Based Crisis Service Before the Introduction of a Mobile Crisis Service, with a Mobile Crisis Service One Year After it Was Developed (Guo, Biegel, Johnsen, & Dyches, 2001)

On July 1, 1996, the county mental health authority covering a "large midwestern industrial metropolitan area" (name not given) centralized delivery of psychiatric emergency services. The new approach included a hotline, a community-based mobile crisis progam, and authorization for state hospitalization under the administration of a single agency. Before this, people in a mental health crisis went to a hospital-based psychiatric emergency room, which had authority to approve admission to the state hospital. The change in service delivery was accomplished by shifting funds from the emergency room to the mobile crisis program with no change in cost to the system.

The study compared a cohort of consumers who received face-to-face hospital-based crisis services during the first 11 months of fiscal year 1995, before the mobile crisis service was developed, with a cohort of consumers who received community-based mobile crisis services during the first 11 months of fiscal year 1997. A data set of 1100 persons in each group was matched on seven variables: gender, race, age, diagnosis, recency of prior service use, substance abuse, and "certification of severe mental disability." Certification is based on having a diagnosis of a severe illness and the degree of dysfunction; 35% were thus certified. The cohort was tracked for 30 days after the initial crisis service.

The mobile crisis service was composed of crisis intervention specialists ("licensed mental health professionals"), nurses, and psychiatrists. Services included diagnosis, crisis intervention, pre-hospital screening, case management, medication, follow up, and linkage to additional community services.

A consumer using the hospital-based service was 51% more likely to be hospitalized than one using the community-based mobile crisis service. Of the hospital-based group, 32.6% were hospitalized; 26% by day 2. Of the mobile crisis group, 24.2% were hospitalized; 18% by day 2.

From day 3 to day 30, 4% were hospitalized in both groups, demonstrating that hospitalization was not simply delayed by the new service. Before the mobile service was created, hospitalization rates of both public and private psychiatric hospitals had been declining by less than 2% per year; in 1996 and 1997, after the service started, rates declined more than 8% per year.

Consumers were more likely to be hospitalized if they were young and homeless, had acute psychiatric problems; were referred by psychiatric hospitals, the legal system, or other treatment facilities; had substance abuse; had no income; and were severely mentally disabled.

Where does this research leave us: to what degree can MCHT replace in patient beds? Writing in 1997, Kluiter summarizes the results of eight randomized controlled trials (he includes the study of Polak, Kirby, 1976, excluded in this chapter because the experimental group were treated in the homes of selected families, paid to provide care, not in their own homes. This is described in Chapter 2).

For an average of 14 months follow up, a total of 610 patients receiving MCHT were studied. 66% avoided hospital admission, and the ratio of days in hospital was 17:60, compared with control care. The generalizability of the target groups in these studies is questionable; those in Stein's and Hoult's studies with their liberal inclusion criteria provided the best basis for policy making. These two studies involved only 125 patients in the MCHT modality. There have been no published RCTs since this was written (but there have been studies comparing different areas and different times—described above).

What about cost saving? Five of the MCHT studies compared costs: Wisconsin, Montreal, Sydney, Southwark, and the Birmingham "Open All Hours" study. MCHT was cheaper by:

- About 0%—Madison study (MCHT cost $797 more—offset by patients earning $1196 more)
- 21%—Sydney study
- 30%—Birmingham "Open All Hours" study
- 40%—Montreal study
- 45%—Southwark study

Kluiter notes that all major psychiatric treatment modalities, including in-patient treatment, are underevaluated. Szmukler and Holloway (2001) describe in-patient care from a research perspective as the "Cinderella of contemporary mental health services," and that "the literature demonstrates a striking lack of clarity behind the purpose of psychiatric admission and the way in which the process is conducted."

Chapter Two

Why Mobile Crisis Home Treatment? How Does It Fit with Mental Health Systems?

> *". . . to hospitalize a patient, is a major decision, which forever after changes the attitude of both the patient and those who care for them."*
>
> (Mendel & Rapport, 1969)

> *". . . even in the most highly evolved system of community care, some in-patient beds are required."*
>
> (Szmukler & Holloway, 2001)

This chapter describes how Mobile Crisis Home Treatment (MCHT) fits in with the mental health system as a whole: in particular, with in-patient treatment, other alternatives to hospital admission, and with crisis intervention and psychiatric emergency services.

MOBILE CRISIS HOME TREATMENT AND HOSPITAL ADMISSION

Mobile Crisis Home Treatment and Psychiatric Bed Reduction

The development of MCHT, its clinical rationale, and outcome research have always been intimately linked to avoidance of hospital admission, reduced hospital stay, and reduction in numbers of hospital beds. The research described in Chapter 1 indicates that MCHT can avoid admission in some patients and reduce length of stay for most, resulting in cost savings for the mental health system. Kluiter (1997) asks to what degree community alternatives can reduce use of hospital beds. To that question can be added: how low can one go with bed reduction? Many clinicians will have concluded that this process has gone too far already. Horror stories of overcrowded

Table 2.1 Historical Changes in Bed Numbers

Country	Interval	Change in beds	Change in beds
England and Wales	1956–1995	–74%	154,000 to 42,000 beds (80/100,000)
U.S.A. state hospital beds	1955–1994	–88%	339/100,000 to 40/100,000
Italy: Emilia-Romagna	1978–1996	–85%	220/100,000 to 34/100,000
Italy: South Verona	1977–1995	–62%	104/100,000 to 40/100,000
Finland	1980–1993	–64%	420/100,000 to 150/100,000
Germany	1970–1988	–29%	160/100,000 to 113/100,000
Netherlands: Groningen	1976–1990	0%	(adults 20–74 years)
Denmark	1978–1998	–50%	
Japan	1960–1993	+300%	95,067 to 362,963 beds

emergency rooms abound. The following discussion is based on Szmukler & Holloway (2001).

Published reports of bed:population ratios are difficult to compare because of differences in the definition of beds. Declines in psychiatric hospital beds may be offset by increases in other forms of residential care, such as group homes, crisis residences, hostels, and nursing homes. For example, in Britain, since 1982, the steep reduction in hospital bed numbers has been almost matched by an increase in such alternatives; some have called this process "trans-institutionalization." Whether there is a substantial private sector adds to the difficulty in interpreting the numbers.

Bed reductions have been rapid in some areas. Between 1994 and 1997, the U.S. Veterans Administration system closed 44% of its beds. In Australia, from 1993 to 1996, psychiatric beds were reduced by 18% overall, 36% in the State of Victoria. There was an overall increase of 55% in community-based funding. See Table 2.1 for examples of historical changes in bed numbers (Szmukler & Holloway, 2001).

The number of acute psychiatric beds in a mental health system is certainly influenced by the creation of an MCHT service. However, numerous other factors influence this, and deciding how many beds are needed is very complex. Szmukler and Holloway describe four groups of factors, that influence the decision.

1. Socio-Demographic

Social deprivation is a term used to describe a complex of social variables, which are linked to psychiatric illness: the greater the social deprivation, the greater the incidence of disorders such as schizophrenia, and the higher is the hospital admission rate. Social variables linked to psychiatric illness and social deprivation include: lower social class, male gender, ethnic groups, unemployment, overcrowding, living alone, living in inner-city areas with transient populations, poverty, and high population density. For example, these variables individually accounted for 71% of the variance in admission rates and in combination accounted for 95% in the southeast Thames region of England. Similarly, in Victoria, Australia, social factors could explain 70–80% of the variation in admission rates in urban areas and 35–48% in rural areas. Social deprivation can result in up to a fourfold difference in the prevalence of mental illness, in the secondary (i.e., specialist) mental health system between the least and the most deprived areas.

One has to take these social factors into account when planning for hospital alternatives. The degree to which beds can be replaced will likely vary depending on local social variables. The effectiveness of MCHT may be hampered for individuals with poor housing arrangements or who are living with few social supports. Crisis residences may be required to give them respite from their environment and/or partial hospitalization to give them a safe, structured, supportive milieu for a substantial part of their day. Community alternatives should not be thought of as an either/or processes. For example, in North Birmingham, U.K., (Ladywood service described in Chapter 3), MCHT is combined with low-level crisis housing.

2. Ideology and Policy

Governments, health departments, the legal system, and third-party payers can all have a major influence on bed numbers: "where there is a will to reduce beds, this usually is achieved" (Szmukler & Holloway, 2001).

Ronald Manderscheid, chief of the Survey and Analysis Branch of the Division of State and Community Systems in the federal government's Centre for Mental Health Services summarizes these influences in America (Lipton, 2001).

> **Legal cases** have resulted in rulings that individuals must be treated in community-based programs if possible; the latest is the Supreme Court's *Olmstead* decision. The L.C. and E.W. v. Olmstead case was brought in 1995 on behalf of two women with mental retardation as well as psychiatric conditions, who were patients in a state psychiatric hospital in Georgia. The treating professionals in the hospital all agreed that they were appropriate for discharge to community programs, but slots were not available. While the case worked its way through the courts, both women were placed in the community where they have been doing very well.

The potential relevance of all this to MCHT provision, is that the State of Georgia asked the Supreme Court to decide whether the federal Americans with Disabilities Act compelled the state to provide treatment in a community placement when appropriate treatment can also be provided in a state mental institution. On June 22, 1991, the court ruled that the state must provide community-based services rather than institutional placement. On June 18, 2001, President Bush directed federal agencies to assist states with Olmstead implementation (Bazelon Centre for Mental Health Law).

- **Consumers** say they want to be in the community, not in the hospital
- **Managed care** diverts patients into less expensive care
- **Medicaid** does not pay for hospitalization of persons aged 21–64 in state and county facilities

The number of people receiving care in ambulatory mental health settings has increased more than 300% between 1969 and 1998, but, Manderscheid says, "that still begs the question of building community systems of care, . . . [Without these] people can't be maintained in the community . . . Just because you offer psychotherapy, [this] is not sufficient. These community resources are becoming more important than ever, he points out, because of the increased number of people diagnosed with mental illnesses in jails and prisons, the increased number of people without access to mental health care, and the decrease in resources to fund private-sector services in the community.

By ideology, Szmukler and Holloway mean a system of beliefs and values resting to a greater or lesser degree on an evidence base. They cite the radical reduction in beds in Italy in the late 1970s, and, in Australia, the creation of a national policy in 1992 to shift from institutional to community care. This was accompanied by strong political support and a large proportion of the budget was "reform and incentive funding" to foster restructuring of mental health services. To these examples can now be added the NHS plan in Britain to establish "crisis resolution teams" (MCHT) and reduce inpatient beds by 30%.

The important point to be made here is that the evidence base for replacing beds with such community alternatives as MCHT is not sufficient to bring it about; without a specific strategy, based on values and beliefs, major change is unlikely. For example, in the Netherlands, the government expected local mental health services to make such changes in the absence of forceful measures such as reducing budgets of large mental hospitals. Between 1989 and 1997, the number of patients treated under "intensive community care" increased threefold; however, in-patient days declined very slowly.

Political pressures can also cause a reversal in these policies. In the 1990s, government in the U.K. became very sensitive to claims that community care had "failed"—fuelled by highly publicised homicides by psychiatric patients. The Department of Health published "discharge guidance" focusing on risk—as a consequence, the length of in-patient stay rose (see the Marks, et al. study in Chapter 1).

3. Factors That Control Flow of Patients into Hospital (Inflow Factors)

This is where MCHT services can influence bed usage; the extent to which different alternatives to hospital are available is an inflow factor: as well as MCHT, partial hospitalization or day hospitals and crisis residences can lead to reduced use of beds. However, gatekeeping of in-patient beds is important if these alternatives are to be fully used. For example, in the "Open All Hours" study (Minghella, et al., 1998), when the original consultant Dr. Hoult left the admission rate rose temporarily. Just because hospital alternatives are available does not guarantee their optimum use; this depends on how well psychiatric emergency staff do their job in assessing whether patients can be steered towards a community alternative and, furthermore, engaging the patient and family to ensure this disposition. Segal, Watson and Akutsu (1996) studied decision making of clinicians in the ER of seven California County general hospitals. They hypothesized that when good quality care was available, less restrictive alternatives are more likely to be used when the patient's condition permits and when other setting characteristics are taken into account. Less restrictive alternatives were available in 61% of the evaluations, used in 39%, and overlooked in 13%. In 8%, available alternatives were considered but not used. The decision to use a less restrictive and less costly alternative was primarily determined by the patient's need, which is related to the severity of the patient's condition. The quality of care also determined whether alternatives were used; a factor associated with overlooking an available alternative was the clinicians ability to adequately engage the patient at a level appropriate to their functioning—the art of care." This was measured using The Art of Care Scale which addresses the patient's perspective (Segal, Egley, & Watson, 1995). It consists of four items measuring the clinicians attempt to engage the patient in a collaborative interaction, elicit information, include the patient in the planning at a level appropriate to their functioning, and attend and respond empathically to the patient's feelings. Being over-involved in the technical aspects of care was associated with a decreased use of alternatives, and it is important to have clinicians with the necessary psychosocial skills.

There is little data showing to what degree MCHT has resulted in actual bed closures. In North Birmingham, beds were reduced from 30 to 16 per 100,000. (Minghella, et al., 1998). In the Newcastle, U.K. area, Stephen Niemiec's home treatment team has allowed the closing of 16 beds out of 120; next year, a further 21 beds will be closed, and in two years, a further 10 beds. This will result in a reduction of the bed:population ratio from 31:100,000 to 21.5:100,000 in Newcastle, and from 29:100,000 to 17:100,000 in North Tyneside (S. Niemiec, personal communication, May 3, 2003). Kennedy and Smyth (2003) report a reduction in admissions by an average of 30% in six cities in the U.K. and Ireland.

Bed:population ratios set by government policy or by professional bodies vary widely.

- Italy—general hospital beds 10:100,000; long-term care residential facilities (small, home-like < 20 beds) 10:100,000 (Burti, 2001)
- Ontario—general hospital beds 18:100,000; chronic beds 12:100,000 (Ontario Ministry of Health, 1993)
- U.K. Royal College of Psychiatrist—general hospital beds 44:100,000 (Breakey, 1996)

Szmukler and Holloway (2001) also consider the actual size of the in-patient unit as an important factor in its ability to cope with variations in the inflow of patients. Planning for admissions is difficult; the rate varies from day to day— some days none, other days many. A mathematical formula using the "Poisson distribution" predicts that a single large unit of 100 beds will buffer the variations better than a number of smaller units e.g.; 5 units of 20 beds each.

4. Factors That Control the Flow of Patients out of the Hospital (Outflow Factors)

Surveys of in-patients in acute beds in England have consistently found that, despite bed occupancy rates of well over 100%, around 30% of patients are placed inappropriately: the chief reason being outflow—not enough residential options for discharge. Outflow control, i.e., control of discharge, is important for MCHT to do its job of decreasing bed usage. In the Connolly, Marks, Lawrence, McNamee, and Muijen, (1996) Southwark, London, study in Chapter 1, it was shown that when the MCHT service lost control of the discharge decision making, the length of stay increased by 300%.

5. Local Customs and Conventions

Clinical teams vary in their practices. Szmukler and Holloway provide examples of otherwise identical teams in Nottingham, Norway, and Australia having variations in their lengths of stay up to threefold. In Chapter 3, some MCHT teams lament how "some of the consultant psychiatrists bypass us." Even a senior consultant complained about colleagues who admit without considering MCHT—"and I'm supposed to be their boss."

Why Avoid Hospital Admission?

Much of the focus of mobile crisis home treatment research is on cost: decreasing hospital admissions usually results in decreased cost. Cost has become a critical factor in the delivery of mental health services and is driving the search for innovative, cost-effective methods of service delivery in the public and private sectors. But, there is more to the issue than economics; in-patient treatment has other disadvantages apart from cost. Like most powerful therapeutic activities, it comes with side effects and disadvantages. See Table 2.2.

What are the sources for the list? Some, such as language barriers (a patient who doesn't speak English) and elderly patients becoming confused, are based on clinical common sense and experience; the rest are extracted from home treatment studies. Stein and Test (1978) express concern that patients don't learn how to deal with their social stressors in hospital, and they are discharged to often highly conflicted family situations where the ingredients for another crisis and

Table 2.2 15 Reasons to Think Twice Before Admitting a Patient

---

1. More expensive than community treatment
2. Psychological triggers of a crisis may not get required attention
3. Disrupts patient's life
4. Patient cannot meet family responsibilities; i.e., childcare
5. Increases chances of being admitted again
6. Social stigma
7. Can cause post-traumatic stress disorder
8. Can foster dependency—"institutional syndrome" in its worst form
9. Relieves pressure on community agencies to develop programs for seriously mentally ill
10. In-patient treatment has an insignificant effect on post hospital adjustment
11. Revolving door syndrome
12. Can cause regression; i.e., in-patients with borderline personalities
13. Patient cannot speak English
14. Can increase confusion in the elderly
15. Patients and their families usually prefer community treatment

---

and hospitalization are omnipresent. Hospital deepens pathological dependency. The more often patients are admitted, the more likely they are to return—the revolving door syndrome (Mendel & Rapport, 1969; Strauss & Carpenter, 1974; and Wynne, 1978). Continued use of the hospital relieves the pressure on community agencies to develop programs for the seriously mentally ill. Hoult (1986) writes:

> Many times the underlying interpersonal stresses which have precipitated the symptoms and sign are ignored or are not adequately dealt with. Doctors working in hospital focus on psychopathology—patient and relatives quickly learn that this is what doctors are interested in and report their difficulties in these terms. Eventually the patient takes on the role of patienthood, community coping skills get lost and relatively minor stresses lead to symptoms which lead to further admission.

McGorry, Chanen, and McCarthy (1991) found evidence of post-traumatic stress syndrome as a consequence of hospital admission procedures for psychotic patients. Such procedures include involuntary admission, police involvement, duress or coercion, forced sedation, restraint and seclusion, and finding oneself in a closed environment with a number of other psychotic or disturbed individuals. McGorry, et al. (1991) followed prospectively 36 in-patients recovering from an acute psychotic episode. Using measures such as the PTSD scale and the Impact of Events scale, they concluded that at four months 45.8% met the DSM-III criteria for PTSD, while at 11 months 34.5% met the DSM-III criteria for PTSD. Symptoms seemed to be linked to the experience of hospitalization, and, less so, to the psychotic experience per se; i.e., recurrent nightmares involving forced sedation or seclusion. McGorry, et al.'s research did not support the hypothesis that PTSD would be more likely to occur after a patient's first admission, or after an involuntary admission, which may cast some doubt on the whole idea; he explains that finding as due to a "ceiling or threshold effect"—that admission for psychosis for a psychologically vulnerable patient is "uniformly an extremely stressful experience."

Apart from cost, a common barrier to arranging in-patient treatment is patient refusal. A fair portion of the clinician's time in acute psychiatric practice seems to be devoted to attempting to persuade unwilling patients to be admitted "for a few days." To many patients, the prospect of psychiatric admission can seem frightening, abhorrent, embarrassing, or, at the very least, downright inconvenient, and they would much prefer home treatment. In the case of more severely disturbed patients, one can resort to involuntary admission, but that can be distasteful to the physician and demoralizing to the patient; or, it may be simply impossible because of stringent criteria in the local mental health legislation. Some of these patients may be receptive to mobile crisis home treatment, thereby avoiding involuntary admission (Dunn, 2001). Compulsory certification rates in County Monaghan, a rural area of Ireland, have more than halved and are currently one third of the average national rate, after the introduction of an MCHT service and an assertive community treatment team (Kennedy, 2003).

In spite of all these caveats, in-patient treatment is sometimes the best option a clinician can offer a patient and his family at a time of crisis. It is a powerful therapeutic activity and will always be a major item in any mental health system. The general indications for in-patient care include: risk of self-injury, dangerousness to others, severely distressing affects or behaviours, and the need for intensive observation for diagnostic clarification and stabilization. (Breaky, 1996).

But, how much risk of self-injury? How distressing the behavior, before one decides to admit? The answers to these questions will vary, depending on the severity of psychopathology, level of support available (both professional and informal), patient's age, personality, the presence of comorbidity, and many other factors. Often, these factors have to be weighed quickly, and yet the decision has widespread implications for health care economics, the future care of the patient, and his role in his family and in society. Allen, et al. (2002), in their definition of a psychiatric emergency (Introduction), highlight certain key elements involved in the decision to admit a patient to hospital in an emergency: the perceived mismatch of needs and resources, for which the emergency service must compensate; the subjective quality of the assessment, the uncertainty, and the lack of supports. This decision making process is eloquently described by Christie (1985) in his article "The Moment of Admission." Christie uses the concept of *insufficiency* to explore how a psychiatrist decides to admit a patient. Generations of psychiatrists have always asked "Why now? Why is this patient requesting admission now?" According to Christie, an honest assessment of these questions not only clarifies the practice at the moment, but also provides an *opportunity to review alternatives to practice—alternatives that may be useful to the patients and clinicians to follow* (for example, MCHT).

> Christie explains insufficiency thus: insufficiency is used to convey the multifactorial sense of collapse, inadequate resources, or marginal controls within a patient and his interpersonal system. Just as cardiac patients are admitted to hospital for cardiac insufficiency, a condition that may grow from problems with diet, exercise, and social supports as well as medications and end organ changes, so the term insufficiency can apply to psychiatric admissions . . . the experienced psychiatrist cognitively and instinctively knows this moment, because he, or she has faced it

Factors Contributing to Insufficiency

- *Patient factors*: sometimes the illness just gets worse, probably for physiological reasons, or because of non-compliance with medication. Certain symptoms or behaviours can set off alarm bells in the psychiatrist's mind, i.e.; command hallucinations, or any actions that might pose a risk to children. Comorbid physical illness, sleep deprivation, or substance abuse can compound the illness.
- *Family factors*: sometimes families have just had enough; they are fatigued, exasperated, or a key supportive member is no longer available.
- *Psychiatrist/mental health system factors*: each practitioner has his or her limitations of time, flexibility, energy, and tolerance. Important professional supports, such as out-patient therapists and day programs can be missing or can change.
- *Psychosocial factors*: the patient's environment may change, such as housing, disability payments, loss of job.

---

many times . . . if the clinician can preserve a reflective consciousness, *this is a time of great opportunity to learn new ways to structure care.* [Italics added]

How is Mobile Crisis Home Treatment an Alternative to Admission?

Allowing acutely ill psychiatric patients to remain in their homes and receive treatment instead of admitting them to hospital is often preferable. But, exactly how is MCHT an *alternative* to in-patient care? What is in-patient care? What do patients receive in the hospital, and can they get it at home instead? How can in-home treatment address the "insufficiencies" of the patient and his caregivers? There is surprisingly little written about what in-patient care provides in concrete operational terms. Menninger (1995) lists the services that in-patients receive, but it is difficult to translate all the interventions in the list into concrete care activities that can be provided by MCHT.

The following list attempts to do just that. It lists every component of in-patient care; exactly what services patients receive on a typical psychiatric ward, enabling one to compare MCHT and hospital treatment and to begin to think how one might substitute the former for the latter. See Table 2.3.

The following is a description of each of these services, accompanied by a glimpse of how they could be replicated in the home and community. Each intervention should be viewed as part of a continuum. The hospital is where care is usually most intense; however, with some creativity, we can provide lesser degrees of it, which may be sufficient to enable a patient to avoid being admitted to hospital. How these interventions are actually delivered in MCHT is described in more detail in Chapters 4, 5, and 6.

Table 2.3 Components of Psychiatric In-Patient Care

1.	Containment
2.	Prevention of self-harm
3.	Prevention of harm to others
4.	Interpersonal contact
5.	On-going assessment
6.	Hotel services
7.	Help with self-care
8.	Drug therapy
9.	Psychotherapy
10.	Electroconvulsive therapy
11.	Assessment of competence in activities of daily living
12.	Structure
13.	Activities
14.	Medical care
15.	Arrangement of community supports
16.	Liaison with the outside world
17.	Daily care by psychiatrist
18.	Daily services of occupational therapist social worker and psychologist
19.	Involuntary treatment, depending on local mental health legislation
20.	Asylum; respite for the patient and/or caregivers

1. Containment

Patients are often admitted because their behavior is too disruptive for their families and immediate community to tolerate. As well as controlling behavior with drugs, nursing staff will contain patients who are highly perturbed, restless, loud, or act inappropriately. This containment is accomplished by restricting patients to a small area, such as their room, by diverting them or by soothing them.

If medications don't calm the patient, home treatment may be difficult, because it is limited in being able to provide containment. In our MCHT service, we have taught families simple methods to deal with mild disruption; for example, a young manic patient allowed herself to be confined to her room when she became overactive (see case of Meghan, Chapter 8). Patients will sometimes respond, especially if they can appreciate that admission to hospital can be avoided this way.

2. Prevention of Self-Harm

Constant observation is the ultimate example of this. Lesser degrees of intervention would be close observation, checking patients and their belongings for "sharps" and other dangerous objects, and, of course, the ability to respond quickly if the patient does something to harm himself. In the home, one can remove dangerous objects and limit supplies of medication and arrange for the patient never to be left alone. Families will sometimes arrange a "shift system" of close friends and relatives to keep the patient safe.

3. Prevention of Harm to Others

The most extreme version of this activity is, of course, physical restraint, or detention in a ward or seclusion room. Prevention of harm to others can also be achieved by such activities as relationship management including soothing an angry paranoid patient, diverting the patient, helping the patient overcome frustration and ventilate feelings, and de-escalation activities.

Home treatment is inadequate when there is significant risk of harm to others. One would obviously do everything possible to avoid putting a family member in a position where the patient might injure them. If, for some reason, such a patient is at home, family members should be coached as to the warning signs of impending violence, avoidance manoeuvres, triggering factors, and how to act decisively by leaving the house and calling the police. Some families, keen to avoid hospital admission, are willing to put up with minor degrees of aggressiveness and can be taught techniques to prevent it and deal with it.

4. Interpersonal Contact

Patients in a crisis sometimes find being alone very frightening; their thoughts and feelings can overwhelm and terrify them, and the mere physical presence of a warm, caring, empathic person can be very comforting. Hospital nursing staff can provide this presence, and, to a lesser degree, so can fellow patients. In home treatment, one can arrange for patients to have someone stay with them, or to go and stay with a friend or family member.

5. On-Going Assessment

One reason for perceived "insufficiency" includes the situation when the patient's psychopathology and behavior become severe and/or change rapidly and unpredictably and cannot be monitored adequately. Admission may be arranged therefore to clarify the diagnosis, to be ready for a sudden turn for the worse; i.e. development of psychotic symptoms, or simply to see what is going on. Home treatment can obviate the need for admission by providing on-going assessment through frequent home visits, regular phone contact, and family coaching.

6. Hostel Services

Sometimes, patients become unable to care for themselves as a result of a psychiatric disorder; their nutrition may be alarmingly poor, their residence a mess. This lack of self-care may be the chief reason for admission. However, hospital may be avoided by providing meals, nutritional supplements, careful monitoring of weight and physical status, or by having patients stay at a hostel or with a relative.

7. Help with Self-Care

A patient's hygiene may be neglected, but nursing care in the home can often adequately address this issue.

8. Drug Therapy

Another common point of "insufficiency" comes when one simply cannot carry on doing pharmacotherapy in the usual out-patient fashion; it becomes obvious that the patient is forgetful and confused about medicines and is likely non-compliant. Or, patients seem to be completely unable to tolerate any drug you try, because they complain of "side effects" and make frequent phone calls to seek reassurance. Home treatment can often alleviate this problem by daily nurse visits, sometimes to actually administer the drugs, or to fill a *dosette box* with a day's supply at a time, and to provide frequent reassurance. Home treatment can also provide close monitoring for toxicity, medical risks, and rapid titration.

9. Psychotherapy

In-patient psychotherapy tends to be short, frequent, informal, and whenever the patient needs it. Often that is all they can tolerate at that stage of their illness. This is easily replicated in home treatment, and, in Western culture, can also be done sometimes by telephone.

10. Electroconvulsive Therapy (ECT)

ECT can easily be provided to out-patients if enough supports are in place; i.e., the nurse may drive the patient to and from the hospital.

11. Assessment of Competence in Activities of Daily Living

Sometimes, one feels one has to admit a patient because of what seems like "impending insufficiency"; one is afraid that the patient will suddenly cease to be able to manage at home due to cognitive impairment, psychotic thinking, or just paralysis, giving up completely. Admission may be avoided in this case by sending someone into the home with the time and flexibility (important because you never know what they may find) to assess functioning.

12. Structure

Most acutely ill patients benefit from having a structured day: a predictable sequence of activities of daily living, household duties, and recreation.

MCHT can help by giving patients a timetable of activities, regular visits, and phone calls to encourage them and motivate them, and sometimes accompanying them or working alongside.

13. Activities

Non-essential enjoyable healthy activities such as walks, crafts, and group projects can be therapeutic and easy to arrange in the community.

14. Medical Care

The more diagnoses the patient has (comorbidity), the more complex their management, and the more taxing the patient's care becomes in an office or out-patient clinic practice. Acute psychiatric disorders can make it difficult for patients to manage their physical health problems adequately, or may even exacerbate them; diabetes is a good example. Conversely, unstable medical disorders can complicate management of psychiatric conditions. However, careful monitoring, and taking a very active approach such as accompanying the patient to the family doctor, or arranging in-home blood tests can prevent admission for these situations.

15. Liaison with the Outside World

Some patients live in chaos, have overwhelming stress, and must deal with a multitude of agencies, including police, child welfare services, lawyers, financial institutions, and employers. They need a great deal of help dealing with these social problems, and home treatment probably shines here; it is likely easier, and more effective, to walk the patient through their particular minefield of social problems in the community rather than at arm's length, while they are in hospital.

16. Arranging Supports in the Community

As above, community supports can be arranged much more effectively in home treatment, with more of a gradual transition from the intensive psychiatric support.

17. Care by a Psychiatrist

Rapid, frequent involvement of a psychiatrist, 24 hours a day if necessary, is a feature of in-patient care. This care can be replicated to a certain degree by making sure the home treatment team's psychiatrist is accessible by phone and that his schedule is sufficiently flexible to enable him to see urgent cases quickly, conduct home visits at short notice, and have adequate time to consult with the staff about his patients; obviously, the method of compensation for psychiatrists' services is a crucial feature—fee-for-service would not enable the above kind of practice.

18. Services of Occupational Therapist, Psychologist, and Social Worker.
These services can all be provided in home treatment.

19. Involuntary Treatment
Even involuntary admission may be available in home treatment in some jurisdictions, although not to the same degree as in a hospital. Community certification is a slowly growing innovation, in which, under the threat of forced admission to hospital, patients can be compelled to comply with treatment.

20. Asylum; Respite for Patient and/or Family
This can be arranged, with MCHT support, by arranging for family members or friends to take turns caring for the patient in their own homes. Or, patients can be admitted to a crisis shelter or a hostel, where the MCHT team continue to provide mental health care.

It is now recognized that there are numerous advantages to avoiding or reducing hospital admission, and we have seen how MCHT can accomplish this: but what are other alternatives to hospital? How does MCHT compare to these, and which one is the best?

HOW DOES MCHT COMPARE TO OTHER ALTERNATIVES TO HOSPITAL?

If there were a competition to determine which is the "best alternative to hospitalization," the other main contenders would be partial hospitalization and residential crisis services.

Partial Hospitalization

Partial hospitalization has been at least as well researched as MCHT. The following is based on reviews by Creed (1995), Hoge, Davidson, Hill, Turner, and Ameli (1992), and Schene (2001). A detailed review of research on partial hospitalization (PH) is beyond the scope of this book.

PH is defined as an ambulatory treatment program that includes the major diagnostic, medical, psychiatric, psychosocial, and pre-vocational treatment modalities designed for patients with serious mental disorders who require coordinated, intensive, comprehensive, and multidisciplinary treatment not provided in an out-patient setting. It allows for a more flexible and less restrictive treatment program by offering an alternative to in-patient treatment. Within the term partial hospitalization is subsumed a confusing array of terms, such as day hospital and day centre.

In the U.K., PH for acutely ill patients is termed day hospitalization; in the U.S., the day hospital/intensive care model. Typical length of stay is 4–8 weeks. The service has a medically oriented staff with a high staff:patient ratio and is usually located close to an in-patient unit.

Randomized controlled studies of PH vs. full-time hospitalization (FTH) show that PH can treat about 40% of patients who would otherwise need admission; there is no difference in symptom reduction, and some show a superior outcome in social functioning for PH. Some show greater patient and family satisfaction. PH costs are lower: 20% cheaper for a day hospital/crisis respite program in the U.S., and almost 2000 pounds cheaper in a British study (Creed, 1995).

It is important to point out that in these studies some patients were not treated only as day patients—they spent some time on an in-patient unit or in a crisis residence. Zwerling and Wilder (1964) attempted to treat all patients presenting for admission, only excluding those with substance dependence, organic brain disorder, or mental retardation. Two thirds were treated in the day hospital, but of these 40% were "boarded" in the in-patient unit for short periods because of risk to self or others. Thirty-four percent of day hospital patients spent one night in hospital, and 22% spent two or more nights. In Creed's (1995) study, about half of the patients spent up to two nights in the hospital prior to randomization.

Creed emphasized that the threshold for admission to day hospital treatment is not fixed, but depends on the nature of the day hospital, particularly how well staffed it is. Staff attitudes are important, especially whether they accept treatment of seriously ill patients. Staff can initially be resistant, thinking that hospital is safer, provides more intensive treatment, and that separation from the family is a good thing. There must be an adequate total number of staff for a disturbed patient to receive individual attention from one member of staff, while groups for the remaining patients continue without disruption. Creed points out that the proportion of acutely ill patients that can be handled varies, and one cannot extrapolate the findings from one day hospital study to another; for example, he studied the day hospital in the nearby town of Blackburn, but, because of lower staffing, the proportion of patients diverted from hospital was less (16%).

Creed emphasizes that more than just day hospital is required to treat acutely ill patients. Some required additional support at home, overnight accommodation in a hostel, and/or help to travel to the day hospital by taxi or minibus. A community psychiatric nurse (CPN) facilitated attendance at the day hospital in Creed's study by helping patients overcome the fear of leaving home. CPN's also were on an on-call rota for telephone support and home visits at the weekend. Day hospital can also be used for early discharge from hospital.

This evolution from "pure" day hospital treatment to day treatment combined with treatment in the home by CPNs at the weekend did not stop there in Creed's program in Manchester. Eventually, in 1997, the day hospital was extended into a mobile crisis home treatment program, operating 24 hours per day, 7 days a week. It metamorphosed into the Manchester Home Option Service, which is described in Chapter 3 of this book. Harrison, Poynton, Marshall, Gater and Creed (1999) describe the reasons for this transformation. Although transportation was provided and some home visits were offered, patients had to attend the day hospital for at least some of their treatment, and it was not possible to engage patients who preferred not to. It was difficult to respond to crises at inconvenient times, like Friday afternoons. There were also conflicting demands on the resources of the day hospital, such as work with less severely ill patients. This service model combines aspects of acute day hospital and home treatment, but patients can receive all their care at home.

This theme, of combining acute day hospital treatment with other alternatives to hospital admission, runs throughout the PH literature. For example, Sledge, et al. (1996) and Sledge, Tebes, Wolff, and Helminiak (1999) compare conventional in-patient treatment for urban, poor, severely ill voluntary patients with an alternative experimental program consisting of a day hospital, which is linked to another alternative to hospital—a crisis residence—a three-bedroom apartment in a middle class residential area of New Haven, Connecticut. This service was feasible for at least 24% of all patients who were candidates for admission. Most patients were excluded because they were not voluntary, others because they required restraints, were intoxicated, needed one-to-one surveillance, or required active medical attention. When the authors excluded those patients for whom this program was not designed and those that could not have been admitted, the feasibility was 83%; outcomes were equal to, and in some measures slightly superior to, hospital care, with a cost saving of 20%.

Schene (2001) lists the therapeutic factors in day hospital treatment. The chief ones, in declining importance are: structure, interpersonal contact, medication, altruism, catharsis, learning, mobilization of family support, connection to community, universality, patient autonomy, successful completion, and security.

Residential Crisis Services

Although a review of the literature on these services is beyond the scope of this book, a thorough discussion of this approach is important because it is an essential partner to the other two alternatives to hospital; both of these are limited in the degree to which they can treat patients who do not have adequate housing and/or social support. Linking them to a crisis residential service can considerably broaden their scope.

Residential alternatives to hospitalization have been used for many years, and have roots going back centuries. They can be divided into two types: those that provide treatment to one or two individuals at a time—most commonly the family-based crisis home—and those that treat patients in groups. Most group crisis facilities can accommodate 6–15 patients and are more common than the individual family-based approach: common labels are crisis houses, crisis hostels, respite houses, crisis respite beds, and crisis stabilization units.

These services

- provide housing during a crisis
- are short term
- serve individuals or small groups
- are used to avoid hospitalization (Stroul, 1988)

Warner (1995) describes the historical roots of these services, which go back to early nineteenth century moral management. Some, such as Polak's family sponsor homes have links to the post-war therapeutic community movement of Maxwell Jones. Others trace their roots back to the experimental treatment environments of R. D. Laing and his associates in the Philadelphia Association in London in the 1960s.

Active ingredients are

- Small, family style and normalizing
- Open door, in residential settings, which allow the user to stay in touch with family, friends, work, and social life
- Flexible, non-coercive, often based more on peer relationships than on hierarchical power structure
- Involve residents running their own environment and using whatever work capacity the patient has to offer
- Pace of treatment is not as fast as hospital—they try to provide a quiet form of "asylum"

These facilities don't usually operate in isolation: they are partnered with a day hospital, some form of mobile crisis home treatment—or both.

Family-Based Crisis Homes

These are also called foster homes and have been used in the Belgian community of Gheel for over 700 years. In the Middle Ages the town attracted many mental patients as a result of the widespread reputation of the Church of St. Dyphna as the site of numerous miraculous healings. The townspeople opened their homes to provide asylum for the mentally ill, who, through participation in the family's daily activities and the assumption of a family role, ultimately became integrated into the family. This tradition of foster care has remained virtually unchanged up to the present (Arce & Vergare, 1985).

A modern pioneer of this method was the Southwest Denver community mental health clinic (Polak & Kirby, 1976; Polak, Kirby, & Deitchman, 1995). The philosophy of the southwest Denver system of treatment was that the primary determinant of admission in 60% of cases was social forces, rather than the patient's illness. The crisis of admission was the final step in a process of interaction between environmental stresses, social system upheavals, the patient's symptoms and the attempt of the social system to adapt. Intervention in the social system crisis was more important for effective treatment and post-hospital adjustment than treatment procedures in the hospital. A major focus, therefore, was treatment in the patient's home setting—essentially MCHT. However, keeping the patient in his own home at all costs can be destructive sometimes, and this is where family sponsor homes came in to play. Originally, in 1970 (Brook, 1973), a crisis hostel was used. This was a surprisingly casual arrangement with a young nurse who worked during the day at a general hospital, who could take up to four patients in her home on the periphery of downtown Denver. She was willing to help with medication, and several neighbours agreed to prepare meals and supervise the residents when she was away. Such was the faith in this arrangement that the in-patient unit was closed, save for two beds for patients who needed to be admitted after 10 p.m. Fifty percent of the residents had schizophrenia, 25% depression; of the 49 patients admitted during the course of a five-month study, 11 had previous psychiatric treatment. During a five-month study, 7 had to be admitted to hospital. The mean length of stay was 5.75 days. Forty-nine residents were compared to a control group—the last 49 persons admitted to the in-patient crisis unit before the hostel opened. At six-month follow-up, 6 of the control group had been readmitted—(3 of them twice), but only 1 of the hostel residents had been.

The residents showed less remission of symptoms than did the control group. This was attributed to the retrospective finding that in-patients received medication in significantly greater doses and more consistently than did hostel residents—thought to be due to staff anxiety at treating people in non-hospital settings. This finding regarding medication indicates the importance of biological factors also, and confirms one of the principles of successful home treatment described in Chapter 6—the need for adequate drug therapy. On other outcome measures ratings were comparable for both groups.

The residence was not formally staffed, but because the neighbours did not follow through on meal preparation and supervision, a nurse from the crisis division of the mental health centre spent several hours a week at the home. It became clear that acutely ill patients needed more formal structure than was available in this loose arrangement, so the strong pre-existing social structures of healthy families was utilised, resulting in the recruitment of six family sponsor homes that could accept up to two patients each. Twenty-four-hour coverage was provided by community nurses, backed up by a psychiatrist on call 24 hours a day. The program also provided an "intensive observation" apartment manned by a psychology student and his wife; patients needing more intensive care could be monitored around the clock. Rapid tranquillisation, another key element in the program, could also be provided.

The family sponsor treatment group were compared to a hospital treatment group in a random controlled trial of 85 patients: only 85 patients were candidates for admission from a catchment area of 100,000 over an 18-month period—a testament to the success of the southwest Denver system of crisis intervention, social systems intervention, and home treatment.

Of the first 48 patients assigned to the home group, 10 could not be treated in the home because of violence or suicidal behaviour. These 10 cases presented mainly in the initial months of the evolution of the experimental service, before the system stabilized. The outcome measures of the two groups after four months favoured the home treatment group, who also had greater satisfaction with treatment. Since the community treatment program began, in-patient bed usage has averaged 286 bed days/year/100,000 population. The authors' clinical impression was that the family sponsor approach was not responsive to the needs of some chronic patients who preferred a more structured, dependent role in an institutional setting.

The story of the demise of this family sponsorship program adds support to one of the principles of successful home treatment outlined in Chapter 6—namely, the need for good supportive administration of these types of programs, and the danger of depending on a "product champion" or "charismatic" leader. Polak left his position as executive director in 1981.

Over the next six years, five directors came and went, hospital alternative treatment got a lower priority, staff turnover increased, the family sponsor homes were increasingly used to warehouse patients, and hospitalization rates soared. Polak writes "it is quite clear that alternatives to acute psychiatric hospitalization cannot survive without continued commitment to the concept by the leadership of the mental health structure in which they operate and both commitment and skill on the part of the clinical staff."

A similar family crisis home program operated in Minneapolis in the 1980s (Leaman, 1987), 80% of patients "considered for in-patient treatment" were referred to the program saving $224,000 and had high levels of satisfaction with treatment.

Dane County, Wisconsin, is also the site of a family crisis home program, part of the Emergency Service Unit (ESU; a form of MCHT), which provides 24-hour support (Bennet, 1995). Forty percent of admissions were an alternative to hospitalization, 40% facilitated early discharge from hospital, and 20% were for a housing issue or "pre-crisis" intervention. Average length of stay was 3–5 days, maximum 2 weeks. Seventy percent of residents were on disability pensions and had diagnoses of schizophrenia, bipolar disorder, or major depression.

Why Does Family Crisis Home Treatment Work?

Bennet (1995):

- The name "home" implies a sense of belonging and safe haven.
- Using private homes. Patients often feel very honoured to be a guest in a private house; in many cases it will have been years (if ever) since they have been in a pleasant living situation and it is appreciated. In such a setting, the principles of normalization are better able to take hold: even a severely dysfunctional patient will rise to the occasion and try hard to be a safe and welcome guest.
- Only one patient in the home at a time. Surveys have shown that patients prefer not to live with other mental health consumers and desire flexible and individually tailored support. Graduated expectations with positive low-key interactions are essential.
- Non-professional providers. These are often immediately seen as an ally and tend not to get into the power struggles that occur with the professionals. At times, non-professionals may have a greater potential to look beyond the various diagnoses and see the real human being.

Group Crisis Residences

Group crisis residences have been established in typical neighbourhood homes, duplexes, and apartments, and in converted motels or office buildings.

Most are located in areas that combine residential or business uses. Crisis residences can be conceptualized as being on a continuum, with 1 being least like a hospital, functioning as respite, and 10 a defacto hospital (functioning as a hospital). Many attempt to minimize the institutional features and strive for a home-like atmosphere; they likely work in a similar fashion to the family crisis homes. Staffing patterns vary widely: some are staffed by an assortment of professionals, including a psychiatrist 20 hours a week, and provide 24-hour nursing coverage. Others rely largely on paraprofessionals who work under the supervision of mental health professionals. Maximum length of stay is usually 2 weeks; some are longer.

La Posada is one example (Weisman, 1985). This program was founded in 1977 and is situated in a two story Victorian mansion in the Mission district of San Francisco. Eight to ten residents live in the house at one time. The program is directed by a psychologist and staffed by a senior counsellor and 9.5 paraprofessional counsellors; 2–3 staff members are in the house at all times. Treatment is provided for acutely psychotic and suicidal patients who do not require physical restraints or locked doors; diagnoses are schizophrenia, paranoia, and other psychoses—20%, bipolar disorder, 16% and major depression, 21%. Thirty percent of patients are hospital diversion, 28% are more seriously disturbed, are early discharges from a short stay locked in-patient unit, and 28% are early intervention patients, not yet needing hospitalization.

This model uses techniques developed in halfway houses to enhance independent functioning and counteract regressive dependent behaviour, accompanied by crisis intervention techniques to facilitate rapid resolution of a crisis. It is a highly structured intensive therapeutic program, linked to an acute day hospital, which most residents attend 9:30 a.m. to 3 p.m. By having residents begin out-patient or day treatment before discharge, La Posada has dramatically reduced the number of referrals to those services that don't follow through. Forty-two percent are discharged to longer-term halfway houses, the rest to independent living arrangements; 6% require hospital admission. Hiring practices are directed at minimizing class, cultural, and social differences between staff and residents.

The cost per day for residential crisis treatment has been approximately one third the cost per day of hospitalization. Weisman states that "crisis-oriented programs can treat almost all voluntary psychiatric patients and can thereby eliminate the need for unlocked acute hospital wards."

My initial question—Which is the best alternative to hospital? was, of course asked with tongue in cheek. It is the "wrong" question. In real life, these hospital alternatives often don't exist in pure form and in isolation, nor should they. We have seen how MCHT is combined with crisis residences. The Ladywood Home Treatment Progam in North Birmingham, described in Chapter 3, has access to a "respite house" with five beds. During my site visit, this house was also used as a kind of day care for a depressed middle aged woman who lived alone; she spent the day at the house, returning to her own home in the evening. The home treatment service of Baltimore Crisis Response, Inc. (Chapter 3), is part of a substantial crisis residence service. Manchester Home Option Service has access to three "crisis respite beds." MCHT is combined with a day hospital, from which it evolved as the Manchester Home Option Service (Chapter 3).

In the research studies in Chapter 1, specific mention is made of combining MCHT with some form of crisis accommodation. Stein and Test (1978) described a specific treatment approach termed "constructive separation," to deal with pathological family relationships, which have contributed to the crisis. The patient is taken from the home and placed elsewhere. The case history of John, age 30, is illustrative. After being accepted for MCHT, John was "constructively separated" from his parents' home and arrangements were made for him to stay at the YMCA. John also immediately started at a sheltered workshop, a form of day care. Hoult's team in Sydney, Australia (Hoult & Reynolds, 1984), use "boarding homes" "if the situation at home between the patient and family appeared untenable." Hoge, et al. (1992) state "future research should focus on the comparative effectiveness of day-hospitalization and intensive out-patient (MCHT) interventions. Such research could identify the types and numbers of acutely ill patients for whom day hospitalization is effective and out-patient interventions are insufficient. This research might also serve to further clarify the essential elements of effective day hospital treatment and the unique contribution of such programs in comprehensive systems of care."

Hoge, et al.'s (1992) question regarding the comparative effectiveness of partial hospitalization and mobile crisis home treatment can be broadened to include crisis residences, which together with PH and MCHT form a *triad* of hospital alternatives. What is the comparative effectiveness of each member of the triad? What are the essential elements of each one, and what is its unique contribution to a comprehensive system of care? Can we identify which types of acutely ill patients are better suited to which alternative, or which types need two of them, or all three? Some may benefit from a sequence of treatment approaches; e.g., mobile crisis home treatment for a week followed by partial hospitalization. The following is a discussion of the strengths and weaknesses of each hospital alternative, with the aim of putting MCHT into the context of a typical mental health system. Each of the three alternatives can provide most of the 20 components of in-patient treatment, some better than others or in a way that suits some patients better. For example, for lonely, socially isolated patients, MCHT can't hold a candle to PH in providing components 4 and 12—interpersonal contact, structure, and activity—at least during the day.

Comparative Advantages and Disadvantages of the Three Alternatives to Hospital

Advantages of Mobile Crisis Home Treatment

- It is the most nimble and versatile of the triad of alternatives. The intensity of intervention can be varied up or down, quickly, responsively, and continuously. All forms of treatment can be mixed and matched at short notice.
- It can treat an infinite variety of patients, from adolescents to octogenarians, non-English speakers, different ethnic groups and social classes, physically infirm, medically ill, blind, deaf, and developmentally disabled.
- It is the least disruptive to patients' lives, allowing them to remain at home with their families and share small household duties. It protects their privacy and avoids the stigma of attending a psychiatric facility and mixing with other psychiatric patients.
- Seeing the patients in their own home is very helpful for assessing the social and family environment and providing hands on practical help with problems of living.
- It can involve the whole family, addressing their concerns, educating them about the illness and teaching them how to cope with it and how to prevent relapse.
- It avoids fostering regression and dependence; patients are expected to behave normally.
- It is responsive to crises at all hours.
- By its assertive approach, it can handle some patients who are unlikely to show up for appointments, don't adhere to treatment, and drop out. It can cope with patients who may be somewhat agitated and disruptive, provided the family can tolerate it and feel competent to cope.

Disadvantages of Mobile Home Crisis Treatment

- It is limited in providing structure, activities, and interpersonal support; much depends on what the family can provide. Lonely, socially isolated patients with little or no social support may need partial hospitalization. Hoge, et al. (1992), writing about assertive community treatment teams (which function similarly to MCHT in this context) state "even staunch proponents of such teams have voiced concern about the team's ability to provide adequate structure and social support for a subset of acutely ill patients. For example, the manager . . . described the practice of having such patients accompany treatment team members in their cars over the course of the workday . . . we have seen such patients sitting in staff offices for the day for lack of an appropriate alternative."

- Patients need to be in a sufficiently stable home environment. Instead they may be in an unhealthy environment; e.g., an inner-city rooming house with dubious characters, lots of substance abuse, violence, and noise, the place in a state of disrepair.
- Patient may need respite from a toxic, abusive family environment.
- If patient is home all day, it can be burdensome to the family.
- Family may be unreliable or incapable of helping the team with monitoring the patient's suicidal thinking, and disturbed behaviour and administering medication.
- While it is helpful to observe patients in their homes, another kind of observation is also helpful; namely, prolonged, over the course of a day, with the patient engaged in various activities with other patients, and perhaps unaware of being observed.

Advantages of Partial Hospitalization

- It can provide interpersonal contact and support for a whole day with staff and other patients.
- It can provide activities and structure for a whole day.
- It can provide respite for the family for a whole day.
- It can provide a day's respite for the patient from an unhealthy social environment.
- It can provide opportunity for prolonged observation of patient.
- It can provide extensive group therapy.
- It can provide close easy access to hospital services such as ECT, neuro-imaging, laboratory (many PH programs are located close to hospitals).

Disadvantages of Partial Hospitalization

- Patients may be too disruptive to the program.
- Patients may have difficulty tolerating being with a group of people for any length of time. At the Hazelglen home treatment program

(see Chapter 3) we have had a supportive low key group—a "tea group" where tea and cookies are served, twice weekly. Even this very low-key supportive group was too much for some patients; they became anxious and restless and asked to leave.

- Patients may have difficulty with frequent regular transportation to and from the day hospital. Creed's day hospital (1995), arranged transportation by taxi or minibus. However, that program served one circumscribed sector of an inner-city area; in N. America, with sprawling suburbs and semi-rural areas (like Wateloo region—home of the Hazelglen program), such transportation assistance may be too expensive and impractical.
- Patients may be unreliable in attendance. There is a high rate of drop out or non-attendance in day hospitals—20–50% (Hoge, et al. 1992).
- Not suitable for patients who cannot communicate with other patients; e.g., those with poor English, deaf, blind, or low IQ. It would not be practical for those who are physically infirm, medically ill, or at the extremes of age groups i.e., adolescents or the very old (unless specifically designed).
- Need a certain critical mass—a large enough daily census for programs to function adequately.
- Disruptive to patient's lives, although not as much as hospitalization. It takes them from their homes, families, and responsibilities that they can still fulfill e.g., simple childcare.
- 20–50% of patients require overnight hospitalization or "guesting" at times, to manage acute symptoms (Hoge ,et al. 1992).
- Unnecessary long lengths of stay raise the possibility that day hospitals can create patient regression and dependence (Hoge, et al.1992).
- There may be a tension between the need for structure and the need for flexibility. Group programs are developed which are suitable for a range of patients. Inadvertently, over time, the program may become "crystallised" into a form that is not suitable for certain kinds of patients, who may get excluded as "inappropriate".
- It is not as flexible as MCHT. Because of census concerns, and group program structure, it may be difficult to vary the intensity of the treatment quickly and responsively.
- It may be difficult to manage crises at inconvenient times.
- Patients may object to mixing with other patients.
- Although less than hospital admission, the experience of being in a day hospital may still be perceived as stigmatizing for some patients.

Advantages of Crisis Residences

- They can provide 24-hour professional monitoring of psychiatric status, medical problems, suicide risk, and progress of drug and alcohol withdrawal.
- They are particularly suitable for patients who are homeless, in an unhealthy environment, or with no supports.
- They can provide respite, asylum and remove patients from harmful influences such as abusive partners.
- They can provide more structure than MCHT.

Disadvantages of Crisis Residences

- They are disruptive to patients' lives and families.
- Some stigma can be associated; many patients don't like having to mix with other mental health consumers, although, in a family crisis home, this is not necessary, because they serve only one or two patients at one time.
- It is difficult to recruit and retain families for family crisis residences.
- They may have some of the disadvantages of hospital; e.g., fostering dependence, especially if the residence is closer to the "de facto hospital" end of the spectrum.
- They may be insufficient as a sole intervention. Residents likely will also need an acute day hospital or a mobile crisis home treatment service for adequate treatment of the crisis.

Working in an MCHT service, visiting places with innovative mental health systems that have a variety of hospital alternatives, and sifting through the mental health services research literature, a picture begins to emerge of a *triad of hospital alternatives,* each one often working in tandem with another, in parallel or sequentially. Together, they can care for up to about 60% of seriously ill patients who would otherwise require in-patient admission (Kluiter, 1997); they can also reduce the duration of hospital stay for some patients for whom admission could not be avoided.

Each of the three types of service is quite different in its method of care and has complementary strengths. PH shines in providing structured activities, interpersonal contact, and prolonged contact with staff. Crisis residences offer a level of respite and asylum close to that of a hospital, but in an informal-home-like setting. These two approaches are still significantly disruptive to the lives of patients and their families and not every patient needs them. In certain areas they may be used extensively, such as very socially deprived inner cities. For the most part, their place should perhaps be as a judiciously

SIDEBAR

What Can a Delphi Exercise Tell Us About Hospital Alternatives?

The Rand Corporation developed the Delphi method in the 1950s for technology forecasting; it enabled the testimony of experts to be combined into a single useful statement. It has also been used to define the essential components of care for schizophrenia and the components of intensive case management.

The Delphi exercise is well established as a method of ascertaining expert opinion in a systematic way that allows free and equal expression of opinion through the anonymity of the procedure. An initial open question generates a range of ideas, submitted by each participant anonymously, and these ideas are then fed back to the whole group, who rate them for their importance. The group then re-rates the items in the light of information about the whole group's response (Burns, et al., 2001). Burns conducted a Delphi exercise with a panel of 12 experts—consultant psychiatrists in the U.K. with an interest and expertise in community-based care. They were asked to list between eight and ten components in response to the question:

> *"In a community-based service that enables people with mental health problems to be treated outside hospital, what are the most important components that achieve this?"*

They developed a list of 97 components in all, and rated them on a scale of 1–5: 1 = essential, 2 = very important, 3 = important, 4 = less important, and 5 = unimportant. A "consensus" was defined as 80% of the participants were within one point of the median; "strong consensus" was defined as 100% were within one point of the median. This exercise was limited in that it was conducted only with psychiatrists. Components rated as "essential" and "very important" were

- home environment (home visiting, assessment and treatment in the home, etc.)
- skill—mix (skilled staff, well trained, community mental health nurses, etc.)
- psychiatrist involvement

- service management (well-organized and managed team, environment that tolerates risk-taking, etc.)
- caseload size
- health/social care integration (attention to social as well as clinical needs, good health and social services liaison, etc.)
- hours (rapid response services access to after hours mental health workers, 7-day service, extended hours, etc.)
- cross-agency working (good links with primary care, knowledge of local support systems, etc.)
- crisis care (crisis availability, etc.)
- housing/accommodation (range of adequate/supported accommodation, high staffed [24-hour] residential accommodation, access to crisis accommodation for those that lack appropriate housing, etc.)
- in-patient policy (team's use of beds should focus on early discharge—"If you want one admitted you need to take one out"—senior psychiatrist involvement in all admissions, etc.)
- caregivers (support for caregivers, etc.)
- day care (sufficient support services; i.e., day care, acute day hospitals, etc.)

The results of this exercise can be viewed as providing some support for the idea that all three hospital alternatives need to be available—mobile crisis home treatment, some form of day care, and crises accommodation, with MCHT being the "default" choice. Most of the components referred to a team providing assessment and treatment in the home and the essential or very important features of such a team. Only two categories referred to day care or crisis accommodation. (See Chapter 4 for further discussion of this research and how it applies to MCHT.)

used addition to MCHT, which, because of its nimble versatility and preservation of the patient's usual family life, may be the best candidate as the *default* (using a computer analogy) disposition for psychiatric emergencies.

The recent mental health policy reports referred to in the Preface, from the U.S., Canada, and Britain, plus the Australian report from 1992, appear to give prominence to MCHT as an alternative to hospital admission. To develop this picture more clearly, more focussed research needs to be done in different types of patients.

MOBILE CRISIS HOME TREATMENT AND SUCH SERVICES AS MODIFIED OUT-PATIENT PROGRAMS AND EARLY INTERVENTION APPROACHES

Some readers may claim that they do mobile crisis home treatment in their services: "we do home visits," or "we see people frequently when they are in a crisis," or "to avoid hospitalization we have a rapid response and crisis intervention." For heuristic purposes, one needs to demarcate very clearly the mental health service one is focussing on; for the sake of clarity one needs to define it clearly, establish boundaries, and provide an operational definition. In real-life practice, however, things are not always that clearly definable—especially in mental health services. To examine how MCHT relates to what *appear* to be similar programs, it is useful to discern and distinguish the two ways in which a mobile/home visiting approach can be used to reduce hospital bed usage: one, the subject of this book is MCHT; the other, which is not dealt with in this book, is early intervention as described in the studies in Chapter 1. MCHT deals with patients in a crisis of such severity that hospital level care is required, and an *alternative* is provided. These studies showed how an early intervention service focuses on patients whose problem has not yet reached the severity where admission is considered. It *prevents* admission by providing rapid assessments, it reaches out assertively to patients who may not adhere to treatment, and the assessment is often carried out at home.

Another mental health service that can be subsumed under early intervention is the South Verona Community Psychiatric Service in Italy, which functions with only a 16-bed psychiatric ward in a general hospital for a population of 75,000, which is a ratio of 21 beds per 100,000. It accomplishes this without any of the triad of hospital alternatives. See Table 2.4.

In practice, many MCHT services have elements of both these approaches, and it is useful to consider them as being on a continuum: between the most intensive, 24-hour specialized service and a non-specialized, less intensive service like Burns's. The degree to which admission can be avoided will vary. Services have various elements of these two related approaches and vary to the degree that they are faithful to any MCHT model. For example, how "mobile" or "home based" does the service have to be?

U.K. services such as Ladywood described in Chapter 1 conduct almost 100% of their interventions in the home. Fenton's study (1982) aimed for 50%, Manchester Home Option service (Chapter 1) encouraged patients to attend the base office. Similarly, the intensity of "24-hour cover" will vary, from teams seeing patients at all hours to providing telephone support and using the local emergency room at night. When accepting a referral of a patient with an acute severe problem, it may be with the

SIDEBAR

THE SOUTH VERONA COMMUNITY
MENTAL HEALTH SERVICE (CMHS)

The "Macro" Approach vs. the "Micro" Approach

South Verona has a population of 75,000 and is one of three catchment areas of the city of Verona (pop. 260,000) in Italy. Its mental health system has none of the usual alternatives to hospitalization for acutely ill patients—no crisis beds, no acute day hospital, and no mobile crisis home treatment—and yet functions well with only 16 general hospital psychiatric beds, and no medium- or long-term beds. Clearly, there are other ways of reducing hospital bed usage. How is it done?

Italy's national mental health plan prescribed the integration of all local mental health and human services under one administrative organization, typically responsible for a population of 150,000. Included were a community mental health centre and general hospital psychiatric wards, no bigger than 16 beds, with one bed per 10,000. (South Verona, because it is a university centre for teaching and research, has a higher bed ratio.) Mental hospitals were closed in 1980.

The service contains functional elements described in this and the previous chapter: including early intervention (as described in Merson's study, Chapter 1); a high degree of accessibility with quick, flexible appointments and some home visiting (as described in Burns' service, Chapter 1); and a very high degree of service integration at all levels—the worker follows the patient. One is reminded of Burns' views on crisis services. He notes that "new assertive services" result in a wide non-specific improvement in services—improved communication and better access, such that crises are much less frequent" (T. Burns, personal communication, Aug. 24, 1998). Crises in mental health are often due to delayed recognition of early signs, unresponsive mental health delivery systems, and difficulty in access; they are rarely emergencies that are a result of uncontrollable biological processes, such as myocardial infarction and dissecting aneurysms.

Home visiting is used, but only when clearly necessary—to visit someone living in a rural area, or who has difficulty leaving the house—or "assertively"; for example, when a patient fails to show up for an urgent out-patient appointment following a visit to the emergency room the night before. Home visiting has declined in recent years, from 1200 a year in 1998 to 750 per year in 2002—about 10% of cases.

The community mental health centre is the linchpin of the CMHS. It is located in an old house near the hospital and is open 8 a.m. to 8 p.m. weekdays, and 8 a.m. to 5 p.m. on Saturday. There are three community teams, each with a staff of 2 nurses, 1–2 psychologists, and 1 social worker. There are 11 psychiatrists plus residents; psychiatrists work part time, due to university commitments.

The worker follows the patient. For example, a psychiatrist may see a patient on a home visit, in the clinic, in the day centre, and care for them in hospital. Appointments are quick, and there is flexibility to see patients the next day and whenever they need. Involuntary admissions are infrequent, because most patients have a good relationship with a worker.

Long-term residential care takes place in home-like communities. There is a group home, 2 apartments, and a 7-bed hostel supervised 24 hours a day. Bed occupancy on the psychiatric ward is 90%, average length of stay is 18 days, with 250 admissions per year.

The first priority of the service is care for the severely ill, and there is a commitment to life-long responsibility to them (the concept of "being in charge" rather than treating.)

In assessing this service one has to take into account local social and cultural factors. Social deprivation is low. Verona is a prosperous city with low unemployment and a stable, predominantly middle-class population. The Italian nuclear and extended family is still healthy and provides accommodation and care for up to 80% of patients.

The Verona approach to reducing bed usage can perhaps be conceived as a "macro" approach, addressing the mental health system of a whole area; in contrast, mobile crisis home treatment can be conceived as a "micro" approach, providing an alternative treatment approach to an individual patient, not that these are necessarily mutually exclusive. Individual patients in an acute crisis are readily admitted. Asked his response to two clinical scenarios, an acute first episode psychosis, and an acutely suicidal middle-aged middle class businessman, Dr. Burti readily replied that he would admit them. It's the way the whole system is designed that reduces bed usage, not striving to avoid admission for a particular patient.

Date of site visit: 27 May, 2003.
Address: Clinical Psichiatrica
Ospedale Policlinico
Yiazzale L.A. Scuro 10-37134
Verona, Italy

clear understanding that they do *not* need hospital level care at that moment—they are *not* candidates for admission, but, if they don't get help within a week, they likely will deteriorate to the point where they will end up in hospital. To only accept patients who unequivocally need hospital now would be inhumane. What would be the point in insisting that they will not be accepted for treatment until they have deteriorated enough in a few days to fit your criteria?

Having acknowledged that some out-patient services may well have elements of MCHT and thereby are able to divert some patients from hospital, I do not want to detract from one of the main messages of this book, detailed in Chapters 4, 5, and 6: that to be an effective *alternative* to hospital, to the degree that significant numbers of beds can be replaced, an MCHT team needs to adhere to certain principles and have all the key elements in place, and that the whole is greater than the sum of the parts.

HOW DOES MOBILE CRISIS HOME TREATMENT FIT IN WITH EMERGENCY PSYCHIATRIC SERVICES AND OUTREACH SERVICES?

Psychiatric Emergency Services

A psychiatric emergency service, as defined in the preface (Stage 4 on the schematic, anatomy of a crisis figure; see Figure 2.1) is the first contact the patient with an acute problem has with a mental health professional.

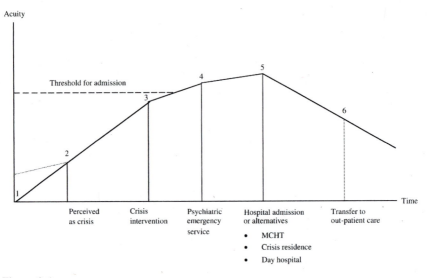

Figure 2.1

   MCHT can interact with a psychiatric emergency service at three points in time (before Stage 4, at Stage 4, and after Stage 4). The most straightforward interaction to describe is after the emergency assessment. Patients assessed by a psychiatric resident, for example, and considered to be a candidate for in-patient level of care, can be diverted to MCHT (Stage 5) instead of being admitted. The MCHT worker receives the referral, usually by phone or fax. They arrange to see the patient, either at their home, or in the psychiatric emergency setting, often the emergency room of a hospital before they are discharged, and may accompany them home. This type of intervention is the subject of the research studies in Chapter 1.

   Psychiatric emergency services are not just assessment and triage services, however. They are also increasingly becoming treatment services as well (Allen, et al., 2002). There are insufficient beds, and patients in need of hospital treatment face impossibly long waits or can't get admitted at all. If they do get admitted, their stay is so short that they often do not receive definitive treatment; i.e., a most complete treatment. For example, a patient with bipolar disorder may simply be treated with anti-psychotic medicine until he is "stable," and then released without mood stabilizing medicine. Patients assessed in emergency rooms and referred for urgent out-patient treatment often fail to connect—only 10% in one study. Forster and King (1994) state: "we are forced to admit defeat and to accept inadequate treatment for our patients, or to recognize the need for yet another reconfiguration of the role of the psychiatric emergency service in the mental health system: as a site for initiating definitive treatment of some of the most seriously ill patients. Recognizing the need for alternatives to hospital treatment for seriously mentally ill persons in a crisis, psychiatric emergency services have taken on new responsibilities as providers of intensive crisis stabilization services, crisis aftercare services, mobile crisis services and crisis case management services." All these terms can likely be subsumed under the term mobile crisis home treatment.

MCHT services can also serve as psychiatric emergency services in themselves; in other words, they may be the first mental health staff to see the patient. For example, primary care physicians may refer an acutely disturbed patient directly from their office, rather than sending him to the psychiatric emergency service at the local hospital emergency room. The team may go to the physician's office and assess the patient there, or more commonly, arrange to meet him later at his home, functioning as a mobile psychiatric urgent service in Allen et al.'s scheme (2002).

MCHT services may also act as a crisis intervention service (Stage 3), and this is the most complex to analyse and describe. For the sake of analysis and clarity, I have been trying to make a clear distinction between crisis intervention and psychiatric emergency service, but, as the reader may observe, it's a struggle—especially when one quotes other authors describing other services; the two terms are used synonymously. But, the distinction is particularly important to make in this context. To reiterate: crisis intervention is the first contact the patient in a crisis has with any kind of professional person, usually not a mental health professional. It can be a primary care physician, emergency physician, police officer, minister, or general social worker or nurse. The main point to emphasize here is that patients at this stage are unscreened; consequently, they may be quite unsuitable for psychiatric treatment in the home. In fact, they may not even have a psychiatric disorder; it could be a housing or family crisis. In other words, a service whose main objective is to divert patients from hospital, may, in exercising a crisis intervention function, be dealing with someone who does not require this level of treatment, or who is too ill for it, and could therefore be conceivably wasting resources. This is the reason why services described as "mobile crisis services" may not show evidence of reducing beds. To cut through the confusion, it is essential to specify what the mobile team's function and goals are. This has already been touched on in Chapter 1 in the context of research studies. For example, a mobile team whose function is to engage psychotic homeless individuals, or maybe transport them to the hospital to avoid alienating them by police involvement, is unlikely to save psychiatric beds; it is more likely to increase their use by finding cases—cases that usually cannot be treated in the community, because they are sleeping on the streets. Why should MCHT services get involved at all in crisis intervention, if their primary purpose is to be an alternative to inpatient care: after all, an in-patient psychiatric ward does not engage in crisis intervention—it just sits there, waiting for patients to come to it. Some MCHT services do almost function that way. The Manchester Home Option Service, described in Chapter 3, only takes referrals from mental health professionals, not from primary care physicians ("we are afraid they will refer inappropriate patients"). But, even that team does engage in a form of crisis intervention, because they accept referrals directly from ex-patients and their families; these individuals, in a crisis, can call and have direct access to the team. Presumably because they are known, the team can quickly and reliably assess whether their problem is one that fits their service. Some MCHT services have no choice as to whether they engage in some crisis intervention of unscreened patients; they are mandated by the funding agency to accept referrals directly from the public. In Ontario, for example, all community mental health programs funded by the province have to accept direct referrals from the public in the interests of accessibility; thus, the Hazelglen MCHT service (described in Chapter 3) treats patients referred by themselves or their families. For these reasons, screening of patients and families is a key element of MCHT (see Chapter 4).

In all communities, a certain number of people will become candidates for hospital admission for an acute mental disorder each year; the proportion will vary, depending on such factors as the degree of social deprivation. Presumably, therefore, all communities could benefit from a mobile crisis home treatment service to divert some of these people from hospital. But, do all communities need a mobile crisis intervention service responding to and going out to unscreened persons? Perhaps not. Persons in a crisis need to somehow be put in contact with a psychiatric emergency service to be rapidly assessed by a mental health professional and to receive treatment, either directly from that service, or by being referred elsewhere. For this to occur, a number of things need to happen. Someone in their social environment, or the person themselves, needs to perceive the crisis for what it is—not ignore it; someone has to have the wherewithal to know what to do and who to call and then arrange for it to happen. In populations where the average level of education and social functioning is adequate, and the medical/social infrastructure is sound, this sequence of events usually unfolds such that people get the help they need. For example, the neighbours recognize the nature of a person's crisis and are not afraid to call the police, or can figure out that they should take them to their primary care physician or the hospital emergency room. They likely don't need a mobile team to come to their home, although it would be very convenient and would save everyone a lot of trouble. Contrast this scenario with one involving an unemployed, poorly educated, socially isolated individual, living in an inner-city slum, where people may be afraid of the police, don't speak English, and many are using drugs. That person may be allowed to deteriorate to an alarming degree before he ends up in contact with a psychiatric emergency service. A mobile crisis intervention team is needed here. It is important to be discriminating about which populations need such a service, because it may be more expensive than the traditional hospital or community clinic crisis service. The following is speculation: for safety reasons, two workers instead of one may be required to go out to see a person in a crisis; the additional time required to travel to their home may double the time the assessment takes; and someone is needed to man the base office while the team is on a call. Conceivably, a mobile crisis assessment could cost up to four times more than an assessment in a conventional, non-mobile crisis service based in an emergency room.

MCHT AND OUTREACH SERVICES

Mobile Crisis Home Treatment, as defined in this book, may be limited in its ability to serve patients who are the usual targets of outreach services. A minimum degree of cooperation by the patient is required for treatment to be successful in MCHT. It is difficult to provide intensive psychiatric treatment in the community to individuals who may also be homeless. One form of outreach service to the homeless that can fit well with MCHT is a shelter or transitional residence; for example, as described by Barrow, Hellman, Lovell, Plapinger, and Struening (1991), where patients have some social stability and support and the shelter staff can help with the treatment. The authors assessed the effects of services on the residence and psychiatric treatment status of homeless mentally ill persons in New York City. They examined the effects of five programs, which included a municipal women's shelter and a transitional residence. One service variable, direct psychiatric services, consisting of on-site services, significantly increased the odds that a patient would be linked to treatment. This fits well with our experience at Hazelglen, where we provide intensive treatment to individuals at two homeless shelters, the House of Friendship for men, and Mary's Place for women; e.g., the case of Ken in Chapter 7.

To understand how mobile crisis home treatment actually works in real life and how it fits into actual mental health systems, the next chapter describes seven services: three in the U.K., three in Canada, and one in the U.S.

Chapter Three
Descriptions of Seven Mobile Crisis Home Treatment Teams

". . . the next task is to learn from other's experiences. Do a lot of background reading, talk to people who have done it—i.e., the service providers. Talk to service users who have experienced it. Consult widely. A lot of the things you want to do have probably been done by others, so you don't have to re-invent the wheel. As you do this, you will gain a lot of understanding of what needs to be done, things you hadn't realised needed to be done, and problems which you hadn't anticipated."

Hoult (1999)

The mobile crisis home treatment services in this chapter were chosen for various reasons. The North American services—U.S.A. and Canada—were the only ones I could find. Unfortunately, this list includes only one U.S. example of MCHT as defined in this book. Undoubtedly there are others, but I was unable to locate them in spite of vigorous efforts. These included canvassing members of the American Association of Community Psychiatrists list-serv group, buttonholing key people at meetings of the American Psychiatric Association and other meetings, calling the few leads that I had, and searching web sites. The reasons for my lack of success are unclear: they likely include the sheer size of the U.S.A.: any such programs may be widely scattered; lack of an agreed terminology: people are not clear about what I am seeking; paucity of recent published literature in the U.S.A. on this topic; my lack of American professional contacts; and the lack of any central organization devoted to such a service delivery model.

In Britain, the St. Albans service was chosen because its catchment area was relatively affluent and suburban, in contrast to the others with which I was familiar, which were located in socially deprived, inner-city areas. Also, it was developed by Neil Brimblecombe, a nurse manager, who has written a book on MCHT from a British perspective (Brimblecombe, 2001). The Manchester Home Option Service is of particular interest because it evolved from a well-researched day hospital.

North Birmingham has been at the centre of MCHT development in Britain, and Professor Sashidharan, who started the Ladywood team, has been a leading figure.

These MCHT services vary considerably from each other; they evolved in different ways and were developed for a number of different reasons. In spite of this, for the most part they contain the key elements and adhere to the principles outlined in the next chapter.

Only one service has achieved the position of gatekeeper to the in-patient beds—the Ladywood service in North Birmingham, U.K.

One of the chief differences in the services is the extent of "availability, 24 hours a day, 7 days a week." "Availability" is defined as "obtainable, or accessible, capable of being made use of, at hand" (Collins English Dictionary, 1991); it does not necessarily mean that staff are actively working in the community or in the office. In this regard, the services vary in two ways: hours of operation—when staff is working, and of course, available; and the extent of, and type of availability after hours (this issue is discussed at length in Chapters, 4, 5, and 6).

The Hazelglen service in Kitchener, Ontario, has the shortest hours of operation; 9 a.m.–5 p.m. five days a week. All the others operate seven days a week, from 8 or 9 a.m. to 9 or 11 p.m.

Two services have no team staff available after hours; in Victoria and Edmonton, patients obtain service at the local emergency ward. Hazelglen service staff are available by phone after hours, and patients are directed to the hospital 24-hour walk-in crisis clinic, which is associated with the service. Patients of the Baltimore Crisis Response program can phone the crisis hotline after hours, and the psychiatrist and the director are available by phone for consultation. If they require face-to-face intervention, they are directed to an emergency room where staff are familiar with the program. The British services have staff who are on call by phone after hours and can also see patients in an emergency.

The services also vary considerably regarding who can refer. The Hazelglen service and Baltimore Crisis Response are the only services that take referrals from literally anybody in the community. All the others take referrals from various combinations of physicians, social agencies, and mental health professionals. Victoria is the most restrictive—referrals are taken from only the 14 psychiatrists at the hospital. Some exclude certain physician groups for fear of inappropriate referrals: Edmonton excludes emergency room physicians; Manchester excludes primary care physicians.

The extent of home visiting varies from 42% in Manchester to almost 100% in Baltimore, Edmonton, St. Albans, and, Ladywood.

Size of services varies, from 3.5 clinical staff in Hazelglen to 14 and 17 in Ladywood and Manchester, respectively.

BALTIMORE CRISIS RESPONSE, INC.

"Nothing is too benign; crises are self-defined."

Edgar Wiggins, Director

This is a mobile crisis treatment service, linked to a crisis residential unit, that was developed, not in response to a bed shortage or to save money, but with the aim of developing a more accessible, flexible, and community-integrated service for the chronically mentally ill who are unserved or underserved by the traditional system.

Baltimore City is the 13th largest city in the U.S. and is located in the State of Maryland on the east coast, 37 miles from Washington, D.C. The population is close to 700,000 (about a third of the metropolitan area of five counties), 60% are African American, and it is home to the largest concentration of poor people in Maryland. It has the biggest population of heroin addicts in the world—about 60,000.

Public mental health services are funded by various sources: Medicaid, State General Funds, and money from Medicare, insurance companies, and cash payments. Prior to 1988, services were mostly office based and, often, individuals lost their clinical service if they refused an appointment, were hospitalised, incarcerated, or became homeless. Services were fragmented and not patient oriented (Baron, Agus, Osher, and Brown, et al. 1998).

In 1986 the city applied to the Robert Wood Johnson Foundation (RWJ) Program on Chronic Mental Illness to enable it to develop a coordinated system of care for those with serious and persistent mental illness. RWJ is the largest private health care foundation in the U.S.A. and this project was its first large-scale mental health initiative.

The city established Baltimore Mental Health Systems (BMHS) to serve as the local mental health authority to develop a coordinated network of care. BMHS has redesigned the delivery system by consolidating providers into lead agencies, expanding services, and creating Baltimore Crisis Response, Inc., to coordinate and provide a full range of services. Numerous problems with the crisis system had been identified by the Crisis Task Force set up by BHMS (Agus, 1991). Five of seven community mental health clinics often referred patients in a crisis to the nearest emergency room; individuals brought to the ER on emergency petitions (assessment for involuntary admission) did not receive an adequate evaluation, resulting in unnecessary hospitalisation; police were the primary source of transportation to the ER. Of the 400 persons with chronic mental illness who were arrested over the course of one year, 116 were charged with a minor offence and might have been diverted from jail had a crisis service been available. A survey of 300 consumers of mental health services were asked to rate what was most important for them when in a crisis: 87% said hospitalization was the least important, while many said 24-hour mental health care was a priority.

Among the guiding principles recommended by the Crisis Task Force were least restrictive treatment, with support to stay in familiar surroundings, and easy access; e.g., a clearly defined point of entry and 24-hour availability. The result was a model which, among other features, included a 24-hour telephone hot line, the initial point of contact with the crisis system; a crisis residence in an apartment block; and a mobile crisis team.

The task force (TF) was committed to using in-patient admission as a last resort. It also recognized that hospitals often desire to fill their psychiatric beds with paying or insured patients and an incentive thus exists for ERs to admit crisis patients unnecessarily.

To remedy this situation, the TF considered whether the crisis service should have the power to authorize all in-patient admissions—to be the gatekeeper of the beds. However, they concluded this was not feasible—clinically or politically—and instead relied on education and suggested that ER staff consult with the crisis service about disposition of patients. The crisis service would act as gatekeeper to state hospital beds.

The mobile crisis team (MCT) and the crisis residence both take up the ground floor of an apartment building in a "poor, drug infested area" in a central area of Baltimore. The MCT takes patients to the crisis residence or treats them in their homes. The idea of home treatment was met with criticism and scepticism at first. When the MCT service first started, they thought it necessary to provide continuous care by a trained lay person, who stayed in the home for up to 72 hours; this has since been found to be unnecessary. The target population is adults with a psychiatric disorder, in a crisis, at risk of hospital admission. They may be exhibiting behaviour that could be harmful to themselves or others, but can contract for their safety; or, they may be experiencing a rapid decline of functioning due to psychiatric symptoms. The catchment area is the whole City of Baltimore; driving distances are 30–40 minutes.

All referrals are channelled through the 24-hour hotline, which is manned by bachelor level staff, which receives 40 hours training. Anyone can refer; 25% are from family, friends, or self; 20% are from emergency rooms; 40% are from hospital mental health clinics; and 24% from other sources. Of the 14,000 calls received by the hotline, about 12.5% (1800) are referred to the MCT. Referrals are not accepted from psychiatric wards for early discharge for fear of "dumps."

Referred patients are seen within 1–2 hours usually, certainly on the same day. Staff always goes in pairs, for safety; a team is made up of a nurse and a social worker. Following a complete assessment, a decision is made as to whether the patient is appropriate and, if so, what level of care would be needed. Sixty percent of referrals are accepted; the bulk of these are admitted to the crisis residence with only 14% are treated in their homes. In 2001, 933 patients were treated in the crisis residence and 152 at home. Of the 40% not accepted for treatment, 37% were inappropriate, 25% refused treatment, 27% were admitted to hospital, and 27% just received telephone support and help.

Length of stay is short: it averages 4 days in the crisis residence and 7–10 days in home treatment, with a maximum of two weeks allowed. Home treatment patients are started on medication and receive supportive psychotherapy, help with psychosocial problems, and family work. Patients can be seen daily if necessary, usually only once by the psychiatrist but more if necessary. No patients are seen at the home base, the address of which is not public knowledge for safety reasons. Of the patients treated in the crisis residence, 58% suffer from depression, 12% from schizophrenia, 17% bipolar disorder, and 4% psychosis; diagnostic breakdown on in-home patients was not available, but likely consist of less psychotic patients—most of these are treated in the crisis residence. The service has space for 12 patients in the crisis residence and 10 in home treatment and is open 8 a.m.– 11 p.m. seven days a week.

MCT staffing consists of 4 staff, 8 a.m.– 4 p.m. shift; 2 staff, noon–8 p.m., 2 staff, 2:30 p.m.–11 p.m. In addition, there are case managers, not part of the MCT, who work on patients' problems accessing services, funding problems, and disposition. After hours, patients can phone the crisis hotline for help, and a psychiatrist and the director are available by phone. If a patient needs more help, they are directed to an emergency room, where staff are familiar with the program. Two psychiatrists work during the weekdays and provide coverage 11 p.m.– 8 a.m.; one of the psychiatrists also works in the detoxification service next door. A number of psychiatric residents also work half-time. Six other regular psychiatrists work both on the team in the evenings and weekends. The psychiatrists work both in the residence and visit patients in their homes. The MCT has 9 full-time masters level social workers and 1 full-time nurse—the rest of the nurses are part time or from an agency; "it's easier to get psychiatrists than nurses."(The nursing shortage is so severe in

Baltimore that a nurse can earn an $8,000 finder's fee for referring someone for a job in the local hospitals.) Most staff are recent college graduates, and there is a steady turnover. There is a policy of hiring consumers, and Baltimore has a facility to specifically train consumers to work in mental health settings.

Baltimore is well endowed with services (including in-patient beds); hence, patients can be quickly referred to a variety of agencies, including mobile treatment teams. These are similar to MCT but are less intensive; in fact, these teams refer to the MCT when their patients need more home visits, particularly from a psychiatrist.

Dealing with patients who are not seriously acute is not seen as a problem; the MCT is used for plugging gaps and connecting patients to services, and this is seen as a legitimate activity. "Nothing is too benign. Crises are self-defined," says BCRI's director Edgar Wiggins, who describes such gap-plugging activity as checking on a mental health clinic patient who was not compliant with medication over a three-day weekend to ensure she took her medication. About 20% of home treatment patients are seen because they could not get a timely enough appointment at a mental health clinic. Every effort is made to keep patients in contact with their existing services and to consult with their caregivers to ensure coordination and harmony of treatment and there is close liaison with the day hospital and Johns Hopkins Medical Center.

Although the catchment area is socially deprived, safety has not been a worry, and there have been no incidents of threats to staff. The service takes precautions, of course: staff always has to go in twos and they ensure guns are removed from the home before the visit.

At the present time, no data are collected to permit on-going evaluation of the service.

Date of site visit: November 4, 2002
Address: Baltimore Crisis Response, Inc.
            5401 Loch Raven Blvd
            Rectory Building Second Floor
            Baltimore, Maryland 21239

CANADA

Hazelglen Outreach Mental Health Service

Kitchener, Ontario, Canada

Kitchener-Waterloo are twin cities, located 70 miles southwest of Toronto. The larger city, Kitchener, has a population of 190,000, and Waterloo has a population of 99,000 with two small universities. Prosperous, with a diverse economy, they have attracted a large immigrant population over the years from many different countries and cultures, most of whom have found work and settled well.

Adult mental health services are provided by a general hospital—the Grand River Hospital: these consist of a 44-bed psychiatric ward, an out-patient clinic, day centre, and a 24-hour walk-in psychiatric emergency service staffed by psychiatric nurses and an on-call psychiatrist located next to the hospital's emergency room.

The history of this service, how it was developed as a response to lack of beds, and its benefit to certain groups such as recent immigrants and the Anabaptist population has already been outlined in the preface. The main stimulus was the lack of beds; we had 44 beds for a population of 300,000–350,000. We could refer "overflow" and longer-term patients to the provincial mental hospital 70 miles away, but availability of beds was unpredictable, and they have been steadily reducing their beds.

A proposal for a mobile crisis home treatment service, similar to Fenton's but slightly larger, was put forward to the provincial government department of health in 1985. Fenton's service had only two staff—a nurse and a social worker, and a half-time psychiatrist; our proposal was for a larger staff, consisting of two nurses, an occupational therapist, a secretary, and a coordinator (a social worker who did half time clinical work) 3.5 clinical staff in total.

Funding was finally approved in 1989, and the service opened later that year; apart from Fenton's Montreal service (which lasted only as long as the research project), ours was the first MCHT service in Canada. One problem soon became apparent. Fenton's service, our template, took referrals only from the psychiatric emergency service in the hospital emergency room. We had envisioned broadening our referral base to primary care physicians, psychiatrists, and out-patient clinics, but still confined to mental health workers and physicians. But, provincial mental health regulations stipulate that any community mental health service must have an open referral system; i.e., accept referrals from anyone, including family and self-referrals. We persuaded the government to allow us to stick to the narrower referral base for up to a year while we got our bearings. As the year unfolded, though, it became clear that we were naïve to expect a steady stream of well-screened referrals from our mental health colleagues and primary care physicians—it just did not happen.

Strange as it may seem, in spite of the shortage of psychiatric beds, staff of the hospital mental health service—of which we are a part—did not refer as many patients as we expected. This apparent resistance to the use of

MCHT has been noted by many writers and is a recurrent theme in this book. Ignorance of home-based treatment and lack of faith in the service's ability to handle acute cases, coupled with anxiety about remaining clinically responsible until we picked up acute patients, seemed to be factors in our system.

With time, and the ever-increasing pressure on in-patient beds, these concerns have been overcome. The hospital emergency room staff and the 24-hour crisis clinic, who work closely together, are the main route to admission, and so it has been especially important to work closely together.

The mandated open referral system has turned out to be a positive feature and our experience of it is illustrative of what are widespread problems of accessibility in many mental health systems. Firstly, without it we would not have received sufficient referrals from the original narrower base. Secondly, very appropriate referrals have been received from such professionals as teachers, general home care nurses, and social service workers. Thirdly, even patients and their caregivers consistently make some very appropriate referrals; we are sometimes left wondering how some of our patients would have received timely help without us.

The Hazelglen office was opened in 1989 in a small shopping centre located in a working class suburban area, about 10 minutes drive from the hospital. Like Fenton's service in Montreal, it is open 9 a.m. to 5 p.m., five days a week. Patients can be seen on the same day of referral if necessary; often they are seen in 1–2 days.

The following figures illustrate how the service fits into the local mental health system:

Figure 3.1 shows pre-existing pathways to admission for an acutely ill patient.

Figure 3.2. shows the alternative option of MCHT.

Figure 3.3 shows how non-mental health professionals and patients and their families have *direct* access to MCHT; an acutely ill patient no longer has to go through their primary care physician or the hospital psychiatric emergency service to receive intensive psychiatric care, in contrast to Figure 3.1.

Twenty-four hour emergency coverage is provided in a number of ways. Patients can phone an emergency pager 24 hours a day, 7 days a week and contact a Hazelglen staff and receive telephone help and support. If the patient needs to be seen, they can go to the 24-hour crisis clinic of the hospital staffed by psychiatric nurses, with access to the psychiatrist on call. If needed, the patient can be transported to the hospital in a taxi. We have a generous taxi budget for this purpose, which is also used to transport patients to the office and to other services such as their primary care physician.

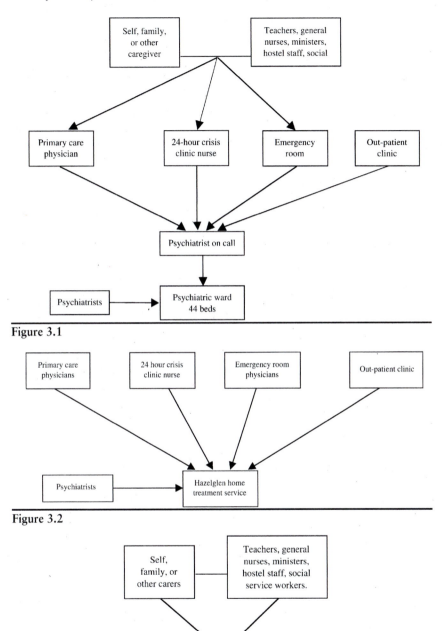

Figure 3.1

Figure 3.2

Figure 3.3

Similar to other services, the need for face-to-face contact after hours is quite rare; the reasons for this are twofold. Crises can usually be anticipated and forestalled by the patient's key worker (called case manager), who, because of the frequency and intensity of contact, becomes familiar with the patients' and families' vulnerabilities. Second, case managers proactively phone patients who are at risk, in the evenings and at weekends, to provide support and early intervention before crises arise. The service psychiatrist is available by pager for telephone consultation from 8 a.m. to 10 p.m. seven days a week—rarely used.

Referrals are phoned in and a screening interview is conducted by phone. Referrals that are not very acute are provided with alternative suggestions for their problem; referrals that are at immediate risk are steered towards the emergency room and/or crisis clinic. The rest are given an appointment for an initial assessment; if possible and if it is safe, we prefer to do this in the patient's home. If they are accepted, patients are then given an appointment with the psychiatrist—for the same day if necessary, usually in the next few days. If there is a clear need, the psychiatrist will see the patient at home; usually because of shortage of psychiatrist time and for efficiency, they are seen at the office.

Some patients we accept don't actually need admission on that day. But, many of these would undoubtedly do so if left without care for the next week or so; they need early intervention, as discussed in the previous chapter. It is a fine balancing act, therefore, to keep the holes in the intake net "the right size" so that we don't spend most of the time assessing patients who are unsuitable. (See Chapter 4 for further discussion.)

Diagnoses of Hazelglen Patients: compared to patients admitted to the psychiatric ward at Grand River Hospital.

Table 3.1

Discharge diagnoses	Hazelglen	Hospital
Depression	50%	38%
Schizophrenia	12%	17%
Mania	9%	7%
Psychosis	10%	15%
Adjustment disorder	10%	15%
Personality disorder	9%	8%

Acuity of Hazelglen Patients

Because the assessment of psychiatric emergencies is subjective, one is never sure in MCHT whether a patient would truly have required hospital admission if home-based treatment had not been available. A scale measuring acuity, giving a score that can be compared to a population of in-patients is therefore helpful, and the Basis-32 serves that purpose.

The Behavior and Symptom Identification Scale (Basis-32; Eisen, 2000) was developed to meet the need for a brief but comprehensive mental health status measure that would be useful in assessing outcome of psychiatric care from the patient perspective. It is a 32-item measure of patient self-reported difficulty in symptoms and functioning that can be administered at appropriate points in the treatment process (typically at intake, termination, and a follow-up point.)

The clinical benchmarks are based on data derived from a normative sample of 500 individuals representative of the U.S. population of adults from ages 18 to 89 and a clinical sample of 659 adults admitted for in-patient treatment at McLean Hospital, Belmont, Massachusetts, from 1996 and 1997. Clinical acuity is rated as severe, moderate, mild, or minimal. The majority (61%) of the in-patient sample scored in the severe range at the time of admission. Eighty-five percent of patients accepted for home-based treatment at Hazelglen had Basis-32 scores in the severe range based on analyses of 54 patients treated April 2002 to January 2003.

Regardless of their discipline, staff function as generic mental health workers, and, because there is no need to work shifts, the patient's care is provided by a single staff member. However, other staff are familiar enough with all the patients to enable them to take over in emergencies when the case manager is not available or to continue treatment when he is on vacation. At the beginning of treatment, most visits are in the home. Not all patients want this, though; some are seen at the office or in a local coffee shop. As in Fenton's service, we aim for an average of 50% home visits.

About 12% of patients require admission to hospital, often for just a brief period. There is little interaction between Hazelglen staff and staff on the psychiatric ward, and we have the usual problems of losing control of the outcome of the hospital admission, with varying results: sometimes we get the patient back at the appropriate time, sometimes we never see them again.

Staff morale is high: of the original three clinical staff, one is still working at Hazelglen, and one left in 2003. The occupational therapist left the area after 1 or 2 years and has been replaced by one who has been there for 10 years.

We have to keep up our guard against being used as a kind of psychosocial "Mr. Fix-it," but much less now since the community have a better understanding of our role. Discharging patients is a continual problem; follow-up services are in short supply with long waiting lists; consequently, we keep patients longer than needed.

Evaluation and Statistics

Mean length of stay is 48 days with a range of 9 to 165
Mean age is 37
Basis-32:

Over 80% of patients significantly improved. Almost half had "very favorable" or "optimal" improvement; i.e., similar to a non-clinical population. The proportion of patients rated as "severe" (85%) was reduced to 35% at discharge.

GAF scores:

Mean score on admission 50
Mean score on discharge 65

Patient satisfaction:

Very helpful 51%
Helpful 37%
Would want help again if they had a problem 100%
Would recommend program 100%
Do you feel this program prevented or reduced hospital treatment?
   Yes 93%
   No 7%
Would you have preferred hospital treatment?
   Yes 7%
   No 93%

Address: Hazelglen Outreach Mental Health Service
         850 King Street West
         Kitchener, Ontario, N2G 1E8, Canada

Acute Home Treatment Program
Capital Health Region of British Columbia

City of Victoria

> *"Repeat episodes are very short—previously, patients would allow their illness to deteriorate, because they didn't want to go to the hospital.*

Now, with home treatment, they are not afraid to ask for help—they call earlier"

"The psychiatrists and in-patient nurses were resistant to the program—but, now, they are starting to come around"

Elizabeth Howey MSc.,N., Clinical Nurse Specialist

The Acute Home Treatment Program (AHTP) is part of the Mental Health Services of the Royal Jubilee Hospital, a general hospital, which serves the Capital Health Region, a catchment area of 350,000. Victoria, with a population of 74,000, is the prosperous capital city of British Columbia. It is a popular retirement destination, but also has some socially deprived areas where chronic psychiatric patients live and who often have drug abuse problems. The program was developed because of insufficient beds in the general hospital, where patients can wait in the emergency room two or three days for one of the 83 psychiatric beds, which operate at "a virtual 104%" capacity.

After a pilot project, the service became fully operational in January 2001. The aim of the program was chiefly to divert patients from hospital, and, also, to reduce length of stay by early discharge. But so far, only 20–25% of patients have avoided admission; most are early discharge referrals. This is attributed to a lack of referrals from psychiatrists who are said to have been skeptical and unenthusiastic. The department of psychiatry of the hospital have restricted referrals to the AHTP to only the patients of the 14 psychiatrists who have admitting privileges, and only if they are willing to follow the patient while they are in the program, which does not have it's own dedicated psychiatrist. The creators of the program had planned to treat patients referred by any psychiatrist or family doctor in the area and had intended to have their own psychiatrist.

Some of the resistance to psychiatric involvement is blamed on the provincial fee schedule, which pays more for care of in-patients, than out-patients, which, in turn, is paid more than staff supervision. Attitudes are changing though; as the psychiatrists become more familiar with the service, they are warming up to it, and some of the strongest skeptics are now championing it. Eight of them have signed letters of agreement that they will follow any of their patients who are admitted to AHTP from the emergency room. They prescribe flexible and pro re nata (as needed) doses of medicine, and are quite accessible to staff; after hours, they can be contacted by pager.

Referrals are made by calling the program any time during hours of operation and completing a one-page referral form. Assessment interviews are carried out in the emergency room, psychiatric ward, or psychiatrists office and, if necessary, can be done within one hour but, sometimes there is a wait of two or three days. Admission criteria include admission to or continuation of hospital treatment would be necessary if home treatment were not available; aged between 19 and 65; patient and family in agreement. Exclusion criteria include imminent risk of harm to self or others; persons who live with patient have history of violence and/or active substance abuse; primary diagnosis is substance abuse; or patient continues to abuse drugs or alcohol.

Patients are cared for by a team of psychiatric nurses, three on the day shift (including the program coordinator) 8 a.m.–4 p.m., and two on afternoon/evening shift, 2 p.m.–10 p.m. There is no key worker—typically, the patient will receive care from three or four staff members. Treatment is focused—target symptoms are decided upon at the initial assessment, and the desired outcomes and discharge criteria are stipulated. Focus charting is used. All treatment is carried out in the home and typically involves three visits per day at first. Visits can last one hour or more and can involve taking patients to appointments or recreational facility, or for a walk.

Most patients have serious, often chronic mental illness and need help with numerous practical problems and in coping with daily life; patients in the pilot project, which targeted psychotic patients, had an average score of 43.7 on the Brief Psychiatric Rating Scale (BPRS) score on admission—cf. mean score of patients in the Southwark, U.K., study, 52 (Muijen, et al., 1994).

Diagnoses

Schizophrenia 49%
Schizoaffective 8%
Bipolar disorder 33%
Depressed, major or unspecified 11%

Psychiatrists must agree to see the patients at least once weekly. Some patients were on Community Treatment Orders (CTOs); failure to comply with home treatment resulted in involuntary admission. Eight percent of patients required admission to hospital during home treatment. Treatment lasted, on average, 25 days, and patients were discharged back to previous caregivers; most patients already had an out-patient case manager and a psychiatrist. The maximum case load is 15.

Safety procedures are unusually elaborate and rigorous. Before a patient is accepted into the service, a safety check is conducted in their home by two case managers, who check all occupants, pets, lighting, acceptable parking, presence of weapons, and even assign a chair for the staff (for easy exit, and never in the kitchen where knives are at hand). Daily staff schedules are e-mailed to hospital security staff, with expected times of arrival and departure and with detailed procedures to be followed if staff don't call in, culminating in police being automatically called if x minutes have elapsed.

Staff do all they can to enhance patients' self-efficacy, by educating them and their families about their illness and involving them in the treatment plan. Medication and treatment adherence is a common focus. Staff often administer medication three times per day, and much use is made of blister packs and dosette boxes, for ease of monitoring. Communication is accomplished through a daily team meeting, a chart containing all workers' notes, a cardex, and cell phones. Staff morale is high, and there is no shortage of nurses for the part-time pool; so far, 19 have undergone the weeklong training session. There are 7 full-time equivalent staff positions; 4 are filled by full-time nurses, 3 by casual staff, from a pool of 19.

The service has been unable to hire a dedicated psychiatrist, but a psychiatrist serves as medical director, meeting one hour every three or four weeks and available at other times for troubleshooting.

The provincial Ministry of Health provides funding for the program, and there is no cost to the patient, most of whom are on provincial disability pensions, which cover their drug costs. The hospital pharmacy provides drugs for some patients, and alternatives are found to pay for other patients' drug costs.

Research Evaluation

The AHTP was evaluated during a pilot project, prior to its permanent setup. The program and its evaluation were based on the home treatment project, developed and evaluated by Wasylenki, Gerhs, Goering, and Toner (1997) (see Chapter 7). Twenty-nine patients were treated over a ten-month period for 37 illness episodes. The target population was any of the 900 patients of the Capital Health Region Mental Health Services, who were having an acute psychotic episode that would otherwise require admission to hospital.

Exclusion criteria were

- Imminent risk to self or others, or history of violence
- Residing with someone who has a history of violence or active substance abuse
- Primary diagnosis is substance abuse
- Actively abusing substances, preventing stabilization of target symptoms

Axis I diagnoses included schizophrenia, schizoaffective disorder, bipolar disorder, paranoid delusional disorder, and major depression with psychosis.

Eleven patient episodes were referred from the in-patient ward for early discharge, 26 from home or a psychiatrist's office. Eighteen out of 29 patients lived with, or had significant family or other caregiver support.

Length of stay in service ranged from 3 to 71 days, with a mode of 32–33 days; the average hours of direct nursing care was 58.4.

Clinical progress was measured by the Brief Psychiatric Rating Scale (BPRS); family burden was measured with the Care Burden Scale for Relatives.

BPRS score—mean 43.7 at admission; 35.6 on discharge.

CBS-R score average 1.8 (0 = no burden, 3 = maximum burden); 0.8 on discharge.

Costs: AHTP, includes nursing salaries, transportation, cell phone—$100.4 per day. Total cost for 33 days = $3301.32.

Hospital cost of average acute episode (average stay 21 days) based on a per diem rate of $230 (this excludes institutional costs of heat, maintenance, laundry, food, etc.): $4830.

AHTP cost was 68% of hospital cost.

The hospital per diem rate that the researchers were given is controversial because it does not include costs of running the institution, the rationale being that these costs would still accrue no matter how many patients were on the ward. Traditionally in this type of research, costs are calculated differently; in Wasylenki's research, a per diem rate of $637 was used; the home treatment costs were similar to Victoria's.

An Attitude Questionnaire (Wasylenki, et al., 1997) showed that patients and caregivers had a clear preference for home treatment—scores of 9–9.4, where 1 indicated preference for hospital, and 10 indicates preference for home treatment.

The Treatment Comparison Questionaire showed significant preference for home treatment. Patients rated their safety as higher in home treatment.

The nurses were positive about their role. They developed as autonomous professionals and gained a clearer understanding of the stigmatization and the interruption in patients' lives associated with hospitalization. They were surprised to discover that they had more effective relationships with patients in the one or two hours a day with home treatment compared to the 8–12 hours spent on the ward. Both settings had a 1:5 staff:patient ratio.

A useful innovation was the use of home treatment to start clozapine treatment for five patients. Because of the close monitoring of vital signs and blood tests required, provincial standards, and manufacturer's stipulations, patients were hospitalized for 10–14 days, typically.

Nurses identified large gaps in knowledge about the illness and medications in the patients and families and spent a lot of time teaching and coaching them, which appeared to have helped some of them function better and stay out of hospital longer after they were discharged. Staff considers the program's operating time of 14 hours a day is adequate; the need for 24-hour care was avoided by adequate assessments, quick response to emerging problems, and contingency planning with patients and families.

Date of site visit: August 6, 2001
Address: Acute Home Treatment Program
         Capital Health Region Mental Health Services
         2334 Trent Street
         Victoria
         British Columbia
         V8R 4Z3

Adult Psychiatric Home Support Team
Edmonton, Alberta

> *"We have evolved into this niche . . . of treating personality disorders."*
>
> Fyfe Bahrey MSW, Team Leader

The Acute Adult Psychiatric Home Support Team operates out of a room located in the psychiatric out-patient department of a large teaching hospital—The University of Alberta Medical Center in the centre of Edmonton. Edmonton, the capital city of the province of Alberta, is a prosperous city with a population of almost a million.

The team is part of the academic department of psychiatry and is embedded in a rich mental health system that has many community treatment programs. These include a mobile crisis service, assertive community treatment team, walk-in psychiatric clinic, day and evening hospital, a first episode schizophrenia program, dialectical behaviour therapy program, and a community and residential drug and alcohol service. It has a number of in-patient units in different hospitals, one of which is a short stay unit, and has a bed ratio of 18:100,000. The mobile crisis service does one-time assessments of psychiatric emergencies.

The service started in 1993 as response to large budget cuts by the provincial government necessitating a substantial reduction in mental health services. This was accomplished by closing a 16-bed unit: valued staff was thereby retained and formed the MCHT service. The team was established by psychiatrist Dr. Richard Hibbard, who had visited the home treatment service in Sydney, Australia, started by Dr. John Hoult.

Staffing consists of 5 full-time equivalents–7 full- and part-time staff, all experienced psychiatric nurses. Two staff work 8 a.m.–4 p.m., and 2 staff work 2 p.m.–10 p.m., 5 days a week. Weekends are covered by 2 staff that work 10 a.m.–10 p.m. Saturday and Sunday.

Like many innovative teams, the interests and expertise of its founder have shaped its identity. Dr. Hibbard has had an interest in borderline personality disorder, and has since left the team to set up a dialectical behaviour therapy service. Consequently, the staff have become competent, comfortable, and effective with patients with borderline and other similar disorders, such as narcissistic and histrionic personality disorders, who often present with self-harm. Crisis survival skills techniques, extracted from the "Skills Training Manual for Treating Borderline Personality Disorder" by Marsha Linehan (1993) have been particularly useful. In some ways, the team finds these patients easier to deal with than those on the in-patient ward. The firm three-week limit to length of stay in the program is very helpful—in limiting dependence and limiting staff's frustration. The patients get more time with staff than on the ward, and it is easier to adhere to a firm, consistent approach and to head off splitting of staff because it is a small, close-knit team. The team approach limits dependence on one person. In hospital, the patients are seen as having little responsibility and "socialize with all their friends." Acting out in the community is less for various reasons. "It's their stuff . . . they are not going to throw their own belongings or trash their own home. They are less likely to run . . . away from their own home . . . what's the point." Firm limits are set, and patients know what to expect; there are consequences, such as discharge if they overdose. At the same time, for three weeks the patients can get a great deal of support when they want it, and validation of their feelings.

However, it should be emphasized that, in spite of Dr. Hibbard's interests, the team has never specifically targeted personality disordered patients; it was designed simply as an alternative to admission for patients with all psychiatric diagnoses, and that is still its purpose.

Referrals are only accepted from physicians—psychiatrists or primary care physicians—but not emergency room physicians, for fear of "dumps." "If the patient looks at them cross-eyed, they straight away say "refer to home support team!"

Referrals are made by fax, sometimes accompanied by a phone call, if there is particular concern, and patients are seen usually within one to two days, but, if necessary, can be seen the same day. All patient contacts are outside the hospital, 85% in the patient's home; however, team leader Fyfe Bahrey questions if it is necessary that all visits be home visits, that when they are improved, patients could come to the office. There is a strictly adhered to maximum length of stay: 3 weeks. Patients are informed of this on admission, and it is seen as preventing unhealthy dependence by borderline and other personality disordered patients. Because there are so many services, referring patients for follow-up without significant delay is not a problem.

Although the service is open until 10 p.m., patients are rarely seen after 7 p.m. The team, does not provide after hours emergency service, from 10 p.m.–8 a.m., not even by telephone; patients are instructed to use the emergency room where there is an emergency psychiatric service with a psychiatrist on call.

Psychiatrist's time dedicated to the team has decreased over the years. Whereas in the past psychiatrists did home visits and residents were part of the team, now the team is served by two psychiatrists who each work about 6–10 hours a week there, don't do home visits, and there are no residents. The two team psychiatrists are responsible for about half the caseload and conduct a supervisory meeting for an hour every morning, going over all the patients. They are not paid sessional money or a salary, but can bill the provincial health insurance plan for supervision of staff. Their contact with patients is billed fee for service, which can make it tricky to predict how much time to keep open for the team with the inevitable fluctuations in caseload. The psychiatrists see the patients in their own offices, one of which is in another hospital, usually a day or two after the patient has been admitted.

The rest of the patients are the responsibility of their referring psychiatrist, of which there are 20 in all. This has presented a number of problems. Many psychiatrists work well with the team, often having done a rotation in it as a resident and understanding its philosophy. Some, though, are difficult to reach quickly; some are perceived as not having sufficient respect for the opinions of the staff and less than responsive to their suggestions.

Another more serious problem is that some of the psychiatrists admit their patients to hospital without consulting the team. The great majority of these patients do not require admission, in the team's opinion, and some of them are well into their course of treatment with the team when it occurs— sometimes without their knowledge, seriously undermining morale. For example, in 2001, 36 patients out of 322 were admitted to hospital, the majority not by the team. A typical scenario is the intake of a self-harming patient with borderline personality disorder, who, sometimes unknown to the team, also gets put on the waiting list for hospital admission at the time of the referral. One or two weeks later, when a bed comes up, the team suddenly discover that the patient has been admitted. All this, of course, confirms one of the principles of MCHT (see Chapter 4)—that having the team's own dedicated psychiatrists, and no more than three, is best.

Team leader Fyfe Bahrey considers the team to be consistently under-used, and notes that patients that could be managed in home treatment are regularly admitted to the hospital, in spite of an occupancy rate of over 100% and a perception that there are insufficient beds. This underutilization has led to a "we take everything approach" to the intake process. Patients are not screened out, except for those who are too sick and need admission (7%), are out of the geographical area, or have a primary problem of substance abuse. In spite of this, the level of psychopathology on admission appears to be appropriately high—an average GAF score of 41.

Consideration is being given to broadening the referral base to non-medical staff; e.g., psychiatric nurses in emergency rooms. However, the future is uncertain, with talk of integrating the home support team with other acute programs.

In spite of the team's comfort level with personality disorders, they still experience them as stressful to deal with and have had their share of dramatic situations. These have included a patient who took a serious overdose half an hour after what was considered a successful home visit; a patient who threatened to shoot her common law partner "when he wakes up"; and a woman who gave her parents a suicide note, then barricaded herself in the bedroom with a knife. All these cases were dealt with firmly with police involvement.

There is no official limit to the caseload; however, when it reaches 25, they notice team functioning becoming more difficult and declining in minor ways.

The average number of visits per patient is 4.2.

Transportation of patients is not optimal. Staff do not drive patients because of concerns regarding insurance, and there is no budget for taxis.

Patients with comorbid substance abuse are not accepted for treatment unless they agree to attend the out-patient drug and alcohol treatment service.

The team regularly accepts phone calls from ex-patients seeking support and provides this. If they want to be re-admitted to home support, though, they need a referral from their psychiatrist or primary care physician.

Diagnoses

Hibbard, et al., (1998) stated that the majority of patients were female with an affective disorder, with over 25% also having an Axis II diagnosis, predominantly borderline—most referred because of a parasuicidal crisis. For many patients the Axis II diagnosis was deferred, suggesting that the prevalence of personality disorder, may actually be higher.

Most recent statistics, from 2002, show 359 patients were treated: 65% had a mood disorder, 16% had schizophrenia or other psychotic disorder, 28% had a personality disorder (about half were borderline personality disorder).

There have been four suicides in ten years.

Date of site visit: July 17, 2003
Address: Acute Adult Psychiatric Home Support Team
University of Alberta Hospital Site
8440-112 Street
Edmonton, Alberta
Canada, T6G2B7

BRITAIN

Ladywood Home Treatment Team

> *"It was falling apart—there was inertia, chaos—it was like an airport lounge. People campaigned outside the hospital to have it closed, but the administration did nothing—the patients asked why they could not be treated at home—eventually, we discharged the patients, transferred those we couldn't, and moved into a shed in the grounds."*
>
> Professor Sashidharan

The Ladywood HT service, which was established by Professor Sashidharan, has three claims to distinction. It serves the 40,000 people who live in Ladywood, an inner city area of Birmingham, a district that is the fourth most socially deprived in Britain. It is one of six home treatment teams that cover the entire catchment area of the North Birmingham Mental Health Trust, 600,000 people in all, and is the only trust providing 24-hour home treatment care for an entire catchment area. And, these teams served as a model used by Britain's Department of Health, for their Mental Health National Service Framework (a ten-year strategy) published in 1999—*The Mental Health Policy Implementation Guide* (Department of Health, 1999). All districts in Britain are to set up "Crisis Resolution/Home Treatment Teams."

The North Birmingham Mental Health Trust is a busy breeding ground of home treatment services. In addition to Professor Sashidharan's Ladywood team, Dr. John Hoult was active in setting up the Yardley/Hodge Hill home treatment team, based on his work in Sydney, Australia, and described in the "Open All Hours" study presented in Chapter 1; and Dr. Christine Dean set up the Sparkbrook home treatment team in the late 1980s, also described in Chapter 1.

When Professor Sashidharan arrived in Birmingham, care for acute psychiatric disorders was mainly provided in an old traditional mental hospital—All Saints Hospital. Sashidharan described the situation. "It was falling apart—there was inertia, chaos—it was like an airport lounge. People campaigned outside the hospital to have it closed, but the administration did nothing—the patients asked why they could not be treated at home—eventually, we discharged the patients, transferred those we couldn't, and moved into a shed in the grounds."

The initiative for the creation of home treatment services was a revolt against the old traditional mental hospital, which was said to serve the ethnic population poorly, especially Afro-Carribean people. Central to the philosophy was giving patients more power. Sashidharan had been influenced by work at Dingleton Hospital in Scotland (which also influenced Burns; see Chapters 1 and 2), and at Trieste in Italy, where all the psychiatric hospitals had been closed down. Although not a philosophy held throughout the rest of the Trust, Sashidharan prefers to de-emphasize some of the medical aspects of psychiatry, such as diagnosis: "we don't use diagnoses . . . diagnoses do not lead to action, they are not reliable . . . can cause stigma. There is a danger of diagnosis trumping everything else, including the leaking roof. We make a problem list with the patient whose problems may be no money, no food; voices may not be a problem."

Ladywood Home Treatment service is located in an old factory, which has been converted into offices. It is essentially one large room containing 14 desks, with a few small side rooms for the doctor, team leader, and the secretary. It is located in the district of Ladywood, which is 45% Afro-Carribean and South Asian, near the centre of the city of Birmingham—in fact, just minutes from an impressive regenerated area for pedestrians on which are situated a recently built theatre and symphony hall, and many other new civic buildings and shops.

Staff consist of a manager, who does some clinical work; seven nurses; six health care assistants, two of whom are service users; one social worker; and a secretary. Medical staff consists of one consultant (Professor Sashidharan), a specialty registrar, and, 9 a.m.–5 p.m., 5 days a week, a senior clinical medical officer (a senior psychiatrist, who has not become a consultant).

Hours of operation are 24 hours a day, 7 days a week, with two shifts: 9 a.m.–5 p.m., 1 p.m.–9 p.m., and an on-call shift, with two team members, 9 p.m.–9 a.m. Staff on night call can be up working 3–4 hours and be on duty the next day; tiredness is acknowledged as a problem, but a separate night shift would be resource intensive.

The target population are people aged 16–65 with a major psychiatric disorder of such severity that they are at risk of requiring in-patient care. The focus is particularly on those with a psychotic illness, both acute and chronic, and those with severe depression; about 60% have a serious mental illness. The service is not primarily targeted at people with anxiety disorders such as agoraphobia, brain damage, dementia, learning difficulties, a primary diagnosis of personality disorder, or recent history of overdose, but who are not suffering from a psychiatric illness, relationship issues, and situations of domestic violence. However, there is not a blanket exclusion of these groups, and each individual case is considered on its merits.

Referrals are not taken from the public directly, except for previous patients and their families. Referrals come from agencies having contact with mentally ill persons and include community treatment teams; hospitals, both in-patient wards (for early discharge) and the ER; family doctors; police; emergency duty team of social services department; and, after hours, the Assertive Outreach Team. During the hours of 9 to 5 Monday to Friday, all referrals to the home treatment team are made to the primary care mental health team, which serves as a single point of entry and gives them a chance to see if they can deal with the crisis first. Referrals after hours are made directly to the team, who are contacted through the hospital switchboard. The service aims to respond within one hour.

The team is the gatekeeper to *all* admissions to the in-patient ward, and they perform this role with dogged determination; Dr. Sashidharan screens all admissions personally, any time of the day or night. The belief is that rapid attention to crises from a wide front is necessary in order to prevent unnecessary admissions. Acceptance rate is 30–40% of outside referrals and 90% from mental health teams, averaging 60% in all.

The assessment takes place whenever possible in the patient's own environment; 97% of contacts are in the home. If possible, caregivers and social network are included. The assessment focuses on the present problem—what has happened that has precipitated action now, rather than last week, or tomorrow—the presenting problem is almost always behavioral. Unsafe or intolerable behavior is the area most likely to be causing community breakdown. The status of interpersonal relationships, i.e., the support network, is crucial, often determining whether the patient can stay at home or will require alternative accommodation or hospital admission.

The service has access to crisis beds and a respite house with five beds; this latter is owned and run by a user group, but funded by the trust ($200,000), who therefore control the beds. The owners staff the house, two during the day, and one at night, and residents do their own self-care and cooking, with support if needed. Sometimes, other patients are sent there during the day for extra support. There is also funding to place patients in furnished apartments, hotels, and bed and breakfast establishments.

Medication is administered 2–3 times a day if necessary, and, in keeping with the principle of empowerment, patients are given the opportunity to select which drug they will take, from a list. Much effort is expended to accommodate patients' needs and wants, even to the extent of paying for faith healers, mediums, and acupuncture. Staff work regularly with priests and Mullahs, and local churches, temples, and gurdwaras are a great resource. Practical help is emphasized and staff go to great lengths sometimes. During my visit, a worker brought in a cat in a cage and proceeded to order kitty litter and cat food, in preparation for taking it to her home while the patient was in hospital. I was told of the case of a Kenyan man, acting strangely in the street, who appeared to be hearing voices and had been apprehended by the police. He said that he was hearing the voice of his sister "from the grave." The team discovered that a relative in Kenya had been trying to reach him—his sister had just died. The team bought him a plane ticket to Kenya; however, he got drunk, and missed it. Eventually, through negotiation, they got him on another plane.

Mainstream medical help is also important; all new referrals are seen by a psychiatrist by the next working day and receive a physical exam and routine blood tests. There is no fixed number of places in the service; at the time of the visit, 40 patients were "on the board," and there have been as many as 60. Even though they have the option of closing the service, they don't; patients are just discharged quicker. The six home treatment teams in the trust get about 250 referrals each month, about 40–50 per team, and accept about 40–50%.

The average length of stay is 3–4 weeks, and three groups of patients identified: 1) "Fast recoverers," who are only involved for 24–48 hours, and usually have a very brief crisis, involving a specific problem to be solved, such as housing or benefits; 2) long-term patients, often with quite complex and intractable problems—some stay six months; and 3) a middle group of patients, acutely ill for three weeks or so. This group is the largest.

The hospital admission rate used to be 20%; now, because of an increase in milder patients, it is about 15%. Even when patients are admitted, the team maintains a link with the family and the patient, who they may take out on a pass to the movies, for example, to maintain social engagement. Hospital admission is only a physical solution to suicide risk, says Sashidharan—it removes access to methods; but, in some cases, it can "energize a dynamic" in which the more restrictions, the more some patients will try—like a game. Suicidal patients are helped by mobilizing social support and networks, which is more difficult to do if the patient lives alone (paradoxically, living alone protects against admission—you don't get pressure from the family). There needs to be an understanding between the patient and the team, that they will call when they feel in danger of self-harm. That, and the promise of rapid access to help, reduces the risk. Maintaining sleep patterns and family education are important. There have only been three suicides in ten years—less than in the hospital. Most at risk for admission are manic patients, because of the need to contain their restlessness and hyperactivity.

It is important that the home treatment team is part of an integrated service model, and, in addition to the in-patient ward; has links to a psychosocial rehab service serving long-term patients at home or in supported housing; has an assertive outreach team, homeless service, early intervention team for first episode psychosis; and has alcohol and drug treatment service. There is a family sponsorship scheme, in which families are paid to care for patients. "If a home treatment service is not part of an integrated service model, it will flounder—it won't be sustainable," says Sashidharan.

Date of site visit: April 16, 18, 2002
Address: Ladywood Home Treatment
          Ground Floor, Morcom House
          Ledsam Street
          Birmingham B168DN

Manchester Home Option Service

"We were notorious for sending out-patients out of the area to find a bed."
"To have both is a luxury" (day treatment and home treatment)

—Fiona Winstanley, option service manager

The Manchester Home Option Service (HOS) is located in the grounds of a university teaching hospital—the Manchester Royal Infirmary—in a spacious single-story building, which used to house the Central Manchester Day Hospital, from which it evolved. Manchester is a large industrial city in the north of England.

The HOS is unusual in that it started life as an acute day hospital intended as an alternative to in-patient admission. Creed, Black, and Anthony, et al. (1990), in a randomized controlled trial, showed that 40% of people presenting for admission could be treated successfully in this day hospital, with few differences in clinical and social outcome. Day hospital treatment is one of the proven alternatives to admission, so why did this group abandon it in favor of home treatment?

Harrison, et al., (1999), in a paper about the Manchester Day Hospital, describe its limitations: some patients were unwilling to attend, even though transportation was offered, patients were left unsupported outside the 9 to 5 operating time, and the broad service offered, such as group work, activities for in-patients, and a drop-in centre, made it difficult to focus on the very acute patients. After 12 years as a day hospital, it was changed to the HOS in March 1997, serving the socially deprived inner-city area of central Manchester.

The impetus for creation of the day hospital, and then the HOS, was lack of in-patient psychiatric beds—many patients ended up being admitted to hospitals in towns miles away; it still happens today, but less.

The catchment area is three distinct geographic "sectors," each with a population of 45,000 and containing many immigrants and students. The number of patients served at one time, is fixed at a maximum of 30 active and 6 ready for discharge. There are 19 staff: 11 nurses, 3 support workers, 2 occupational therapists, 1 occupational technician, a secretary, and a manager. Medical staff consists of 3 consultants, each 2 half days per week, a full-time senior house offficer (junior resident), and a half-time senior registrar (senior resident). Occupational therapy staff work 9 to 5, but occasionally do a late shift or the night call shift and take on a key worker role. They act as generic workers, but have one day per week for assessments.

The service operates 24 hours a day, seven days a week; the team base office is open 9 a.m.–11 p.m. and two staff members are on call at night by phone. Referrals can be made any time and are only taken from psychiatrists, community mental health teams, emergency rooms (psychiatrist on call), and community psychiatric nurses; all referrals have to be OK'd by a psychiatrist. Referrals are not taken from family doctors because of concern that many of them would be considered inappropriate. Referrals are taken from the in-patient wards for early discharge, providing they are still acute, but they don't get as many of these as they think they should, although the HOS is accepted by the consultants because beds are so tight. The service does not serve a gatekeeper role.

The target group is all adult patients aged 16–65 presenting with acute psychiatric problems that would otherwise require in-patient treatment; also (unusual for home treatment programs), patients with dementia are accepted for short-term assessment of care needs. Excluded are those detained under the Mental Health Act, those at risk of harming themselves or others, those who could not return to a safe home environment, or those whose primary diagnosis is drug or alcohol abuse.

Intake assessment from 9 a.m.–5 p.m., is done by a staff person, designated the assessment officer for that day, whose schedule is freed up for the purpose. Screening is done by phone, but often a face-to-face interview is needed. The initial assessment focuses on identification of risk, compliance with the service, support networks, and home circumstances. Wherever possible, caregivers are included in this process, and sometimes the decision to accept is delayed until the family is contacted. Initial assessments are usually done at the base office, but sometimes in the home, and, at night, usually in the emergency room. Once a patient is accepted, treatment begins immediately, including taking patients home and giving medication, if indicated. Initially, the emphasis is on engagement, safety, reduction of symptoms, and daily functioning. A wide variety of treatments is used: family therapy, cognitive behavior therapy (CBT) for psychosis, cooking and activity groups, anxiety management groups, and individual psychotherapy. Two staff members are designated for each patient as the key worker, and co-key worker responsible for the treatment plan, and whom the patient gets to know best. If patients are already known to a mental health worker, that person is expected to continue to work with them during the home treatment episode. Staff communicates through three handover meetings per day, the chart, and the use of mobile phones and pagers.

The HOS does not have the same emphasis on *home* visits and treatment as one finds in other MCHT services; it is really a combination of the original day hospital, plus a home treatment team. "To have both is a luxury," said manager Fiona Winstanley. Attendance at the base office is encouraged and provides respite for the family and structure for the patient. Transportation is provided by three cars belonging to the service. Patients are seen between one and three times a day, depending on the level of risk and the need to supervise medication. Most are seen twice daily—once at the base office, and once at home in the evening. A survey of activity showed that 49% of patient contacts were at the base office, 42% at home, and 9% at other locations. Medication is handled in a number of ways, including dosette boxes and daily visits to administer them directly to the patient. There are problems melding home treatment medicine administration with dispensing regulations; a common theme, in which institutional rules don't keep pace with the move of care into the home. Much use is made of PRN (as needed) doses of medicine to avoid the doctor having to prescribe over the phone in an urgent situation, which is not allowed.The HOS has access to three crisis respite beds. Sixteen percent of patients require admission, which can be a difficult process, involving admitting out of the area, paying for beds in a private hospital, or "swapping" patients. Once admitted, patients are usually lost to the service, finishing their treatment in the hospital and eventually being discharged to a community team—a common problem in home treatment. There have been no problems with safety of staff or patients. Staff visit patients' homes alone, but not for the first visit, and not at night. If there are safety concerns, patients can be seen in the emergency room.

Staff have learned to develop clear boundaries regarding what they do and the types of patients they can help. For example, they used to take patients with long-standing personality problems, which were always suicidal and would not tell staff where they were. Home treatment seemed to make them worse, giving them more opportunity and attention for this type of behavior. Now, they make sure that there are clear, tight expectations of what patients and staff expect from each other.

Survey of Service Activity (Harrison, et al., 1999)

During the first year of service, 349 patients were referred and 61% were accepted. The most common reasons for non-acceptance were unwillingness to cooperate (23%), not ill enough (24%), and needing admission (24%). Commonest sources of referral were ER (40%), followed by out-patient department (25%).

Diagnoses were 40% schizophrenia or related psychotic illness, 29% depression (including 7% who were psychotic), 15% bipolar affective disorder, 11% anxiety or adjustment, and 6% other.

Out-of-area admissions were reduced from a total of 290 in 1996/1997(pre HOS), to 78 in 1998/1999.

In 2000/2001, the median length of stay was 33 days; 75% of patients were discharged before 80 days, a few stayed up to 200 days. The budget is 507,764 pounds.

Comparison with an In-Patient Sample

During the first 10 weeks of the new service, details of consecutive admissions to HOS (43) and the in-patient (37) unit were collected, and staff rated all patients using a modified version of the Social Behavior Schedule (SBS).

In-patients were most likely to be rated as demonstrating attention-seeking behavior, bizarre speech content, incoherent speech, socially unacceptable habits, and over-activity, whereas HOS patients were more likely to be rated as having problems with eating and drinking enough or posing a suicidal risk. In-patients were more likely to have adverse experiences such as involuntary admissions, custodial sentences, and homelessness. HOS patients had fewer problems with relationships and daily occupation and overall, were less sick.

The median length of stay is 33 days; 75% are discharged before 80 days—a few stay 200 days.

User satisfaction surveys gave the service a high rating: 57% very satisfied, 22% fairly satisfied. Service features giving most satisfaction were support from staff, flexibility of contact, and "kept me out of hospital."

Users wanted more opportunity to talk, contact with doctors, and a broader range of activities.

Case Histories (Marshall & Harrison, 1998)

Alison

Alison was referred by her consultant after attending for an out-patient appointment. The assessment officer saw her immediately in the out-patient department. Diagnosed with bipolar affective disorder in 1972, she had been admitted to hospital six times since then: four times with depression, and twice for hypomania. She had been a patient at HOS a year ago, when she was depressed.

She was now presenting with hypomania: irritable and demanding behavior, eating and sleeping poorly, and strained relationship with her partner. She had stopped taking her lithium (a mood stabilizer) and was in poor physical condition.

Alison was reluctant to come to the base office unless absolutely necessary and she had a good working relationship with her community psychiatric nurse (CPN). She agreed to be seen twice a day, and her CPN would continue to see her weekly, also occasionally with HOS staff, and she would come to a weekly team meeting.

Alison was quite needy, often calling after hours, sometimes requiring a home visit at these times. After three months, contact was reduced to once every other day and finally to two visits a week, one from the team and one from the CPN. After four months, her symptoms and medications were stabilised enough for her to be discharged to her CPN.

Shirley

Shirley is 43 and lives with her husband Eric and their two sons, both in their early 20s. She was referred one Saturday afternoon by the duty psychiatrist at the hospital ER, where she had gone complaining of increased depression and suicidal ideas. The assessment officer went to see her at home two hours later.

Shirley had begun to feel depressed and anxious about four months earlier, had seen her family doctor two weeks prior, and had been prescribed an antidepressant, but was now feeling worse. She was not eating or sleeping, was neglecting herself, and was talking about suicide. She was very distressed, confused, and frightened. There was no previous psychiatric history, and there were no obvious precipitating factors.

Although she talked about self-harm and suicide, the assessment officer thought she could be managed by home treatment, which Shirley preferred, not wanting to go to hospital. She was immediately taken to the base, where she was given a physical examination by the duty psychiatrist and medication was prescribed. She was then taken back home, given the emergency telephone number. The plan was to see her key worker at least twice a day, once in the morning, and once in the evening, to monitor her mental state, administer her medication, and give support to her family.

On Monday, she was reviewed by the interdisciplinary team, seen by a team psychiatrist and prescribed antipsychotic and antidepressant medicine. Her key worker introduced her to relaxation techniques and engaged her in some cognitive behavioural therapy.

After one week, visits were reduced to once daily; after three weeks, to alternate face-to-face and telephone contacts, and she was taking her medicine without supervision. After four weeks she was almost symptom free, and she was discharged to her family doctor after five weeks.

Yousseff

Yousseff is single, 37, unemployed, and lives alone in a public housing apartment. He was referred by the consultant at the local hospital, where he had been admitted involuntarily to the psychiatric intensive care unit.

He has suffered from schizoaffective disorder since 1981 and had been admitted to a secure facility, usually involuntarily, many times. He often presented with disinhibited and threatening behavior and paranoid delusions. He usually responded to medication, would be discharged on oral or depot medication, which he would stop taking and become ill again. He had a case manager and a social worker.

At the time of the referral he had stabilized, but he had some residual symptoms. He was allowed home on a "Section 17," which means that if he refused treatment he would be admitted again involuntarily. He attended the base for his medication daily and was visited at home in the evening for the first week, but then began to refuse his medicine, and his mental state deteriorated sufficiently to warrant return to hospital by police.

Two days later, he was again given "Section 17 leave" under supervision of HOS, and this time adhered to treatment; he was discharged from home treatment after six weeks, with few symptoms.

Date of site visit: April 17, 2002
Address: Central Manchester Healthcare NHS Trust
          Department of Psychiatry
          Home Option Service
          Rawnsley Building
          Manchester Royal Infirmary
          Oxford Road, Manchester, M13 9WL

St. Albans Community Treatment Team

> *"When beds are full, we are used more appropriately."*

> *"It was a mistake when, at first, to get known, we took all referrals; when we got more restrictive, people didn't like it—they were very offended that we didn't take their patients."*

Sue Smith RN, manager

The St. Albans Community Treatment Team (CTT) serves an affluent, mixed urban and rural area 15 miles north of London. St. Albans is an old Roman town, built around a cathedral. For 70 years, the Hill End Hospital, a psychiatric hospital built on the edge of the town provided the bulk of acute psychiatric care. In 1993, in line with the general policy of closing large institutions, it was decided to close it, and psychiatric services were redesigned using a service model with a strong community focus, including home treatment as an alternative to admission; two "community treatment teams" were created as a result.

The St. Albans CTT, funded by the West Hertfordshire Community Health NHS Trust, serves a catchment area of 145,000—the towns of St. Albans, Harpenden, and surrounding villages. The team is located in a small, separate building in the grounds of a modern, free-standing, 24-bed psychiatric admission unit, Albany Lodge. There is a large room, plus a few smaller offices. The target population is those adults who are suffering from an acute psychiatric disorder or an acute exacerbation of an enduring psychiatric problem severe enough to warrant hospital admission. Excluded are patients younger than 16 and those suffering from an organic disorder.

Staff consists of 8 nurses, 1 support worker, and 1 part-time manager (who manages both CTTs). Medical staff include a full time senior house officer (junior resident), a specialist registrar (senior resident) three days a week, and a consultant one day a week, who is also available at other times. Hours of operation are 9 a.m.–9 p.m., seven days a week, 9 p.m.–11 p.m. for emergency referrals from the emergency room. Between 9 p.m. and 9 a.m., there is a staff on call, and, if necessary, patients can be seen at the inpatient ward. Shifts are 9 a.m.–5 p.m., 1 p.m.–9 p.m., and 9 p.m.–11 p.m.

Referrals are taken from users, caregivers, family doctors, and other agencies from 9 a.m. to 5 p.m. through the Community Mental Health Centre, who do an initial screening. The staff person who is duty assessor for that day then screens all referrals. Mental health professionals can refer direct from 9 a.m.–11 p.m.; family doctors and police can refer direct after 5 p.m. Referrals are also taken from the in-patient ward for early discharge; sometimes these are not very acute, but are accepted because beds are saved. Sometimes, the team will assess for suitability for home treatment by supervising in-patients' passes home from the ward; this can last for up to a week. Patients can be seen within two hours if necessary, usually on the same day, occasionally within two days. Acceptance rate at the time of the site visit was said to be 40%, although it had been about 62% in an earlier study of the service. Assessments are done by the nurse and the team psychiatrist during the day, and the on-call community psychiatrist is used after hours. They are conducted preferably in the patient's home (75%) and can last 0.5 to 3 hours, but usually average 1 hour. Patients' community mental health workers are encouraged to be present, and their involvement is encouraged throughout the course of home treatment. Medication can be given immediately, but this can be problematic, as it is dispensed by retail pharmacists, and staff may have to drive around looking for one that is open; sometimes patients cannot afford the 6 pounds prescription fee (another example of medication practices not being as smooth and efficient as those in a hospital).

Patients have a named nurse responsible for the treatment plan, and usually they will meet at least three staff during the course of their treatment, although they prefer to interact with just one. Patients are seen at least daily at first, sometimes 2–3 times a day. Telephone contact is used frequently. When they are more stable, they are encouraged to come to the base office. The total number of patients at the time of the site visit was 25; they almost never close for admissions, but "if it got to 50 we would have to close." Safety has not been a problem; if in doubt, staff visit in pairs or see the patient away from the home. The manager did recall one incident in which she was threatened with a knife and escaped through a window; however, she did not perceive much of a danger from the patient, who had a personality disorder. The team provides anxiety and stress management, brief therapy/problem-solving approaches, family work, assistance with problems of daily living, intensive short-term counseling, support and advice to caregivers, and help connect patients to other services. Patients are supposed to have a physical examination, but this has been difficult to achieve for all patients.

The team is also supposed to be a gatekeeper to the psychiatric ward, except for admissions after 11 p.m., and certain administrative exceptions such as patients who are from out of the catchment area or transfers from secure beds. A survey that took place in 1996, reported in Brimblecombe (year ????) suggested 17% of admissions meeting home treatment criteria were bypassing the team; however, a more recent informal audit of admissions in 1998 showed just 6–7% could have been taken on for home treatment.

Lessons learned include greater confidence treating manic patients, with an emphasis on liberal use of benzodiazepines for rapid sedation, and "holding our anxieties and having more faith in the team." Borderline personality disorder patients can be treated if there are contracts, firm limits, and boundaries, and if "everyone sticks to the same agreed approach." Patients with post-partum disorders do well, particularly if care of the baby through family involvement can be arranged, so the team can concentrate on the mother.

Statistics

Diagnoses

- Schizophrenia and other psychoses 22.8%
- Mood disorders 53.8%
- Neurotic, stress related, and somatoform
    disorders 10.6%
- Disorders of personality 9.1%
- Other 3.5%

Mean length of stay 44 days
Median length of stay 30 days
Budget 230,000 pounds
Referral rate to CTTs equated as 295 per 100,000 population per annum
Eight percent of assessments were referred as in-patients; they were more likely to be less acute
Most community referrals were from psychiatric services (45%) and family doctors (28%)
Twenty-one percent were admitted at some time during home treatment after a median period of 13 days (mean = 41)

Research

Brimblecombe and O'Sullivan (1999) studied the influence of diagnosis on acceptance rates and admission to hospital.

During one year, 318 people were assessed and 61.9% were accepted by the CTT; 69.2% of schizophrenic patients and 74.6% of mood disorder patients were accepted for home treatment, but only 37.5% of patients with personality disorder were accepted. Diagnosis also influenced admission rates at the time of the assessment: mood disorder patients were less likely to be admitted (7.0%), whereas 25.0% of those with personality disorder were admitted. Fifty percent of those with mood disorder who were admitted were hypomanic, even though they constituted only 14.2% of total number of mood disorders assessed; 18.5% of schizophrenic patients were admitted.

After home treatment had started, 18.9% of those diagnosed with mood disorder were admitted, 15.6% of those with schizophrenia, and 22.2% of those with personality disorder. The most common reasons for admission were risk to self (43.2%); risk to others (16.25%), and patient preference (27%). These findings appear to accord with research by Tyler R. Merson, (1994; see Chapter 8), showing patients with personality disorder were not as successfully treated in MCHT as patients with other diagnoses.

Case Histories (Brimblecombe)

John, 19—psychosis, likely drug induced

John was referred by his family doctor after being brought to the office by his mother. John, 19 years old, had been acting bizarrely since returning from a holiday in Spain two weeks previously. After a discussion with the Community Mental Health Centre duty worker, the referral was passed to the CTT, who saw John at home later that day.

John was distracted and unable to give a clear account of what had been happening; at times, he appeared to be listening to voices, but declined to answer questions about this. His mother said he may have taken drugs while on holiday, but she did not know what type. He did not appear to be a danger to himself or others.

He was accepted for home treatment and was visited twice daily at first. A urine drug screen was negative. Although ambivalent at first, he agreed to take medicine administered by staff, but developed side effects; the CTT doctor adjusted his medicine immediately. Support was given to his mother, who continued to be anxious about her son. After two days, John became more friendly and communicative to staff, but still would not talk about what he was experiencing. After three days, visits were reduced to once daily, and he and his mother were responsible for administering the medicine. Within two weeks he appeared "nearly back to normal," but he could remember little of the previous few weeks. Contact was reduced further to every two days, and John began to discuss what happened on holiday: he revealed that he had taken some drugs, but was unsure what type. After a further two weeks of phone contact, he was discharged, with a follow-up appointment in the out-patient department a month later.

Jane, 43—depression and suicidal plans

Jane, a teacher, was referred by her family doctor, who wanted her admitted after she had told him that she planned to kill herself. She was assessed that same morning in her home, where she lived alone. She was tearful and agitated, and had been off work with depression for three months, related to work problems where she had been disciplined for poor performance; recently, she had been told that the school was unwilling to have her return. Jane had few friends and had taken an overdose in her late teens after being jilted.

Jane continued to express a wish to take an overdose, but agreed to give the CTT a chance to help by visiting her twice daily and holding her medicine; she also allowed staff to remove other tablets from her home. She was introduced to some day care facilities that the CTT had immediate access to in order to lessen her social isolation and give her some meaningful activity. Initially, she was driven by staff to the day care, but soon began to go by bus. After an initial period of supportive counseling, a more focused approach was taken by staff, who adopted a problem-solving approach, based on her setting small daily goals; e.g., going shopping, and contacting her union advisor. After two weeks of home treatment, she called the team at 7 p.m., saying she had taken an overdose. An ambulance took her to the emergency room, and she was reassessed by the CTT next morning. The overdose had been small and seemed related to further negative news about her work future; she recognized that this was not helpful to her, and returned home.

After several weeks of gradually reducing contact, she was discharged to her family doctor and was awaiting an assessment for cognitive behavioral psychotherapy. By this point, she had accepted that she would not be able to return to work and had started a computer course.

Michael, 29—chronic paranoid schizophrenia; home treatment and hospital admission

Michael was referred for home treatment by his community psychiatric nurse (CPN) because he had become increasingly psychotic recently and had likely stopped his medication. The CTT, together with his nurse, assessed Michael during which time he gestured bizarrely and gave monosyllabic answers. He acknowledged that he might be forgetting his medication occasionally, and that it did help him "think more clearly" when he took it. He appeared to be eating poorly and had no food in his apartment. In the past, Michael had been assaultive when unwell, but denied any angry feelings towards others currently.

After taking Michael out to buy some food, the CTT made plans with him to visit twice daily, and the CPN would continue her visits. However, he was often out, and staff sometimes visited several times before finding him at home, or they sometimes found him at a day center he attended. All visits were done in pairs, due to the risk of him would becoming aggressive. As well as providing medications, the team encouraged him to cook and took him shopping. His mental state remained unchanged during the first week, even though his medication had been increased, a view confirmed by the day center staff, who found him "odd" but not threatening.

After one week, the CTT was informed that the fire brigade had been called to Michael's apartment the previous evening. They visited him immediately and found a large burn in the middle of his carpet; he said he had "burnt some things" but did not explain further, nor did he seem to recognize the dangers of his actions. Because of concern that he might be a risk to himself or others, he was admitted to hospital under the Mental Health Act.

Jane, 30—threats to commit suicide; neither home treatment, nor admission

Jane had sporadic involvement with mental health services in the past; previous diagnoses included depression and personality disorder. She presented at a local psychiatric unit at 8 p.m. requesting admission, saying she would kill herself if not admitted as she could no longer cope with her abusive boyfriend and her debts. She was assessed by the CTT duty assessor and the duty doctor of the unit and was found to be distressed, but had no evidence of clinical depression. After a long discussion about her difficulties, Jane reluctantly agreed to stay with a friend overnight and return the next day to discuss her problems with a worker at the community mental health centre; she would also re-contact the Citizen's Advice Bureau for financial advice. She was not accepted for home treatment because her problem was not one that would otherwise require admission.

Harold, 63—possible alcohol withdrawal; hospital admission at initial assessment

Harold had a long history of alcoholism and depression and lived in a group home. He was referred to CTT by his home worker, who said he had been up all night "talking rubbish." An urgent assessment revealed that he was very agitated, sweating profusely, had rambling speech, and was poorly oriented. Staff said he was a heavy drinker, but did not know when he had his last drink. Because of concerns that he was in alcohol withdrawal he was taken to the emergency room, admitted, and the CTT played no further part in his care.

Jean, 72—chronic recurrent depression, many admissions; extended assessment

Jean was well known to psychiatric services, having a 50-year history of "depressive episodes," with many admissions to hospital. She lived in sheltered accommodation and was referred by her community mental health social worker on a Friday afternoon. The warden of the sheltered apartments and her family doctor were worried about her and thought she needed to be in hospital. Her social worker said she generally coped quite well, but sometimes became extremely anxious and demanding and was difficult to cope with.

The CTT assessed her with her social worker; she presented as mildly depressed but very anxious, repeatedly saying "I cannot go on like this," which appeared to be related to the recent death of an acquaintance. The warden was very anxious that Jean might harm herself over the weekend when she was not there. Jean was negative about her future, but had no specific suicidal thoughts or plans. Due to concern that her level of anxiety might precipitate an admission to hospital over the weekend, the CTT agreed to carry out an extended assessment for that period.

The CTT visited twice daily and allowed her to express her feelings of anxiety and grief. On Monday, the social worker returned with the team, and care was handed back to her, although the availability of CTT after office hours for advice or reassessment was emphasized.

Date of site visit: April 22, 2002
Address: St. Albans Community Treatment Team
Albany Lodge
Church Crescent
St. Albans, Herts AL35JF

Chapter Four
Key Elements and Principles of Mobile Crisis Home Treatment

"A critical challenge for the mental health field is to facilitate the wide-spread adoption of research-based practices in routine mental health care settings so that persons with severe mental illnesses can benefit from services that have been shown to work."

(Torrey, Draker, Dixon, Burns, Flynn, & Rush, 2001)

After seeing the evidence in favor of MCHT and learning about various successful examples in different countries, readers may wish to try their hand at starting their own program; but, they will likely encounter many obstacles on the journey, such as the Valley of Faint-Hearted, Uninspired Planning and the Slough of Conflicting Values (to borrow from John Bunyan).

"Why don't the knuckleheads use common sense?" asks Gary B. Melton, who attempts to answer the question why innovative services have not become conventional . . . if an innovation is cheaper but more effective than current practices, why wouldn't it be quickly and widely adopted? (Melton, 1997). He says policy makers are influenced by values that conflict with the innovative program, such as a desire to maintain institutional jobs, third-party payers not reimbursing policy holders, and a preoccupation with symbolic issues (e.g., focusing on who has the authority to decide about treatment.) Also, planning and implementation are inadequate in many ways. There is a failure to differentiate between individual and aggregate effects (the hue and cry that ensues from a few cases going sour obscures an aggregate benefit to the community as a whole). Although ideas underlying innovative service design are often simple, implementation is complex because of the ripple effect throughout the whole health care system. Demonstration programs are usually small scale and treatment flexibility cannot always be maintained as programs grow and become bureaucratized. Administrators have a desire for certainty and want additional replication of research on new service models even when the relevant research is already much stronger than for traditional institutional models. They are reluctant to take risks—conventional practices are the norm, and they don't want to attract condemnation or civil liability. New treatment models require new money, usually from institutional programs, where the lion's share of the budget is. But downscaling facilities may not result in savings; costs of buildings are largely fixed (unless closed), and they are so overcrowded that merely giving adequate care to the remaining patients may consume any money saved. Of particular concern to managed care companies is that the availability of new, less restrictive programs may widen the net to serve patients previously not served by institutional services (Kwakwa, 1995).

These difficulties in translating evidence-based practice research into everyday clinical programs have prompted a series of papers that describe the Implementing Evidence-Based Practices for Severe Mental Illness Project, which is sponsored by the Robert Wood Johnson Foundation, the National Alliance for the Mentally Ill, and others (Torrey, et al., 2001). The authors introduce the concept of an implementation toolkit for effective practices, which includes written material such as practical workbooks. These next three chapters are written in a similar spirit, and with a similar intention. If the reader wanted to set up an MCHT program, what features should they include? What are the essential elements and principles of MCHT, and how faithful to a putative model should a program be?

We don't know the essential elements of MCHT, as critics point out; further research is needed. (It can also be argued that the essential elements of psychiatric in-patient treatment or day hospital treatment are unknown.) No feature of MCHT is unique; for example, staff in a conventional out-patient clinic may carry out home visits, and their patients may have access to 24-hour emergency services. But conventional out-patient care, no matter how good, is unlikely to contain all the elements of MCHT, combined in quite the same way, and, as in so many other endeavors, the whole is likely greater than the sum of its parts. A well-functioning community mental health team can *prevent* admissions, by early intervention, for example, but cannot usually provide an *alternative* to hospital. See Chapter 2 for discussion.

The next three chapters could be described as a manual on how to set up and operate a mobile crisis home treatment program, and it is with some reservations that I approach this task. There are few precedents; is there a single manual on how to set up and operate a psychiatric in-patient unit? The one treatment delivery system most akin to MCHT is the program for assertive community treatment (PACT). Recently, two PACT manuals have been developed (Allness & Knoedler, 1998; Stein & Santos, 1998). Compared to MCHT, the faithful dissemination and replication of the PACT model is far advanced. Fourteen American state mental health authorities have made ACT programs a core strategy in their plans. The National Alliance for the Mentally Ill (NAMI) and the founders of PACT have established Programs of Assertive Community Treatment, Inc. (PACT, Inc.), a national non-profit organization that offers training, monitoring, certification, and management information services to sponsors of provider organizations seeking to replicate the PACT model (Santos, 1997).

In contrast, MCHT programs have been scattered at random, even in Britain, with little systematic communication between them. It was only in 1999 that the first Good Practices in Home Treatment Conference was held at the University of Wolverhampton in the U.K. The situation in Britain is about to change rapidly, and recent publications that describe the key elements and principles of MCHT will be used in this chapter: the *Mental Health Policy Implementation Guide* (Department of Health, 2001) and the Sainsbury Centre for Mental Health's Locality Service in Mental Health (Wood & Carr, 1998). The Australian *Guidelines for Psychiatric Crisis Teams and Extended Hours Services* (Department of Health, NSW, 1987) will also be used.

In spite of these reservations, I think it is reasonable to attempt this task of writing a manual of operations, based on an analogy with psychiatric in-patient treatment. Even though there may be no single manual that tells you how to set up and operate a psychiatric ward, there is a collective body of knowledge, clinical wisdom, and set of skills that enable mental health professionals to travel far afield and function well in psychiatric units all over the world with what they have learned through formal training, reading, and, most of all, from experience.

Similarly, as I work in MCHT, read about it, talk to people, and visit programs in different countries, there is evident a collective body of knowledge, skills, and experience that can now be written down. Certainly, the principles and essential elements of MCHT outlined by Hoult (1999) based on experiences and research in Australia and the U.K., appear very familiar to those of us in MCHT in Canada, and fit well with those found in Fenton's (1982) Montreal study.

As seen in the previous chapter, there are obvious but not fundamental differences in programs—depending on the setting, the target population and, in particular, the resources available. Psychiatrist Christine Dean's account of studying Urdu at evening classes, conducting assessments in Urdu, and arranging for Pakistani music and food in her inner-city program in Birmingham appear novel from a southern Ontario perspective (Dean, 1993).

The research described in Chapter 1, and the experience gained in MCHT programs, all point to a series of interconnected essential elements and principles of home treatment (Brimblecombe, 2001; Sainsbury Centre for Mental Health, 2001; Department of Health, 2001; McGlynn & Smyth, 1998; Department of Health NSW, 1987; Hoult, 1999; J. Hoult, personal communication, April 23, 2002; Smyth & Hoult, 2000). See Tables 4.1 and 4.2.

In his paper *How to Set Up a Home Treatment Service,* Hoult (1999) suggests that one learn from others' experiences, by talking to people who

Table 4.1

Key Elements of Mobile Crisis Home Treatment	
Availability 24 hours/day, 7 days/week	Lengthy assessment
Mobile/home visiting	Screening of patients and families
Rapid response	Designated named worker
Small caseloads	Teams work as a unit
Involvement of doctors	Telephone contact
Rapid access to medication	Support for social network
Intensive intervention at the beginning	Practical help
Frequent contact	Brief hospitalization when necessary/ close links with in-patient unit
Social system intervention	Stay on until crisis resolved
Links to other agencies/link patient to other agencies	Supportive administration
Handover to on-going care	

Table 4.2

Principles of Mobile Crisis Home Treatment	
Patient attitude/approach to the patient	Family's attitude/approach to the family
Staff autonomy	Assertive approach to engagement
Time-limited intervention/ focused care plan	Gatekeeper to the hospital

have done it, and it is in that spirit that the Hazelglen program in Ontario, Canada (described in Chapter 3) will be used to flesh out the list of key elements and principles. This is not to suggest that Hazelglen is a paragon of MCHT programs, and, as was made clear in earlier chapters, it has not been the subject of any research. It is cited as a common or garden service. Hazelglen is a practical model to use; it is North American, it is small (i.e., cheap), based on a well-known study—Fenton's Montreal study—part of the "golden triangle of Montreal, Wisconsin and Sydney" (Smyth, 1999) and one of only five studies suitable for inclusion in the Cochrane Library review (Joy, et al., 2001). Also, it was not set up as a special research project, and after 13 years is no longer a novelty. The disadvantages are that it has not been thoroughly evaluated in a research project and, being small, with limited hours of operation, it does not reveal the full potential of MCHT as one might see, for example, in some of the large U.K. programs.

ESSENTIAL ELEMENTS OF INTENSIVE HOME TREATMENT

Availability, 24 Hours a Day, 7 Days a Week

In-patient treatment is available around the clock, and any service intended as an alternative should provide some care 24 hours a day, 7 days a week. How much care, and what form it takes, though, will depend on a number of things: these include size of budget, characteristics of the patients, the acuity of their illness, degree of family and caregiver support, and what other after hours emergency services are available.

Minghella, et al., (1998) questioned whether a full 24-hour, 7 days a week service was necessary. Minghella's North Birmingham service found that only 5% of their actual face-to-face contacts were at night, even though almost half their patients were psychotic. An on-call system was necessary, but rarely operated as full "waking" 24-hour care. In a survey of 22 MCHT services in the U.K. (Orme, 2001), 13 services operated 11–14 hours Monday to Friday, with a variety of opening times weekends and civic holidays. One operated on an on-call basis from 5 p.m. to 9 a.m., 7 days a week. Only one service operated through a 24-hour period without using an on call staff.

Hazelglen operates similarly to Fenton's Montreal service, 9 a.m.–5 p.m. Monday to Friday (95.6% of home visits took place during regular hours in Fenton's study), with a telephone on-call service after hours and at weekends. Face-to-face emergency clinical intervention is available at a 24-hour walk-in crisis clinic, which is part of the same hospital mental health service and shares the same manager. It is situated by the emergency room of the general hospital and is staffed by senior psychiatric nurses, who work closely with our staff and with backup by a consultant psychiatrist, which has rarely been needed.

Mobile, Including Home Visiting

Home visiting is a sine qua non for MCHT. The patient's home is the alternative to the psychiatric ward, the setting where treatment takes place. Fenton, et al., (1982) considered it essential to establish rapport quickly with the patient and his family, to help them establish guidelines for behavior, and to enable them to assume some of the tasks normally performed by experienced staff.

It is more effective to work with the patient and family if they are seen together in the home; one gets to see all the family, including the children, in their natural environment. They are usually impressed with the presence of one or more mental health experts coming quickly to their aid in their home, and it develops a close therapeutic bond. The case manager can assess the strengths and weaknesses of the family and the home environment, and the social factors contributing to the crisis can become clearer. Failure to care for oneself is a common reason for referral, and we can see for ourselves what is lacking. Many of the 20 components of inpatient care listed in Chapter 2, can only be adequately provided by actually going into the patient's home.

There may be no alternative but to go to the home; the patient cannot be relied upon to come to or be brought to the office if they are too ill. They cannot drive or negotiate the bus system, or might be too anxious to even leave the house. Overt psychotic behavior can make it impossible for a family to bring the patient. Even if patients can come to the office, it's not unusual for them to miss appointments due to poor memory and confusion, or slowness in getting going.

However, not every encounter with the patient needs to be in the home; about 50% of visits in Fenton's program were in the office, and we aim for the same proportion, for a number of reasons. As the patient improves, it is good for them to get out of the house, and how they accomplish that is a helpful measure of their functioning. Home visiting takes up more of the staff's time than an office visit. Psychiatrists' time for example, may be particularly valuable in some settings (e.g., Canada) because of severe manpower shortages, and it may not be the best use of that time to routinely see the patient in the home unless it is clinically necessary. Home visiting by psychiatrists is more likely to be a routine, if residents are part of the team (as in British teams described in Chapter 3). In some settings, safety concerns make office visits of patients impractical; for example, the address of the MCHT program of Baltimore Crisis Response is not publicized.

The program needs to be mobile in more ways than one. Workers need to be able to get to the patient's home quickly, at short notice; we follow and recommend the policy suggested by Fenton of a maximum driving time of 30 minutes. Patients need to be mobile too. In order to get to the office, they may need a taxi; many are not well enough to drive or negotiate the public transport system, or may be too poor. Patients also may need transportation to other caregivers, such as a family doctor or the social welfare office. Policies need to be in place so workers can transport them in their vehicles. We recommend a generous allowance in the budget for patients to use taxis.

Rapid Response

MCHT cannot compete with hospital treatment in this regard; help is instantly available in a well-functioning psychiatric unit. Some patients are so severely ill that they don't recognize they need help or they reject it and nurses have to monitor their behavior and symptoms closely, anticipate their needs, and be ready to respond quickly. But not all patients who get admitted are like that. Some have never required instant help and even more don't require it after one or two days hospital stay; these are the patients who can be treated by MCHT. For example, a study of psychiatric in patients in the Province of Saskatchewan, Canada, showed that many stay in hospital longer than necessary; 38% were never acute when admitted, and only 18% were considered to be acute after two days, but, there were no alternative services available (Driver, 2001).

MCHT staff with few scheduled appointments, with large chunks of unstructured time, and the capacity to be mobile can respond quickly to patients' urgent needs. This element of rapid response is linked to the next essential requirement of home treatment: small caseloads.

Small Caseloads

Although Hoult, (1999) Fenton, (1982) and the Department of Health (2001) do not mention this key element, it is of crucial importance. Rapid response and frequent visiting would be impossible without a low staff:patient ratio. An MCHT service is, in one respect, like a fire station: staff are sitting around, doing routine tasks such as dictating reports, and can, at a moments notice, drop everything to attend to a patient who has just called in a panic.

The optimum ratio will vary, depending on such things as the seriousness of the patient's illness and the length of stay. A service need not always stick to a fixed ratio; it can vary with circumstances. However, one does need a target, in order to budget correctly and hire the appropriate number of staff, but there are almost no guidelines. A ratio of 10:1 is recommend for assertive community treatment teams (Stein & Santos, 1998), but the acuity of MCHT patients in some services may be greater; by definition, they are all in a crisis of a severity to warrant admission. MCHT services in the U.K. appear to operate with a ratio of 5–6:1; in the Hazelglen service, we operate with a ratio of about 10:1.

Involvement of Doctors

One would not think of attempting to conduct hospital treatment without doctors, so any MCHT program without adequate medical input will not be a convincing substitute for in-patient care. Other key elements, such as rapid access to medication and admission to hospital, are dependent on doctors. They are usually powerful voices in health care organizations and their role as a "product champion" for home treatment is important (Brimblecombe, 2001b). The addition of a psychiatrist to a mobile psychiatric crisis intervention team in Michigan resulted in a sharp decrease in hospital admissions. The admission rate rebounded when the services of the psychiatrist were terminated (see Kalamazoo County study in Chapter 1) (Reding & Raphelson, 1995).

The program should have its own psychiatrist(s), attending at least 40–50% time, to provide the full range of medical services. These include diagnosis, physical assessment, drug treatment, mental health act certification or sectioning, staff supervision, and psychotherapy. There are MCHT programs that manage with less than this; staff has to rely on the individual patient's psychiatrist, who may work in a totally different setting—for example, the Victoria, B.C. service in Chapter 3. It can work adequately, but teams usually prefer to have a program psychiatrist; as a *principle* or *key element*, a program psychiatrist is recommended.

Rapid Access to Medication

This requirement is one of the reasons patients get admitted to hospital, so an MCHT program has to find some way to provide it. Rapid treatment with calming medicines is one of the single, most effective ways to prevent an admission; so often severe anxiety, agitation, or psychotic thinking and behavior are what prompt demands for hospital treatment.

Treatment guidelines for Axis I psychiatric disorders include pharmacotherapy.

The psychiatrist has to ensure procedures are in place so that a drug can be quickly prescribed, dispensed, and administered and that the dose of that drug can be quickly adjusted or discontinued. The staff needs to ensure that medication quickly gets to the patient; this may require frequent visits to give the medicine or coach the family to give it.

Intensive Intervention at the Beginning

Home treatment should not be attempted unless this can be guaranteed. When hospital admission is being considered by the patient, family, and health care providers, there is a "multifactorial sense of collapse, inadequate resources, or marginal controls within the patient and his interpersonal system" (Christie, 1985)—"insufficiency," as described in Chapter 2. The situation is unpredictable, disturbing, and potentially hazardous; hospital is considered because it gives everyone a sense of security—that whatever happens can be taken care of.

MCHT, to provide a credible alternative, must be arranged so that the situation does not get out of control and the patient and his family develop faith, trust, and hope that treatment is adequate and will be successful; hence, the need for intensive involvement in the first week or so of treatment. For that to happen the workers' schedules need to be free and flexible enough, which is related to other key elements like small case loads and after hours care.

Frequent Contact

In-patients are in contact with a nurse or other staff anywhere from once a day to receiving constant observation. How closely should one attempt to replicate this level of care; how frequent is frequent? In the acute stage, some patients may need to be visited twice daily, usually once daily is sufficient.

Lengthy Assessment

When a patient is admitted to hospital, one need not conduct one's initial interview all at one time; it may be more convenient to split it up into smaller segments. The patient is always available and may not be able to tolerate a full interview. One does not have to predict every possible adverse clinical outcome; if the patient's condition does suddenly deteriorate, the ward nurse is able to quickly intervene.

This won't work for MCHT, for obvious reasons. When the initial assessment is completed, you have to have established the following: whether this patient can be handled by the team, whether the family and social network can cope, and what the patient needs to get through the next 24 hours. Then you have to set up the necessary interventions, and teach the family how to cope, so you have to be prepared to spend sufficient time on the initial assessment, not necessarily continuously, but certainly before the day is over.

Screening of Patients and Families

In the research studies of MCHT in Chapter 1 patients were usually assessed in an emergency room as to whether they required hospital admission, and those that did meet the criteria were randomly assigned to a home treatment team. In everyday clinical life, matters are not so tidy. Referrals can arrive from many different sources, depending on local policies. It is important to only treat patients who are acute enough, who otherwise would require hospital admission. Treating less acute patients wastes resources, making it less likely that the program will be able to reduce bed usage. Similarly, accepting referrals of patients who are too ill for MCHT is also a waste of resources; the team may then be stuck with the responsibility of arranging hospital admission, which may thereby be delayed. Eligibility criteria should be as clear as possible, so that the team does not have to spend a lot of time on screening out inappropriate patients.

These issues are illustrated by the experience of an MCHT program in Cornwall, U.K. (Kwakwa, 1995). So much time was spent on assessments that there was insufficient time to provide an intensive service, and, in addition to the original targeted group, psychotic patients, a whole new group of patients who would not previously have presented for admission were treated.

Designated Named Worker/Ability of Team Members to Work as a Unit

If the service operates after hours and at weekends, a shift system is needed so each patient will receive care from more than one worker. In the Hazelgen program, because it operates from 9 a.m.–5 p.m., the patient has only one worker. This enables a strong therapeutic relationship to be quickly developed with the patient and the family, and the deep level of awareness of the patient's situation allows the worker to be able to anticipate and head off most emergencies. It may be difficult for a patient to get close to numerous workers in a short space of time; the optimum number of workers in contact with a patient and their family is not clear, and likely will vary with each patient and their clinical situation. In the Cornwall, U.K., MCHT program described by Kwakwa (1995), more than half of the patients who completetd a satisfaction survey said they did not like the fact that so many staff provided care, and they felt this was therapeutically disruptive. On the other hand, a qualitative research study of patients, and caregivers, experience of treatment received from the Intensive Home Treatment Team in south Leeds (U.K.) showed that "because users saw the IHTT operating as a team, the fact that they might see or speak to someone other than their key worker did not prove problematic. In part this stemmed from their experience of contact. When they telephoned the on-call service, the worker had some knowledge and understanding of who they were and their problems. But it also reflected the level of distress they felt, that they were desperate for support" (Godfrey & Townsend, 1995).

However the team is set up, two things are necessary. The team must work as a unit: there needs to be a rapid response to a patient with an urgent need, even though their worker may not be available that day; therefore, all team members need to be aware of all patients and their major problems, to some extent. In a well-functioning MCHT program, the staff seems to naturally know each others' whereabouts, problems, and needs. Second, there needs to be someone who takes responsibility for the care plan and continuity of care, someone accountable to the patient, family, and others—a designated named worker.

Telephone Contact

In Fenton's Montreal program, the research showed that phone contact with patients was often as acceptable as face-to-face contact. The team contacted each patient or family, or both, an average of 21 times. Of these contacts, 87% were made within regular working hours. During the first week of treatment, each patient or family member, or both, had an average of two phone conversations with a staff member during office hours; a third of patients or family members had at least three conversations.

Quick access to the team by telephone, can be very important for patients. It enables them to get help in a hurry and gives them a sense of security. Telephone usage will depend on local customs; in the U.K. it may be used less because local calls are charged by the minute. In Ontario, phone contact has recently been more difficult to arrange because an increasing number of patients cannot afford a phone due to cutbacks in social welfare services. We are experimenting with loaning patients cell phones.

Support for Social Network

A principal of MCHT is that the patient's family, friends, and neighbors play a major role in their care, taking the place of hospital staff and services to the extent that is possible. It is essential to provide support to the people involved, which can take the form of reassurance, explanation, encouragement, and education. For example, an apartment superintendent can be a key figure in our experience and can be helpful in keeping us informed about problems, monitoring a patient's behavior, and providing informal support to patients.

The case of 80-year-old Lydia illustrates this principle. This woman had recently been widowed and had become acutely psychotic, afraid to sleep in her bed, and refused to let any health care providers into her house; only the family and the next-door neighbor were allowed. This latter person had been providing some support already, by taking in food and visiting regularly. The case manager arranged for her to be paid by the family to increase and sustain this care, thus relieving the family of some burden and avoiding admission to hospital.

Practical Help

Psychosocial stressors such as threatened eviction, financial worries, child care pressures often are a major cause of the patient's crisis. An acute psychiatric illness can make daily functioning almost impossible, leading to the sense of "multifactorial collapse," described as insufficiency in Chapter 2. MCHT is well placed to address these problems and much of a case manager's work can be devoted to that. Two components of in-patient care previously described are hostel services and help with self-care. Nothing is too trivial. We have changed fuses on cooking stoves and arranged for care and disposition of household pets. Staff need to be able to find their way about the social welfare benefit system, know how to intervene at the patient's place of employment and with their insurance company, and know how to work with landlords.

Social Systems Intervention

As the field of view widens from practical problems that need solutions, social system issues come into focus. The worker needs to be able to think conceptually and ecologically about the dynamics in the patient's social system and environment—turbulence in it may have helped to trigger a breakdown, and support from it can foster recovery.

For example, a patient had a big problem with his church group. A member of the Jehovah's Witness faith, the congregation was his life, apart from his work. His illness had resulted in some behavior that threatened to jeopardize his continued acceptance by the church. His case manager sat down with the elders to explain the matter, gain their support, and work out a solution with the patient. Other important social systems in which one may need to intervene are universities, high schools, and neighborhoods.

Brief Hospitalisation when Necessary

If an MCHT program is targeting the acutely ill patient accurately, then a certain proportion of them will require admission to hospital; often, for only a brief period. At the Hazelglen program, we admit about 12%; Brimblecombe (2001b) noted a range of 11% to 34% in the U.K. Admission should not be seen as a failure; in fact, if very few patients were admitted from a service, one would suspect that it was not targeting the seriously ill.

If one considers the continuum of severity of illness, its fluctuations, and the unpredictable changes in a patient's stresses and supports, it is not surprising that some patients in the higher range of acuity may need hospital from time to time. Ideally, there should be full consultation and cooperation between the MCHT staff and the hospital staff. This is linked to another important element.

Close Links with a Psychiatric Unit

This is necessary in order to safely deal with the most acute patients, whose clinical condition may change quickly; an established procedure to quickly arrange admission should be in place.

Patients and families should be given a choice of MCHT or hospital at any time during the course of their treatment, and this needs to be made clear to them at the beginning. However, that does not necessarily mean it is always the MCHT staff's responsibility to arrange it. Patients and families sometimes desire admission unnecessarily in the opinion of their clinicians. MCHT staff should be able to tell them that they have the right to seek admission but should not be obliged to arrange it if they don't agree.

Sometimes families and patients are understandably nervous about accepting MCHT instead of hospital. A useful approach here is to tell them that MCHT can be tried first, and then, if they are not satisfied, they can be promised admission.

There should also be an established procedure to discharge admitted patients from MCHT programs, in which the two teams share information about the how the patient has fared in hospital, and when and how home treatment can safely take over.

Link Patient with Agencies/Program Linkages to Agencies

The hospital provides everything for the patient, from snacks and clean bed sheets to sophisticated psychotherapy and medication. The problem is that they only do this for a very short time; after an increasingly early discharge, the patient's well being is dependent on a mix of out-patient or day hospital care, referral to social agencies, and family support.

MCHT never sets out to provide everything, and uses the principal of "functional equivalence"; this means a focus on what support functions are required and the idea that communities can devise different strategies to provide them—the case manager will use whatever is available to provide the services the patient requires (Ontario Ministry of Health, 1988). Good MCHT case managers can be amazingly inventive and keep their ears to the ground, always on the lookout for community services to help their patient; e.g., enthusiastic church outreach program for the poor, or a tolerant drop-in center. Close links with the patient's primary care physician are very important.

All this requires cultivation of well-forged links with community agencies. These links are also necessary for the well-being of the program. The launching of an MCHT program creates a ripple across the pond of social and mental health services. These are impactive, unconventional, and poorly understood entities, which can be seen variously as turf competitor, added burden, source of new referrals, or salvation for many agencies.

Stay on until Crisis is Resolved/Handover to On-going Care

For a patient, leaving hospital can be like falling off a cliff; supports are lacking for the (increasingly early) discharged patient. MCHT can provide a much smoother transition through this phase of their illness, and some programs such as Fenton's Montreal program and Hazelglen deliberately combine the in-patient acute phase and the sub-acute follow-up phase.

The patient should be sufficiently recovered to move to the next, lower level of care, be it primary care physician or out-patient clinic, without them relapsing within the next few weeks.

Supportive Administration

Burns, (T. Burns, personal communication, August 24, 1998; Burns, et al., 2001) have raised the issue of whether MCHT programs are sustainable. They emphasize the high stress on staff and the often pivotal position of an influential innovator who started the program and nurtures it, so that it's vulnerable if he departs.

MCHT programs may not fit well with hospital and medical rules and beliefs. They can drift from their original purpose if other demands are made or financial and staffing support wanes. All this adds up to the need for a high level of empathic administrative support; they need an administrator that "gets it." As mentioned above, administrators may have a strong need for certainty and can be reluctant to take risks. MCHT is innovative, and often policies have to be developed on the fly; existing policies for the rest of the organization may not fit. For example, the need for flexible staff roles and hours may conflict with union rules; hospital regulations meant for an institution may not fit a service based in a shopping plaza, where staff may be on the road and in patients' homes most of the time. For example, policies concerning taking charts out of the office or medication may conflict. The administrator of the program needs to be a strong advocate, therefore, to the rest of the hospital to explain how MCHT works and why policies need to be modified.

Because the MCHT service is so accessible—no waiting list, with patients seen the same day—other parts of the health care system may demand access; for example, a hospital may demand that the service follow discharged in-patients. The administrator needs to protect the program from these outside pressures.

PRINCIPLES OF INTENSIVE HOME TREATMENT

Patient Attitude/Approach to the Patient

In the real estate business, there is a saying—"location, location, location"; in MCHT, its "attitude, attitude, attitude." Without the right patient attitude, MCHT's chances of success are diminished; with it, they are greatly enhanced.

What is "the right attitude?" It includes patient awareness that at some level that he is ill; a perception of the team as benign experts who can be trusted and are potentially helpful; and an understanding that to get better, they have to do certain things such as take medicine, let workers into their house, or telephone them. It does not include a strong belief that the only way to get better is to go to the hospital, or that one deserves a good rest away from all one's stresses.

While modern in-patient treatment encourages patients to be active partners in their treatment, hospital routine can still engender passivity. Patient's lives are regimented by the routine of meal times and medication times, smoking restrictions, and privileges. An active patient and/or family are key ingredients; the case manager orchestrates the activities needed to get the patient well, but actively provides few of them. The patient has as much say in his treatment as is possible and, to the degree that autonomy is not practical or possible, the family fills in the gaps

This staff/patient/family partnership starts at the initial meeting, particularly with education. Patients need to understand the illness and what is needed to get better and what role they can play, all of which requires a big education component in home treatment. Education extends to helping the patient maintain as many of their activities as possible; helping to care for children and washing the dishes can help offset any added family burden of MCHT.

The Approach to Families

The family's attitude is also vital. If the family are exhausted, and frustrated through coping with the patient's illness, they are likely to want the patient admitted to hospital, instead of being treated at home. I am reminded of a talk I gave to a Family of Schizophrenics group about our new mobile crisis home treatment program and being surprised at the cool reception. These families had been through so much that they could not conceive of deliberately choosing to cope with a psychotic son or daughter at home instead of having him or her admitted. Other families are quite the opposite; they may have been so traumatized by the process of seeing their child involuntarily admitted—the physical restraints and forced injections—that they will do anything to avoid that happening again.

Sometimes families can feel shut out of the process of the patient's treatment in hospital; this is not so in MCHT, where they are a vital part, taking the place of staff to some degree, where they provide the components of in-patient care as listed in Chapter 2. So they are coached, supported, educated, and empowered. However, MCHT is not always a family love-in redolent of *The Waltons* TV show. Family interpersonal problems are a common contributor to mental illness, and family members themselves may be psychiatrically ill. Previously independent patients don't always adjust quickly to parent or spouse suddenly adopting a caregiver role. The family may want to impose some of their own notions about psychiatric illness and treatment, based on ethnic beliefs and different cultural practices.

In an Australian study of individuals presenting to a mobile crisis home treatment service with a first episode psychosis, it was found that treatment was not as successful if family support was rated low (Fitzgerald & Kulkarni, 1998; Brimblecombe, 2001).

Staff Autonomy

An important principle is the hiring and development of staff that can function with a high degree of autonomy and responsibility. They need to be able to cope in novel, quickly changing circumstances where they have little control and without instant access to medical advice and intervention.

Safety

One of the first questions of prospective staff is about their safety; many have come from an in-patient setting where "codes" are a regular feature. The need to address the safety of staff is a fundamental principle of all MCHT programs. Training and protocols need to be in place. However, experience in this field suggests that safety is not as much of an issue as one would anticipate. While they took safety seriously, and all had well-developed policies, none of the services I visited (see Chapter 3) perceived it as much of a problem.

This is likely due to the following features:

- Patients are willing to some degree to receive treatment; otherwise, they would not be in the program.

- They have much more control than in hospital; you are on their home ground, as an invited visitor. If they don't like what you are doing, they can tell you to leave. They don't have to conform to the many rules and restrictions of a hospital and are in their own familiar surroundings.
- They are with their families and neighbors, where normal behavior is expected. Any disruptive behavior is going to affect their friends and loved ones, not some anonymous professional whose job it is to deal with it.

Gatekeeper to the Hospital

This is an admirable principle if you can set up your program this way. But, given the tenuous relationship many MCHT programs have with in-patient units, where most of the money and power reside, this is not often possible.

Why is it important? In an ideal world, patients would receive the least restrictive and cost-beneficial form of treatment at each stage of their illness, moving easily along the continuum of care. All patients in the lower two thirds of acuity of illness, conventionally treated in hospital, with adequate social support would be treated at home (or in other alternatives such as partial hospitalization); any patient of MCHT who needs brief hospital admission would stay in hospital for the minimum required time before being discharged back to the team. Having the MCHT service as gatekeeper to admission would enable this to happen. For an MCHT service to have the maximum impact on bed utilization, it needs to be the gatekeeper to the hospital for its catchment area (Hoult, 1989).

In reality, this is rarely the case. Many psychiatrists may not refer to home treatment, preferring to admit patients; home treatment patients, who are admitted for what should have been a brief period, may find their caregivers reluctant to quickly discharge them, perhaps not having sufficient faith in home treatment's capacity to handle their illness. Quick discharge, may result in more work for the in-patient staff, which provides a disincentive. Rapid discharge results in a higher turnover of patients, which means more assessments have to be done, and likely, a higher overall acuity level of patients.

The alternative to being the gatekeeper is an exquisite level of finely tuned cooperation between all levels of care. More common scenarios are insufficient referrals; referrals of less acute patients; hospital admissions of patients that can be treated by the MCHT team; and loss of the team's patients to the hospital system, ones who may have only needed admission for a few days.

Throughout this book and the home treatment literature runs the theme of resistance to change and the hegemony of the hospital (Brimblecombe, 2001b). Friedman, Beck, & Weiner (1964) describes a mobile crisis home treatment service in Boston in the 1960s where eventually a policy had to be enforced that all referrals for admission had to go through the home treatment service. Education may not be enough, and clear policies about admission and appropriate use of alternatives are essential. In the 1990s Hoult worked with a home treatment service in Sydney, Australia, where the admission rate was halved. After he left, the admission unit was moved from the local mental hospital to a teaching hospital, where the new doctors did not routinely call the home treatment service; admission rates and bed usage reverted to the previous level.

At the other end—discharges from hospital—it is similarly important that the mobile crisis home treatment team have a strong influence over when their patients should be discharged. In the Daily Living Program of the Maudsley group (Audini, Marks, Lawrence, & Watts, 1994; see Chapter 1), when the responsibility for discharge of their patients was transferred to the ward team, the length of stay tripled.

While it may not be possible to control admissions and discharge, it is very important to do everything possible to exert maximum influence on these hospital activities.

Assertive Approach to Engagement

One reason that patients are admitted to hospital is because they are too ill to engage with out-patient care (these resources have become inadequate—part of insufficiency, described in Chapter 2). Acutely ill, perhaps they cannot get themselves out of bed or don't answer the phone. They may be too paranoid to go outside or cannot use public transport. They may not absorb the simplest instructions about medication or may misuse it in various ways. Hospital takes care of all that; secure and contained, the patient can be given the necessary treatment.

For these patients to be treated out of hospital, a passive, "patient takes responsibility, attitude is not going to work; an assertive approach to engagement is necessary. This can mean, for example, that one bangs harder on their door, or calls them on the cell phone from the driveway if they don't answer, when you make a home visit, which, in a profound state of depression or in a suspicious psychotic state, some don't.

Time Limited Intervention/Focused Care Plan

Many severely ill patients have chronic multiple problems. Their illnesses, personality problems, pathological family relationships, many psychosocial stressors, medical problems, difficulties with medicines, comorbid substance abuse, and other conditions all conspire to produce a crisis, to which hospital admission is seen as a necessary solution. Because of pressure on beds, publicity about the limitations of hospitals, and because most patients are glad to have a short stay, discharge is often accepted willingly. Ward staff and patients have limited expectations of hospital—you stay until the crisis is over—at least, enough to go home.

This is not so in mobile crisis home treatment. A case manager becomes very close to the patient and his family, becoming intimately aware of their lives and its many problems firsthand. To the patient and the family, preserving clear boundaries between home treatment and conventional out-patient treatment in the interest of focusing scarce resources may not seem as obviously important as the difference between being in or out of hospital.

For these reasons it can become difficult to know when treatment should finish or, even, if you do know, to exit gracefully. Sometimes, just as the present crisis is about to be resolved sufficiently to discharge the patient to out-patient care, another problem pops up that, at least in the patient's mind, appears to warrant your attention.

It is therefore important to be focused, from the beginning, about what home treatment is supposed to achieve, and to be open and clear about this with the patient and the family. Using written explicit goals and continuously monitoring progress is helpful. Targeting symptoms and behaviors is also helpful.

SIDEBAR

What Can a Delphi Exercise Tell Us about the Key Elements of MCHT?

Burn's Delphi exercise (Burns, et al., 2001; see Chapter 2 for description) provides support for the above list of key elements and principles.

Home Environment

Home visiting (and the capacity for frequent home visits) and assessment and treatment in the home environment were both rated as essential, with 100% and 91% consensus, respectively.

There was consensus that "flexibility of contact frequency" was essential (91%) and that "visiting possible up to four times weekly" was very important (100%).

Home-based care with home-based assessment from a psychiatrist were rated very important, with 91% consensus.

The idea of "a team dedicated to intensive home treatment" was rated as very important but failed to reach consensus (73%), ranging from 1 to 4.

Skill Mix

There was 100% consensus that "skilled staff, well trained" and "community mental health nurses" were essential, and that having a "team with broad range and special expertise" was very important. There was also 91% consensus that it was essential for the service to be a "multidisciplinary team."

Psychiatrist Involvement

There was 100% consensus that having a "psychiatrist as a member of the multidisciplinary team," and "experienced community oriented psychiatrists" were essential for the service.

Service Management

There was 100% consensus that a "well-organized and managed team" was essential, and that "good gatekeeping and prioritization" and "an environment which tolerates risk-taking" were very important. There was consensus (91%) that "strong leadership" was essential and that "regular multidisciplinary review" and "comprehensive systematic physical, social and psychological assessment" were very important.

Caseload Size

There was 100% consensus that having "reasonable case loads" (less than 1:25) was very important. Having still smaller caseloads (key worker with caseload of 1:15 maximum) was rated only important, with a consensus of 82%.

Health/Social Care Integration

There was 100% consensus that "attention to social as well as clinical needs" was essential, and that "good health and social services liaison" was very important.

There was consensus that a "care plan to address social, housing, benefits, etc." was very important (91%).

Hours

There was 100% consensus that "rapid response services" and "access to out-of-hours mental health workers" were very important. The idea of a "7-day service, extended hours" was considered very important, with 91% consensus.

"Flexible working hours (6 a.m.–9 p.m.; not 24 hours)" reached weaker consensus (82%).

"Available 24 hours to a defined patch" (consultants catchment area) was rated only as important, and two specific comments by participants challenged the need for 7-day, 24-hour services.

Crisis Care

There was 100% consensus that "crisis availability" was very important. The consensus about having a specific crisis focus— "crisis elements of team" and "crisis services" was weaker (both 82%), but both were rated very important.

Housing/Accommodation

There was 100% consensus that "housing" (supported and unsupported), a "range of supported accommodation," and "high staffed" (24-hour) residential accommodation were all very important.

There was also 91% consensus that "access to crisis accommodation for those who lack appropriate housing" was very important.

In-Patient Policy

There was consensus (82%) that it was very important that "the team's use of in-patient beds should focus on early discharge—if you want one admitted you have to take one out"; and "senior psychiatrist involvement in all admissions" was rated important, with 91% consensus.

Caregivers

There was 100% consensus that "support for caregivers" was very important, and consensus that "attention to needs of informal caregivers" was very important.

There was strong consensus that "family/caregiver focused education/information" was important.

"Supportive families" was thought to be important (91% consensus).

Day Care

There was 100% consensus that "sufficient support services" (day care) was very important, and "acute day hospital" was rated as important (91% consensus).

Having discussed the key elements and principles of MCHT, the next two chapters discuss how these are applied to setting up and operating a service and conducting the day-to-day clinical activities.

Chapter Five

How to Set Up and Operate a Mobile Crisis Home Treatment Service

> *"It is quite clear that alternatives to acute hospitalization cannot survive without continued commitment to the concept by the leadership of the mental health structure in which they operate and both commitment and skill on the part of the clinical staff."*

> (Polak et al. 1995)

In the previous chapter, supportive administration was identified as a key element of MCHT programs. At the risk of sounding effete and elitist, the case will be made here that MCHT services require special attention; unless their unique needs and vulnerabilities are recognized and dealt with, they will not thrive. In Britain, where MCHT is becoming well established as part of the mental health system, these concerns may be less valid. However, where it is less established, they should be addressed.

My experience, and that of others, has been that, although it is perfectly clear to those of us in MCHT services how these services work and what can be accomplished, it seems difficult for some to understand and become convinced; consequently, the administrator has to be a very credible and convincing communicator. Potential referrers, such as primary care physicians, ER physicians, and psychiatrists, may be sceptical about what level of risk can be managed and nervous about the medico-legal liabilities that may ensue from choosing MCHT over hospital for a patient. Administrators, too, may be uneasy about risks and unconvinced that cost savings can be achieved.

Referrers can accept that an in-patient unit is "full"—there are, after all, only a finite number of beds—but it may be difficult to accept that an MCHT team is "full," especially given the low caseloads, and there may be pressure to accept one more patient. The rapid accessibility to treatment, so crucial to MCHT functioning, makes it a sitting duck for all kinds of demands to fill gaps in the local service; it is so supple and versatile it can get used as a sort of Swiss Army knife for any pressing need. As well as fending off inappropriate referrals, referrals that are too sick or too mild, and demands to take more patients than the service can handle, administrators can have the opposite problem: being by-passed by psychiatrists, who continue to admit patients suitable for home treatment. Thus, the nature of MCHT requires a lot of interaction and forging of agreements and linkages, all conducted with firmness and diplomacy.

Although morale is usually high in these services, staff need a lot of support in their role, which will be new to many of them—operating in ambiguous unstructured settings, having a great deal of autonomy, with an unusual degree of responsibility on their shoulders compared to more traditional mental health settings. When things go wrong, such as patients attempting suicide, they will need to feel supported by their manager.

STARTING UP A MOBILE CRISIS HOME TREATMENT SERVICE

The First Six Key Decisions to Be Made

The most important decisions to be made in starting a service are six in total.

1. Target population
2. Catchment area
3. Hours of operation
4. Sources of referral
5. Size of team (determined by the size of the budget)
6. Model of assessment used: will the service act as a "crisis" assessment service, or will it only accept patients who have been already seen and screened by a mental health professional.

The six key issues in starting a team are, of course, interrelated; each issue influences the others. For example, the hours of operation and degree of crisis resolution function will heavily influence the amount of money required. But, in mental health planning, the amount of money available to start a service may be limited from the outset, and one has to accept what one is given and plan accordingly; i.e., the budget can determine the level of service.

THE FUNNEL MODEL

The analogy or model of a funnel is useful to illustrate the function of a mobile crisis home treatment service in a mental health system, and to discuss the above six issues. In the introduction, at Stage 3 in the anatomy of a crisis figure (Figure 1), four common help-seeking pathways that patients and families take when they face an emergency situation were identified. They turn to:

- emergency room of a general hospital
- primary care physician
- police
- community-based crisis service/social worker

Individuals who are already in the mental health system can, in addition to the above four pathways, seek help from two others: their psychiatrist or an out-patient/community mental health team.

These six services (serving a "crisis function") act as a filter, and refer the most acute cases for hospital admission to a psychiatric ward (in practice, there are usually only five; police, unless they have their own crisis staff, usually take the individual to the emergency room). In other words, there is a "funnelling" of urgent psychiatric patients to the hospital from six sources as shown in the following figure:

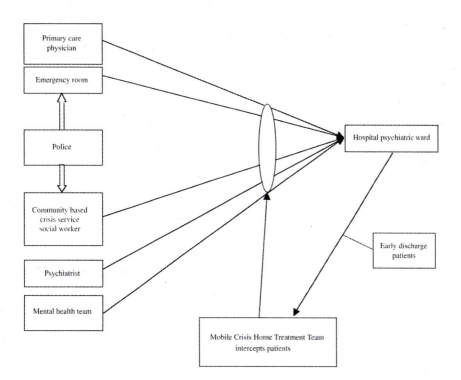

Figure 5.1 The funnel model.

The aim of a mobile crisis home treatment service is to *intercept* these patients destined for the psychiatric ward and divert them to home treatment.

Ten Factors That Determine Success in Intercepting Patients, Destined for Hospital Admission and Saving Beds

The success of this endeavour—intercepting patients and thereby saving beds, and, more specifically, the number of patients intercepted in a day or a week, depends mostly on a total of ten factors:

1. *How quickly the MCHT service can assess the patient.* A seriously ill patient cannot be left waiting in an ER for very long, and yet may not be well enough to be discharged home to wait for the team to make a home visit later that day. The team may need to go to the ER at short notice, take over the patient's care, and accompany them to their home.

   A primary care physician with an acutely ill patient in the office wants a quick response from the team, either to come and meet the patient or see them at home within a few hours. Otherwise, the doctor will deem it safer to send the patient to the hospital for admission.

2. *Hours that the service is open for referrals.* This is self-evident; if you are not open, you can't intercept patients (except see next section). Although a service may be open in the evening for their own patients, they may not accept an urgent referral only a few hours before the end of the shift, because there would be insufficient time to finish an assessment and treatment plan.

3. *Opportunity for after hours referrals.* An ER physician, for example, may think that it is safe to discharge a patient home in the care of their family in the evening, provided that they and the family can be assured that the patient will be seen the next morning. Some MCHT services arrange for referrals to be made to the staff on call, who are familiar with the commitments of the day shift, to make that guarantee.

4. *Intensity of service that you can provide.* Obviously, a very sick patient or one with no social supports will require more visits, and longer visits per day; some may be hours in length. If you cannot provide that, hospital admission will be required.

5. *Scarcity of hospital beds.* There is a strong relationship between service provision and service use, similar to the economic relationship between supply and demand; where psychiatric beds are available, they will be filled, whatever the quantity of provision (Thornicroft & Tansella, 2001). Lack of beds forces clinicians to be creative and look for alternatives.

6. *Presence of incentives to admit to hospital.* These are numerous, and can include financial incentives, in a private hospital; beds saved by a psychiatrist who refers to MCHT may get used by another psychiatrist, so there is an incentive to "keep your beds full, or else you will lose them to somebody else"; fear that if beds are not used, hospital administration will want to close them.

7. *Availability of other alternatives to hospital.* Respite beds and a day hospital can serve as alternatives to admission. Also, some well-functioning mental health teams may be able to see the patient immediately and may have a home visiting capacity, so that the crisis can be dealt with adequately.

8. *Distinct features of the target population.* Home treatment is less successful with certain categories of patient; for example, those who are homeless or live in chaotic social situations without supports from family or caregivers, and those with severe substance abuse problems. The level of social deprivation in the catchment area will have an influence on the number of acutely ill individuals who are potential patients and the intensity of service required to be able to keep them out of hospital. Levels of psychosis can be 3–4 times the average in inner city areas (Wood & Carr, 1998).

9. *Attitude of referrers, hospital psychiatrists, working relationships.* This is a broad category of variables, containing many elements. The attitude of referrers means the degree of interest they have in seeking alternatives to admission and the degree of understanding of and trust they have in the MCHT service. It also includes whether emergency room clinicians have the skills to engage the patient and their family and be able to steer them towards a community alternative (see Chapter 2, study by Segal, et al., 1995). Another key factor is the attitude of hospital psychiatrists: whether they have a mental health systems orientation, or are just interested in their own bailiwick (do they want to save beds in this

manner); whether they trust patients will get adequate care; and, with reference to early discharge referrals (not included in the funnel model), if they see a point to reducing the length of stay on their ward. (If the psychiatrist on the in-patient ward was also the MCHT psychiatrist, it would help to ensure appropriate referrals.) Broader forces, such as the prevailing ideology about mental health delivery, also influence these elements. To some degree, these factors may be modified by the next factor:

10. *Success in developing relationships with referrers.* "Anyone attempting to establish a new MCHT service is likely to have to overcome the fact that previous experience or lack of experience of home treatment may narrow the perception of what constitutes an alternative. Essentially for many clinicians, direct exposure to the benefits of home treatment services may be needed before they see it is a real alternative" (Brimblecombe, 2001b).

The quality of the linkages to referring sources is vital; without sufficient suitable referrals, the service will flounder. MCHT needs to be sold, and sold repeatedly, to referring clinicians, and needs to be integrated as much as possible into the local mental health system. In our experience in setting up two services, this process can take at least three years for the service to really find its place; there needs to be a continuous loop of communication to and fro, often regarding specific cases.

Of the 10 variables that influence how successful the team will be in intercepting patients (and therefore saving beds), four of them are structural features of the local mental health system, and therefore outside the team's control: scarcity of beds, availability of other alternatives to hospital admission, distinct features of the target population, and incentives to admit patients (some of these may be modifiable).

Four of the variables are under the control of the MCHT team and depend on its size and how it is structured: how quick the response to the referral, hours the team operates, after hours referral, and the intensity of the service. The bigger the team, the more one can intercept patients who would otherwise be admitted.

The two remaining factors are dynamic and depend on attitudes, culture, and political factors in the local mental health system, and on the kinds of relationships and influence developed by the team, both at startup and on going.

Target Population

The goal of MCHT programs is to provide an alternative to admission for patients and divert them from the local in-patient facility. The target population, therefore, is usually the same as that of the hospital service that serves the same catchment area, except for those patients who are too suicidal or dangerous, whose symptoms or dysfunction are too severe, who lack adequate social support, or who are unwilling to be treated at home. Also usually excluded are patients with primary diagnoses of substance abuse or organic brain disease.

The target population of the Hazelglen program, for example, includes patients with:

- acute psychoses, including first episode schizophrenia
- relapses in patients with severe and persistent mental illness such as chronic schizophrenia
- hypomania and mania
- major depression
- psychosocial crises in patients with personality disorders, moderate psychiatric problems, or drug and alcohol problems
- psychosocial crises with no previous psychiatric history, presenting with threats of suicide, self-harm, or severe disabling symptoms of anxiety and depression

Planners will have to decide the age range to be served and whether they accept patients with drug and alcohol problems or those with developmental disabilities and severe learning disabilities. Mobile crisis home treatment has been used for children (Fassler, Hanson-Myer, & Brenner, 1997), but most services so far, have been developed for adults, defined as 16 or 17 and above. It is perfectly suitable for older adults (over 65), but sometimes they are served by a different part of the local mental health system. MCHT services do not usually accept those patients with a primary diagnosis of substance abuse, but it is recognized that psychiatric patients with comorbid addiction problems are often ill served by regular addiction services. Patients with developmental disabilities may have their own service but, if not, in our experience, can be well served by home treatment, enabling them to remain with their specialized caregivers while receiving intensive psychiatric treatment.

Catchment Area

In order to decide on the catchment area to be served, one could simply define it as within a reasonable radius from the base office, in order to ensure mobility, home visiting, and rapid access to help, which are the hallmarks of MCHT. We use a maximum half-hour drive as a practical guide, derived from Fenton's Montreal study (Fenton, et al., 1982). In Britain, mental health services are sectorized and an MCHT catchment area would be defined by the "patch" of the consultant to the team; typically, one consultant serves a population of 40,000. As described in Chapter 3, for the MCHT service in Ladywood, which has one consultant and does serve a crisis function in one of the most socially deprived areas of Britain, the catchment area is 45,000. The Manchester Home Option service, serving an inner-city area and without a significant crisis function, has a catchment area consisting of the total of the three consultants patches, each 45,000–135,000 in total. The St. Albans team serves 145,000, mainly suburban and rural, without a large crisis function. Orme (2001), in a survey of MCHT in the U.K., found populations served ranged from 57,000 to 230,000.

Some catchment areas are designed to harmonize with that of the local hospital, which is often city-wide. In Canada, the catchment area population of the three services described in Chapter 3, is the same as that of the local hospital; 350,000 in Victoria, B.C. and about 300,0000 in Kitchener, Hazelglen, service, and almost a million in Edmonton.

Sources of Referral

This will be influenced by the team's origins: who started it, what problems it was designed to address, source of funding, what organisation it is part of, and who and what services are covered by third-party payers. From the five or six common pathways that patients and families take in an emergency, as shown in Figure 1, referrers fall into three groups: mental health service providers; primary care physicians and ER physicians; and others, which includes patients and families. Teams take referrals from mental health professionals with varying degrees of selectivity: psychiatrists, mental health teams, crisis services, emergency room staff, and in-patient wards for early discharge to home treatment. For example, in Edmonton, referrals are not taken from emergency room physicians; in Victoria, only psychiatrists at the hospital can refer. Some, but not all, take referrals from primary care physicians; Manchester Home Option Team, for example, did not, because of concern they would refer inappropriate patients. Many teams confine their referrals to the above, but some will take referrals from previous patients; for example, the Manchester Home Option Team. The Hazelglen service takes referrals from anybody, including self-referrals, because of the provincial Ministry of Health's open referral policy. The mandated open referral system has turned out to be a positive feature, and our experience of it is illustrative of what are widespread problems of accessibility in many mental health systems. Very appropriate referrals have been received from such professionals as teachers, general home care nurses, and social service workers. Even patients and their caregivers consistently make some very appropriate referrals—we are sometimes left wondering how some of these patients would have received timely help without us. We agree with Burns (1990) who, discussing his home-based community service (described in Chapter 1) wrote "All the staff involved (including quite senior clinicians) remarked that the sheer variety of pathways by which patients found their way into psychiatric care came as a surprise to them." The usual pathways to acute care as shown in Figure 5.1 sometimes don't work as designed. Primary care physicians sometimes can be hard to access quickly, are unresponsive, or don't grasp the seriousness of the situation; for example, a general home care nurse referred a profoundly depressed and agitated elderly person to Hazelglen after having no success in alerting the primary care physician. Some patients are reluctant to go to their physician with a psychiatric problem, seeing them as unskilled or uninterested in this area, or, they are embarrassed to confide in them about an aspect of their life that they are ashamed of and imagine might diminish them in the eyes of their doctor. Increasingly, in Canada patients don't have a primary care physician due to manpower shortages.

Primary care physicians have a great deal of difficulty carrying out their role in response to a crisis. Busy primary care practice may not allow sufficient time to conduct an adequate assessment and start psychiatric treatment at short notice. An urgent psychiatric consultation can be difficult to obtain; emergency consultations are often available at general hospital emergency rooms, but sometimes the only rapid treatment intervention is admission; rapid out-patient treatment is not feasible due to waiting lists. The only other outcome of sending a patient to the emergency room may be a consultation report of varying timeliness and utility. Some patients, because of a disturbed mental state, previous experience with the mental health system, or personality, are reluctant to accept an urgent referral by their doctor to an unknown person for a psychiatric assessment. They may only be persuaded to accept this by a trusted helper, such as a school guidance counsellor, occupational health nurse, or religious leader; hence, the value of accepting referrals from them.

At the beginning, it may be prudent to confine referrals to a small group of providers, and expand as experience is gained. On the other hand, if referrals are not forthcoming to the new service, due to the slow acceptance of MCHT, one may need to cast a broad net from the beginning—just to get enough patients to keep it going.

The model of assessment, hours of operation, and size of team are interrelated and depend on the budget.

Model of Assessment

This refers to the two models of MCHT described in the introduction (Brimblecombe, 2001b), how much the team will function as a "crisis assessment" service itself and conducts the majority of urgent assessments in the catchment area. Or does the service only take referrals from psychiatrists and other mental health workers after they have done the initial assessment? This issue is complex, and the ideal way of operating is not yet clear. On the one hand, acting as front line crisis service can waste a lot of time with assessments of unsuitable patients; in one U.K. consultant's experience, only a third of crisis assessments resulted in a referral to home treatment. On the other hand, it is argued that if the service is to effectively serve as the gatekeeper to the in-patient service, it would have to assess all urgent cases referred from ERs, mental health teams, primary care physicians, and other sources, and the in-patient ward would have to agree to only accept admissions screened by the team. In practice, this appears to be an ideal that may be hard to achieve (only seen in one service described in Chapter 3).

In practice, some teams may be a hybrid of the two models. At the Hazelglen service, for example, we might get an urgent referral from a family or a patient, to which we respond within a few hours, thereby providing a direct crisis service as the mental health service of first contact. Similarly, services such as the Manchester Home Option Team accept direct referrals from previous patients of the service.

Hours of Operation and Size of Team

The larger the team, the more impact it will have on decreasing the need for in-patient beds, because it can provide more intensive treatment, can provide more crisis function, and be open more hours each day. For a team to have maximum impact, it should operate from 8 a.m. to late evening, with two staff on call after hours, be open seven days a week, and have a significant crisis function; for such a team, experience in Britain and Australia indicates that a clinical staff of 12, with 1 manager and clerical support, is required.

Hoult (personal communication, April 23, 2002) recommends a team of 12 clinical staff, consisting of "mostly nurses," with 2–3 social workers, 2 support workers, plus a manager and clerical staff; this would serve a catchment area that generates about 400 admissions per year. The Yardley/Hodge Hill MCHT service profiled in the "Open All Hours" study

(Minghella, et al., 1998) in Chapter 1 has a staff of 1 team leader, 8 RNs, 2 social workers, 2 support workers, 0.4 psychologist, and an administrator. The Ladywood team consists of 6 RNs including a team leader, 6 health care workers, and 1 social worker. To enable adequate communication between team members, so important for MCHT, teams should not be bigger than 14 or 15.

If one is given carte blanche financially to develop an MCHT team, then the Hoult model should be adopted for maximum impact. However, if the budget is limited one may have to develop a more modest plan, especially at the beginning. Don't be discouraged; an MCHT team does not necessarily have to have 12–14 staff; even if it only operates from 9 a.m.–5 p.m. five days a week (as in the Hazelglen service), considerable numbers of patients can be intercepted and admissions avoided. Team size and budget can be planned to fit somewhere along the spectrum between the two extremes: the most expensive Hoult model and the cheapest Fenton model. In Fenton's Montreal study, 53.5% of patients who presented for admission between 9 a.m. and 5 p.m. on weekdays were deemed suitable for MCHT. Hazelglen, based on Fenton's model operates from 9 a.m. to 5 p.m., five days per week and has a clinical staff of 3.5—2 RNs, 1 occupational therapist, and 1 social worker, who is also the manager—and has half the usual caseload. The Victoria, B.C., MCHT team (Chapter 3) consists of 1 manager and 7 RNs and functions 8 a.m.–10 p.m. seven days a week, with no on-call function (that service is assumed by the hospital emergency room).

Sometimes, in starting a team, the hours of operation are modest at first—it may be a pilot project, or the budget is small, but, as it proves itself, is allowed to expand. The St. Albans team (see Chapter 3; N. Brimblecombe, personal communication, April 21, 2002) has a staff of nine nurses. This level of staffing took two years to achieve due to financial restrictions. The team developed slowly, gradually extending its hours of operation, until they reached the full complement and could be open 9 a.m. to 11 p.m. seven days a week.

Whatever the hours of operation, provision must be made in even the cheapest service for a 24-hour on-call emergency component. This component can be mainly carried out by telephone contact; face-to-face interventions conducted by the on-call staff or provided by a separate service (such as the local emergency psychiatric service, which usually operates out of the general hospital, as in the Hazelglen, Edmonton, and Victoria teams) are needed infrequently. Whatever the budget, you have to cut your cloth according to your pattern.

The source of funding for the team's budget can be "new money," say, from a grant, or it can be derived from other services that the team is designed to reduce or replace, such as from the downsizing of a local mental hospital. Planners may want to deliberately close a psychiatric ward to free up money for an MCHT service, but even this kind of plan needs an infusion of new money to "prime the pump." Minghella, et al., (1998) describes how MCHT can be funded through a careful incremental reduction in in-patient beds, provided that the MCHT service really does focus on the most seriously ill patients who have been occupying those beds. The degree of change from an in-patient–oriented acute treatment service to a community-based service has to be great enough to close a whole ward— but it has to be done in a staged and planned way. It is not possible to cut the beds one day and start the community service the next; bridging funding is essential. The following British example makes it clear how this can be accomplished.

In 1994, The Sainsbury Centre for Mental Health invited mental health services across the U.K. to bid for a share of 3 million pounds, to establish innovative services for people with severe and long-term mental health problems. Eight sites, selected from over 300 applications, were awarded a three-year grant as pump priming to get their services up and running. The North Birmingham group were awarded 500,000 pounds over a three-year period—about one pound per person of the adult population, or an additional 2% on top of the current mental health expenditure. There was a planned reduction in in-patient beds from 41 on two sites to 20 beds on 1 site at the end of the project—from 30 beds/100,000 to 16 beds/100,000. The cost of the Yardley/Hodge Hill service was 481,373 pounds for staff, supplies, overhead, and capital in 1997.

Once the six key decisions regarding catchment area, target population, size of team (and budget), hours of operation, model of assessment, and sources of referral have been made, one can then proceed with planning the team.

Should the MCHT Service be a Separate Team or Integrated?

The MCHT services described in this book are all stand-alone, separate teams. MCHT services can also be developed as an integral part of a conventional community mental health team or out-patient clinic. Here, the service is not the responsibility of a separate team, but of the staff who undertake all aspects of mental health work with people who may or may not be acutely ill. The advantages and disadvantages of both structures are summarized (J. Hoult, personal communication, April 23, 2002; Sainsbury Centre for Mental Health, 2001).

Separate MCHT service advantages

- Staff develop a high level of skills
- Teams can deliver care more flexibly since staff don't have permanent cases
- Easier to provide a rapid response since this is the sole responsibility
- Staff are recruited to work in a 24-hour service
- Fewer problems of handover as care plan is known to whole team
- Able to plan interventions as a team
- More consistent response to patients
- On-going training achievable for whole team
- Specialised service attractive to staff

Separate MCHT service disadvantages

- Expensive
- Problems of critical mass for holidays/vacancies/sickness
- Potential lack of integration with other services
- Continuity of care may suffer when patients are referred on
- Patients have to relate to a number of professionals at a difficult time
- Yet another interface involving criteria, boundaries, handover of patients
- Loss of opportunity to practise MCHT "crisis" work for rest of mental health teams; affects development of skills

Integrated MCHT and standard mental health team advantages

- Same staff working with all patients; easier continuity of care
- Less likely that patients would "fall through the net" since no need to refer to another team

Integrated MCHT and standard mental health team disadvantages

- Stress on staff if they have to work both 9–5 and after—hours shifts
- Crisis cases will be potentially disruptive to long-term case work of service
- Difficult to maintain contact with crisis patients when dealing with long-term patients

Staffing

The service should aim to have enough staff to cover 2 shifts per day, 7 days a week, while team size should be kept manageable enough for communication purposes—between 10 and 15. For a team that operates 8 a.m.–10 p.m., seven days a week, two shifts, 8 a.m.–4 p.m., with 4–5 staff, and 2 p.m.–10 p.m. with 3–4 staff are recommended; plus, Hoult suggests 2 staff from evening shift remain on call. One wonders, though, how practical and sustainable that arrangement would be. A practical concern is the unattractiveness of such a shift to senior staff, who at their career stage are likely to be looking for a position with no shifts at all. In some settings, such as Canada and the U.S., there is considerable competition for experienced psychiatric nurses. Doubts have been raised concerning the sustainability of MCHT teams with particular reference to on-call duties (Burns, et al., 2001; T. Burns, personal communication, Date). Other, more palatable on-call arrangements may need to be considered, such as having one person providing telephone emergency advice and support, and using the hospital emergency service on the rare occasions that the patient needs to be seen in the night. Two handover meetings are required; at 8 a.m. and when the second shift comes on at 2 p.m. There needs to be adequate staff to manage the treatment phase; a good rule of thumb is to plan for a maximum of two daily visits. There should be sufficient resources to allow for daily visiting for one third to one half of the patients depending on the acuity and average length of stay (although, as explained in Chapter 6, this is not always necessary). One should also be able to manage three times per day for some very ill patients. This is assuming that not all patients in the program are in the acute stages of a crisis. Some will have moved beyond this stage, and yet others will be almost ready for discharge to an out-patient clinic. Traditionally, community-based services don't ensure that they are always fully staffed; absences through illness or vacation are usually covered by existing staff, unless prolonged. Because MCHT is an acute service functioning as an alternative to in-patient care, this approach is less satisfactory and services should take a leaf out of the psychiatric ward manager's book and develop a roster of staff that can be called in when the regular staff would find it difficult to fill in. The Victoria, B.C., home treatment service has just such a roster of nurses who have been trained in the method.

In many settings, staff will likely be experienced psychiatric nurses: comparatively more of them have the requisite skills and experience with acutely ill patients, they can give injections, are familiar with medications, and are able to assess patient's physical health. But, there are certainly social workers, occupational therapists, and psychologists who also have this experience and many of these skills, and in some settings are more available than nurses (e.g., Baltimore, Maryland, in Chapter 3). The Hazelglen team includes nurses, a social worker, and an occupational therapist. Social workers have particular skills in working with families and dealing with social problems; occupational therapists are often used to conduct functional assessments in the home; and psychologists usually are used to conduct tests, help with diagnostic assessments, and conduct psychotherapy. However, we find that no one discipline routinely has all the skills and knowledge for this kind of work; mental health workers should be seen individually for what they have to offer and the team's manager should adopt a philosophy of hiring the best person available for the job. This gives the service the flexibility to adapt to the local labor market and the ability to snap up any suitably qualified individuals of which there may be a shortage. All staff should provide the core services to patients and be able to function as the key or named worker. Many teams also hire less professionally qualified individuals, such as the equivalent of a health care aide, who can help patients with their practical problems and activities of daily living. These workers can work on shifts, supervised by more professional staff.

Some teams, in keeping with the philosophy of achieving the best fit between patients and the service, have a policy of hiring a certain number of individuals who have been treated for serious mental illness—termed "users" in the U.K., and "consumers" in North America. Baltimore Crisis Response does this, as does the Ladywood, North Birmingham, service (see Chapter 3). Another similar consideration is the intentional hiring of some staff who share the language, ethnicity, and culture of certain prominent patient groups; e.g., Asians in the U.K.

The ideal worker should be flexible, confident in novel, unstructured situations, and able to make quick decisions on their own, but also be able to work in a team. They need to be clinically practical, able to zero in on the essence of a crisis, focus on target symptoms and behaviour, and not get bogged down and overwhelmed by all of a patient's problem. They need to be warm, empathic, with a sense of humor, and able to rapidly engage patients in the home setting and negotiate with them and their caregivers. Some community experience will be helpful, and they should have at least three years' experience in working with acutely ill patients. They need to be willing to "roll up their sleeves" and help patients with mundane problems that may be defeating them; it may not be psychotherapy, but it is a powerful way of engaging individuals.

Provision needs to be made for overtime pay that might be required, if staff have to deal with a patient shortly before their shift is over or if they are called in after hours.

The team will need some administrative support, and secretaries are important members; they are often the first person that referrers, patients, and families speak to and, especially in a small team, may be only person in the office at times, so they need to be carefully picked for their personality style, experience, and ability to respond to urgent situations.

Psychiatrists

In the previous chapter, a key element was the team having its own psychiatrist(s). It is recommended that no more than three psychiatrists be part of a team. Having a psychiatrist dedicated to the service allows for the development of close working relationships so important in such work. For staff to have the necessary autonomy and level of responsibility for the decisions they make in the community, there has to be a sufficient degree of trust and faith between them and the medical staff.

The psychiatrists help to set the tone of the service, and when setting up the team one wants to ensure that they accept the philosophy of home treatment. What does this mean in practice? It means that they should be willing and comfortable going on home visits to the lowliest of dwellings, conducting an interview with a number of friends and relatives present, and taking into account their opinions about what should be done. There is no room for a "medical" authoritarian approach of the doctor knowing what is best. Staff need to take part in the patients' interviews with the psychiatrist to feel that their opinions count and be able to interact assertively. Although one may not want a medical maverick on the team, one prefers a doctor who is not excessively legalistic and hidebound about risks and procedures and who sees the value in trying to develop novel solutions to keeping sick patients in their community.

Premises

The MCHT office should be centrally positioned in the catchment area. If patients come to the office regularly, it should be located on one or two bus routes and be physically accessible. Some inner-city offices do not allow patients to visit the office, security is high because of the neighbourhood, and its location may not be public knowledge (e.g., Baltimore Crisis Response). Ample and accessible parking space is required.

To encourage staff interaction so that everyone knows what is going on with staff and patients most of the time, the office should have an open plan, with few individual offices. Staff should be all in one large room, with enough desks and shelves for at least the number present during a shift. There should be a kitchen where staff can eat together and a large room for the daily staff meeting, family meetings, group therapy, and community meetings. Two single offices should suffice for interviews. The secretary's office should be large enough to store files and office supplies and should serve as a reception area, connecting with the waiting room. Safety features can include a plexiglass screen at the reception window and a strong door with locks.

Medication should be kept in a locked cupboard. There should be a stock of medicines, and one may have to rely on drug company samples, because hospitals, while providing drugs free to in-patients, often refuse to do this for out-patients, a common example of how hospitals and third-party payers have not adjusted to the new reality of more treatment taking place in the community.

Equipment

Fax machine
Photocopier
Computers
Videocassette recorder
Medical equipment such as stethoscopes, sphygmomanometer, ophthalmoscope
Communication equipment such as cell phones, pagers
Toy box for small children accompanying their parents

Communication

In a well-functioning MCHT team, staff have a sixth sense for what is going on with patients and staff. They know which patients are brewing a crisis or need extra attention. They know which staff are experiencing difficulties with patients, and they know which outside agencies, staff, or doctors are currently being a thorn in the flesh. This level of awareness is the result of the type of people they are and the culture of the team. Of course, aids to communication are required. Most teams rely on daily team meetings, log books of activities such as intake experience with referrals, patients' charts and a central display of patient names, clinical information, caregiver names and addresses, and medication. Often this information is written on a large white board or, as in Hazelglen, on a typed list that everyone carries around.

Transportation

Budget for patient bus tickets, taxi vouchers
Staff drive their own vehicles and have insurance to cover transportation of patients or drive vehicles owned by the team. Whatever the method, rapid, trouble-free mobility of staff and patients is essential.

Partnerships and Linkages

Throughout the process of planning and setting up the team, the manager and medical staff will need to meet regularly with community agencies, hospital staff, physicians—anybody who is a stakeholder. Most important are potential referrers, such as emergency room physicians and staff, primary care physicians, mental health teams, and psychiatrists. You cannot meet too often with these groups. They need to be given written descriptions of the target population, criteria for acceptance, exclusion criteria, and how to make a referral. Of course, this seeming simple transaction will usually have to be supplemented with dollops of diplomacy, marketing of the service, and on-going problem solving.

Other important groups include psychiatrists and staff on the in-patient ward and other services to which patients will be referred. Letters of agreement may need to be written for these groups. It is particularly important at the outset to determine how patients will get admitted in an emergency, who will be responsible for them in the hospital, and how the team can get the patient back; once patients are admitted, if there is not significant clinical input from the team, ward staff may be reluctant to discharge them soon enough. The opinions of users/consumers and families also need to be taken into consideration.

What will be the referring agency's role vis-a-vis the patient? Sometimes after MCHT becomes involved all the other support services melt away, assuming the team will assume responsibility for all of a patient's care. What the team's role is and what the of the community case manager or the patient's regular psychiatrist is needs to be spelled out ahead of time. One of the great advantages of home treatment is that, unlike in-patient treatment, the patient does not lose all their regular mental health providers and team staff usually want to share the clinical care with those already involved. At the same time, one likes to preserve the right of the team staff to act rapidly in an urgent situation, which, after all, is what made home treatment necessary in the first place. Similarly, we have found it necessary to have all psychotropic drugs be the sole responsibility of the team psychiatrist; acutely ill patients often cannot wait for a response from outside community physicians, whose practice may not be set up for such rapid communication.

As mentioned in Chapter 4, it is recommended that the team serve as the gatekeeper to the in-patient ward. In practise, this key element is rarely possible and is likely to be a non-starter politically in many settings. For example, Baltimore Mental Health Services considered this at the planning stage but concluded that it was politically not feasible (see Chapter 3). Even if one could obtain this level of agreement among the players in the local system, it would take up much of the team's time to process and assess all the referrals of patients that somebody thinks should be admitted to hospital, unless it was a small catchment area.

What may be a more practical goal is to educate the main referrers to the point where, as a policy and procedure, they would regard mobile crisis home treatment as the "default" selection for disposition of patients in an emergency. Of course, if other alternatives to admission also exist, such as crisis residences, this would have to be factored in to any agreement. To achieve this goal would take a continuous effort, which is often best focussed on discussion of specific patients; for example, if MCHT staff could be part of a weekly in-patient team meeting to discuss patients that would be suitable for home treatment.

Evaluation

You need to decide a system of evaluating what data will be routinely collected before you start the service.

Managers of MCHT services need to collect data in order to answer the following questions:

1. Are we treating our target population?

    The level of acuity is of special interest: are our patients sick enough that they would have likely required admission to hospital if we didn't exist?

    How does the acuity of our patients compare to that of patients in our local psychiatric inpatient facility?

    Common acuity measures are GAF, BPRS, BASIS 32 (see Appendix for details). These scales are administered around the time of the initial assessment, and at discharge.

    Diagnosis is also relevant to target population, so a standard system of recording this is required, DSM-IV or ICD 10.

    There may be particular groups in your area to be targeted; e.g., how many homeless people or people from certain ethnic groups are we treating?

    Are we dealing with chronic patients? Number of previous hospitalisations is a good measure.

2. Are we getting referrals from the right sources?

It's hard to miss a theme running through this book: reluctance of clinicians to divert hospital-bound patients to MCHT. So you need to keep track of numbers of referrals, where they come from and, their appropriateness (some clinicians might use the service for the wrong reason; e.g., a quicker out-patient consultation, or follow up of discharged in-patients who have received substantial treatment in hospital). These data point to which referrers need a diplomatic visit and a discussion of barriers, attitudes, and problems, and, perhaps, a re-education session.

3. How many referrals are inappropriate, and what proportion of patients is not accepted?

    This question relates to how much time the service spends assessing patients vs. actually treating them (Kwakwa, 1995).

4. How many patients do we admit to hospital, and at what stage in their treatment; how long do they stay, and do we get them back?

    A large proportion of patients who, at the assessment stage, are found to need hospital admission would suggest referrals are inappropriate because they are too ill for home treatment; the referrer is not screening properly, and time may be wasted on doing many assessments that don't lead to treatment at home. On the other hand, some mobile crisis teams assess and arrange admission for hard-to-engage patients such as homeless individuals, and this may be quite appropriate, if that is a goal of the service. The availability of a crisis residence would lower the rate of admission, of course, because of the alternative it provides.

5. How long do patients stay in home treatment? Are we confining ourselves to the acute, and maybe sub-acute phase of the illness— just dealing with the crisis, or are we using valuable resources treating patients in the "out-patient" phase, perhaps because of inadequate community resources—nowhere to refer patients on to?

6. Are we responding quickly enough to referrals?

    Feedback from referrer satisfaction surveys will help.

7. What are we doing with patients?

    This includes number of visits and their location—home, office, or elsewhere—psychiatrists' visits, telephone contacts, after hours contacts.

8. Are we working with families according to the principles of home treatment?

   Are we meeting the people in the patient's support network—family, roommates, or even people such as apartment superintendents? Are we assessing caregiver burden and providing support and education?

9. How are families coping with having the patient at home instead of in the hospital?

   Family burden assessments need to be done. (See appendix for ratings scales.)

10. What is the effect of our treatment?

    This has to do with degree of improvement on scales of symptom severity and functioning, drop out rate (and reasons), and client satisfaction rating. (See appendix for rating scales.)

11. Are we reducing hospital admission?

    This may be difficult to measure because there are so many factors influencing this. Admission rates, bed occupancy, and number of involuntary admissions may give some indication.

12. Keep track of untoward events.

    These include suicide attempts and completed suicides, harm to others, police involvement, being a victim of violence, harm to staff.

13. What is the cost of the service?

Staff Training

It is assumed that staff will have adequate experience dealing with patients with acute psychiatric disorders. Most staff will likely have come from an institutional setting and need to be inducted into the model and philosophy of mobile crisis home treatment. The most important set of skills to learn is:

1. comprehensive assessment, particularly risk assessment, in the home setting
2. how to rapidly engage and form an alliance with the patient and the family, and negotiate a treatment plan, with specific reference to self-harm, harm to others, unwilling patients, demands for hospital admission, and substance abuse

To continue other important learning topics are

   3. how to do a home visit

   4. safety procedures

   5. difficult situations:
  - a. Hostile, threatening patient, or patient refuses help
  - b. Family—demanding hospital, hostile, denying illness, anti-psychiatry, unable to or refuse to help

   6. assessments of daily functioning—self-care, physical care, social functioning, food preparation, money management, and childcare

   7. needs assessment—food, shelter, finances

   8. determining level of care—admission, number of home visits per day

   9. family and social network assessment

  10. practical knowledge and skills—be able to provide assistance with self-care, diet, money management

  11. local resources—how to link patients, preferably by visiting agencies and meeting key people

  12. how to identify target problems, symptoms, and behaviors

  13. how to intervene in family and social situations

  14. how to help solve patients' problems with welfare authorities, managed care, Medicaid, employers, insurance companies, and child welfare authorities

  15. medication management, including monitoring, adherence, side effects, and overcoming reluctance of patient and family

  16. how to arrange admission to hospital

  17. how to work with patients who self-harm

  18. how to deal with actively psychotic patients in the community

  19. how to deal with specific ethnic groups: what they prefer, what they don't like, attitude to mental health, how they typically present with illness

Having set up the mobile crisis home treatment service and gotten it running, the next chapter deals with the clinical day-to-day operation and how MCHT manages specific psychiatric disorders.

Chapter Six
Daily Program Operation

"There now exists a store of experience and skills in this area built up, frankly, largely by trial and error over the early years of home treatment . . ."

(Brimblecombe, 2001b)

Intake

The goals of the intake process are

- to be quick to respond and, user friendly as possible
- to determine if degree of acuity is appropriate and look for any safety risks
- to exclude cases in a pleasant, constructive, helpful manner, suggesting alternatives

In order to gain and retain credibility from referrers, the process should be as quick and as hassle free as possible. Those making the referral are likely to be concerned and anxious to deal quickly with the patient, who is in a crisis, and they may be tempted to admit them to hospital or send them to the emergency room if the MCHT process does not work smoothly. If you are fortunate enough to be the gatekeeper, as Hoult suggests, you don't have that worry.

A telephone line dedicated to intake is the most user friendly, and should be manned by a staff member responsible for intake that day. Hazelglen cannot afford to have a worker who only does intake; they each have their own caseload and are sometimes unable to answer the phone, so the referrer is asked to leave a message. Some services mainly use a fax for referrals.

After hours, referrers such as ER staff can refer through the person on call; the patient in the ER can then be given an appointment for the next day, and the name of a contact person. An advantage of being open after hours is that one can assess cases referred in the evening without any delay, thereby extending the range of acuity your program can handle.

Determining the right degree of acuity has already been identified as a crucial issue in MCHT services. Studies report a high proportion of patients screened out: 38–48%. Harrison, Alam, and Marshall (2001) studied the referral and intake process in the Manchester Home Options service (described in Chapter 3). In spite of a relatively narrow referral base (no primary care physicians, only mental health staff, and emergency room staff), 48% of referrals were deemed unsuitable. The main reasons were lack of cooperation (23%), not sufficiently ill (23%), or too ill (21%). Referrals from junior doctors and emergency rooms were least likely to be accepted; further training of junior doctors regarding the role of MCHT was suggested. Brimblecombe and O'Sullivan (1999) report 38.1% of patients screened out in the St. Albans service (described in Chapter 3). Ford, et al. (2001), in the "Open all Hours" study (Chapter 1) report referrals being taken from any source and 42% of patients screened out and referred elsewhere. An experienced staff with knowledge of the local community will often be able to make a good estimate of suitability after a 15-minute phone interview. Sometimes, if the referral comes from the potential patient or their family, it can be difficult to assess acuity on the phone, and, if there is doubt, the patient is seen for a screening interview. Past history and response to treatment are helpful, and referrers are requested to fax previous and current reports. A degree of skepticism is required for the job; referrers can omit damning information and become adept at learning the right "open sesame" phrases such as "I was thinking of admitting this patient to hospital."

You need as complete a picture as possible of the current urgent situation to avoid blundering into a messy crisis that may already involve other agencies and may be quite different, in reality from that described by a well-meaning but unwitting referrer. So—who else is involved, and what are their roles. What does the potential patient and their family think is the problem, and do they want the help you are offering? This also presents an opportunity to educate referring agencies about home treatment and what it does best. Even though the referrer may be anxious that his patient be seen soon, it can be surprisingly difficult to contact newly referred patients; they may not share the same sense of urgency as the referrer, or their lives may be so chaotic that just to reach them and negotiate an appointment may be an achievement—some patients lack telephones. Its important to document on the referral sheet all the calls made and messages left, with the times. Make a copy of the original referral sheet, and take only the copy to the home.

To help assess acuity, we developed the Hazelglen Acuity Rating Scale, HARS (see Table 6.1). This was adapted from a similar scale developed by Bengelsdorf, Levy, Emerson, and Barile (1984) for the purpose of determining if patients presenting in the emergency room needed admission to hospital, in an attempt to standardize clinical decision making. The HARS has proven quite useful, but has not been tested for reliability or validity.

SIDEBAR
Hazelglen Acuity Rating

A. Symptom Severity

0	1	2	3	4	5
Extreme symptoms that will lead to imminent danger	Syndrome with loss of reality, agitation or uncontrollable behavior	Syndrome (as per DSM-IV	Symptoms (subsyndromal)	Some emotional upset	No complaints or symptoms noted

B. Functioning

0	1	2	3	4	5
Extreme change in functioning and impairment will lead to imminent danger	Major changes in functioning and lack of ability to care for self	Change in functioning affecting patients ability to function outside the home	Some changes in life functioning affecting employment and relationship functioning	Some change but normal activities of daily living	Carries on in daily activity with no change

C. Risk to self or others					
0	1	2	3	4	5
Clear imminent danger to self or others is extreme	Danger to self or others (not imminent)	Potential danger	Some risk with barriers to suicide, self-harm, or violence	Some risk factors of suicide or violence present, but no thoughts	No risk factors

Decision Guide (total of scores from A, B, C)

Hospital	Mobile crisis home treatment	Out-patient treatment
0–2 .	3–7	Above 7

This rating scale is used only as a guide to intake decisions; clinical common sense overrides when necessary.

If the source of referrals is restricted, to, say, just psychiatrists, you may not have these problems in determining suitability; but, if your net has to be wide, a significant number of people will have to be turned away, and how this is done is important. Leave the patient and family with a sense of being listened to respectfully and with empathy and try to give them some suggestions as to where the best place to get help is. Educate referrers diplomatically about why you did not accept their patient. Use the intake procedure to develop a reputation for being savvy and helpful. Suggest other, more suitable places to refer their patients to, so that they have gotten something out of the phone call. Intake is your front window; make it look good.

Initial Assessment

The initial assessment is best carried out in the patient's home unless it is not considered safe or the patient objects.

How to Do a Home Visit

Is it safe to go? This can be assessed by looking at the referral information— is there a past history of violence, hostile attitude, or substance abuse? Much can be determined by the initial phone contact with the patient. Ask who will be there: the patient may be an apparently harmless elderly lady; however, she may have her 24-year-old, drug-using, antisocial grandson living there. If there is reason to be concerned, arrange for family or other suitable support person to be present (these people may not live with the patient), or go in pairs, with a male staff member if possible; at least tell other staff where you are going and when you should be back. Or you can arrange for the patient to come to the office in a cab. Consider whether it is in a dangerous part of town and how easy it will be to get to your car quickly if possible.

Does the patient have any objections? Make sure they understand the reason for it and the conditions; e.g., confidentiality. It is very important to show respect for the patient's and family's boundaries; you are on their turf. If the patient refuses, gently enquire why and try to overcome his reluctance if possible; e.g., by indicating an understanding and non-judgmental attitude to their embarrassment about the state of their house.

Phone shortly before you set out—patients may forget you are coming or they may be in the habit of not answering the door because of paranoia; you may need to phone from the driveway if there is no response.

Act like a visitor—indulge in warm and friendly small talk and greet all who are present, such as small children. Follow the patient's lead as to whether they prefer to be interviewed alone or with family present; they usually prefer the latter. You can always find an opportunity later to pursue more private issues. Go with the flow; interruptions from dogs, children, neighbors, and phone calls are not unusual, and are all grist to the mill.

Be prepared: take your cell phone and some medication, which can make the difference between success and failure of home treatment. A patient's anxiety, agitation, or insomnia can quickly tip the balance in their ability to cope out of hospital; a benzodiazepine drug (anti-anxiety) or atypical anti-psychotic drug can work wonders.

What you do in the home depends on the purpose of the visit. All MCHT patients receive some home visits. Some patients are only seen at home, such as the elderly, physically infirm, or those too distraught to come to the office. Home visits are an essential component, but there is no need for 100% of visits to be in the home. In fact, as patients get better, getting them to negotiate a trip to the office can be an aid in assessment and rehabilitation.

After the intake screening, the referral information is given to the case manager, who usually does the initial assessment in the home.

This assessment is a different kettle of fish to the hospital assessment interview. Patients behave differently in their own home; they are more relaxed, less formal and deferential, and may be involved in their daily activities in the middle of your visit. They attend to children's runny noses, answer the phone, and may have to deal with the refrigerator repairman in between answering your questions. Other people may be present—such as spouse or parents who have their own questions and concerns. There may be some practical problems that need urgent attention e.g., Elise, a 50-year-old eccentric woman with paranoid schizophrenia lived alone, except for 15 cage birds whose care had completely overwhelmed her. For the sake of the birds and the patient, urgent disposition of these pets was called for and the resourceful case manager made some kind of an arrangement with a local pet store.

All this adds up to the fact that sailing smoothly through a full psychiatric history, and mental examination may not be possible; and, that flexibility and creativity are needed often. You may have to obtain some information by a more indirect approach.

The first few minutes are very important. The novelty of home-treatment, coupled with the absence of hospital structure and routines may leave the patient and/or the family with some doubt as to who you are, and what is going to be your plan. It is important, therefore, to be ready to explain things, to convey competence, and an air of being in charge of the situation. You need to set priorities—e.g., Who needs to be settled first—the patient or the family? What are the patient's immediate needs? Are they willing to accept home treatment—if not, what will be your next step?

Never assume anything.

Of course, at the end of the day, the psychiatric history and mental examination should be no less complete than would be obtained in the hospital. A full account of the presenting problem, recent history, past history and treatment, personal and family history, medical history, and mental status are required. It is particularly important to establish, who initiated the referral, whose problem is it and why are they seeking help now.

In the section on principles in chapter four it was recommended that sufficient time be taken at the first visit—some programs stayed 2.5–3 hours. At Hazelglen, we find 1.5 usually sufficient. In the second half of the visit, you need to address what degree of symptom control is necessary—e.g., severe agitation left untreated, even for 12 hours can wear out a patient and family, who, unable to tolerate any more, may demand hospital admission. Some severely disturbed patients may fluctuate in their ability to cooperate—the home visit, perhaps with supportive family present, may provide only a short window of opportunity in which to administer antipsychotic medication—e.g., in the form of a zupenthixol injection. (an antipsychotic drug which lasts about 48 hours)

What immediate practical problems need addressing for the next 12–24 hours? These can include having no food, no one to look after the children, being unable to stay alone, having no money, and being unable to afford medicine. The case manager may need to arrange a trip to the food bank, enlist the help of friends or relatives, and get urgent social service assistance. The concept of insufficiency described in Chapter 2 can be useful in organizing a treatment plan. The reason the referrer wanted the patient in hospital gives a clue as to what is a priority: suicidal risk, being unable to follow treatment instructions and comply with medication regimes, unable to get out of bed or care for self, disturbing behavior—in short, what crises may erupt in the next 12–24 hours?

It is important to engage the patient and family in a therapeutic alliance—or at least the family; it may take 1–2 days to engage the patient in the treatment plan. It is sometimes possible to avoid involuntary admission with MCHT; even quite resistant disturbed patients can be gradually persuaded to accept treatment. For some unwilling patients, such as an 18-year-old with first episode schizophrenia, it may be more productive to temporarily dispense with most of the formal psychiatric assessment and concentrate one's efforts in forging an alliance. It can be helpful to find something the patient wants help with; e.g., to get a part-time job. After one or two visits, one can bring the conversation around to their current psychiatric problems and, one hopes, develop a treatment plan. Of course, in an urgent situation you don't have much time, and a decision needs to be made quickly; to close the case whether or proceed to involuntary admission. In closing the case, do it in a friendly way, leaving the door open.

The case manager usually does the initial assessment, but in some cases, the psychiatrist is also present at the first visit. In the U.K., where junior trainee psychiatrists are more available, or in academic settings where there are residents, they are often present for the first visit, which is obviously preferable. It is particularly important for the psychiatrist to be present at the beginning, if involuntary admission is anticipated, or if the case is particularly acute. The assessment is written on a form and an appointment with the psychiatrist is arranged. Because the psychiatrist's time is at a premium due to manpower shortages at Hazelglen, most cases are seen at the office. Common clinical reasons for psychiatrist home visits include: patient too distraught or disorganized to make it to the office, elderly or physically infirm, or, simply, unmotivated.

Medical Assessment

In some MCHT programs, the psychiatrist carries a medical bag, and every patient gets a physical examination and laboratory tests. Because of the risk that psychiatric symptoms can be caused by undiagnosed medical problems, some centers feel very strongly about this, particularly if there is much concern about medico-legal liability. It is prudent to follow medical practices, geared to the local situation. For example, chronic patients in inner-city areas of large U.S. cities are found to have a high frequency of physical disorders and very poor primary health care. In Ontario, it does not appear to be necessary for all patients to have an initial physical assessment. Most patients have a primary care physician and often they have seen them recently. Psychiatric in-patients in Ontario no longer routinely require a physical examination. If a significant medical problem is suspected, the case manager and psychiatrist make more systematic enquiries and, if necessary, refer the patient to their family physician. Patients who have not see a physician recently are requested to do so. The case manager may need to accompany the patient to the doctor's office and the laboratory if they are too disorganized or unmotivated. We forge close links with primary care physicians, keeping them informed by phone, and sending them our reports and discharge summaries.

Hospitalization

Common reasons for hospital admission include: family exhaustion and anxiety, inability or unwillingness to help with treatment, development of suicidal urges or psychotic symptoms that cannot safely be managed by MCHT, poor cooperation, lack of treatment adherence, and tumultuous social situation.

The process of hospitalization is often the least satisfactory feature of MCHT; the optimum smooth admission and discharge of patients, especially discharge, does not happen. The in-patient staff may not have faith in the MCHT program and may keep the patient longer than is necessary, deeming them too ill to be managed by home treatment. Ideally, the MCHT and in-patient team are part of the same organization and share the same philosophy, and sufficient influence can be brought to bear on both teams to cooperate.

Sometimes, though, it's just the nature of the patient's illness that determines a long in-patient stay—the disease process is too rapid and quickly gets out of control and these patients may continue their downward course after admission.

Medication

Being able to get the right medication quickly and reliably into a disturbed patient is where MCHT shines and where it is distinguished from less intensive services, which may aspire to or even claim to provide the equivalent service. In this regard, the aim is to replicate pharmacotherapy as closely as possible, as it is delivered in hospital. This means it is fast, flexible, and closely monitored to achieve the desired results.

To achieve this, staff need to have a sophisticated knowledge of psychiatric drugs; sufficient autonomy to make quick, sometimes creative decisions on the spot; and rapid access to the psychiatrist. At the initial assessment, the patient may be in urgent need of medication if they are to remain at home. Sometimes there is only a narrow window of opportunity in which the patient will accept medication on the day of the initial assessment. In the case, of Mary a 49-year-old woman with chronic schizophrenia in a psychotic relapse (see Chapter 7), the case manager reckoned she had better seize the moment when the patient said "give it" (meaning an overdue injection). Another patient, Ken, a 42-year-old man with chronic schizophrenia who had been psychotic for a long time living on the streets (see Chapter 7) would only listen to the police about such things as medication; he regarded them as the only people he could trust. Somewhat reluctantly, two police officers who knew him were persuaded to talk to him in order to convince him to accept an injection of fluphenazine decanoate (a long-acting depot anti-psychotic drug); that was a turning point in his care—he subsequently agreed to live in a hostel for men and gradually accepted more psychiatric and practical help.

Obtaining medication must be made as easy as possible. Practical help may be required to get a prescription filled; e.g., help with getting a social services drug benefit card or transportation to the pharmacy. Unfortunately, regulations and benefits concerning medication have not kept pace with the move from hospital to community care. In Canada, for example, drugs are free in the hospital, but not for patients in the community. Some patients cannot afford drugs, have no private drug coverage, and are not eligible for social service assistance. Drug company samples have proven very helpful until other arrangements can be made. Some hospitals will provide free drugs to MCHT programs.

Medicines can be given daily to the patient by the case manager or the task can be delegated to a family member. Medicine boxes with a space for each dose (dosette boxes) are invaluable and are provided by our program. Also, "blister packs" prepared by the pharmacy can be helpful, although rapid, frequent dose changes can be difficult to arrange. The case manager checks the boxes regularly to determine whether the patient is adhering to the medication regime. Patients are not just uninformed, passive recipients of medicine, as can occur in hospital. They are required to take more responsibility and an active role in their care. Consequently, they end up learning a lot more about the medicines than they knew before.

Pamphlets and videos are used to educate them and their families. Some flexibility is allowed with dosing, using PRN as-required doses, the timing and rationale all carefully explained and spelled out for the patient and family.

Adherence to medication treatment is a concern, and the degree of control over this is less than in hospital. Sticky notes are plastered on fridges and bathroom mirrors and patients are phoned with reminders to take their medicines. Dose regimes are kept simple, to fit in with the patient's schedule; if necessary it may not be done "by the book"; e.g., a medicine normally given twice daily may be given once a day, if that is what it takes to get the medicine into the patient. A phenomenon we have learned to watch out for is drug sharing; in some families, it seems to be accepted that you can take each others' medicines. If necessary, staff can visit two or three times daily to administer medicine.

Patients may be resistant to taking medicines and may not see the need for them. The rationale for a drug may need to be couched in terms they can relate to in their current mental state; e.g., they may be persuaded to take an antipsychotic for sleeplessness or for "stress." More accurate explanations can be given later, when they have more insight and are thinking more clearly. They may be fearful of side effects, a fear noticed especially with elderly patients. We often give very small doses at first to avoid the slightest possibility of an adverse effect that might prompt the patient to reject further help; some won't give you a second chance. One severely ill housebound woman with obsessive-compulsive disorder had intense fears about putting any medicine in her mouth, even fears of dying. At the start of treatment, before she would take her medicine, she insisted that her husband had to take one of her fluvoxamine tablets—"if he doesn't die I guess it's safe." Even then, we had to allow her total control—she literally would lick the pill, or shave off minute doses. Eventually, she got up to a small therapeutic dose and her outcome was good.

For safety, small amounts are prescribed and dispensed, and we encourage patients to allow us to dispose of all their extra pills left over from previous prescriptions.

Managing Suicide Risk

Very depressed patients with strong suicidal urges don't always jump at your offer of admission to hospital; instead of grateful acceptance, you may face painful negotiation and need all your skills of persuasion. They are often angry, demoralized, hopeless, and ashamed; you, their care provider, can be frustrated, anxious, and in a dilemma—do you add to their misery by admitting them involunarily, or live with an unacceptable risk? Home treatment offers an alternative for some of these patients.

How does one assess whether the patient, who is clearly too much at risk for conventional out-patient management, can be safely managed in a home treatment program? Will the extra support, monitoring, 24-hour emergency coverage, and home visiting be good enough? It is assumed that the reader is familiar with suicidal risk assessment in general, and the factors that heighten or diminish the dangers. The following account highlights those determinants most germane to MCHT.

We want to know whether there is a family member, or other caregiver who is willing and able to help: how important is it to them that the patient avoids hospital admission, and what is their perception of the suicidal risk? Two cases illustrate this. Two middle-aged men, both depressed and suicidal, presented within days of each other, providing an educational contrast. One had been admitted to hospital before with serious depression and frightening suicidal thoughts; his wife made it very clear that she wanted him admitted again but the patient himself was ambivalent. The other man was severely depressed for the first time and had never been in hospital. He and his wife were alarmed that he might require admission. She said she would do everything possible to keep him out of hospital, including arranging 24-hour surveillance by her and other family members.

The lessons here are that previous admission increases the chance of subsequent admission, and a family's willingness to accept and share the risk and shoulder some responsibility are important factors in one's decision to accept the patient into home treatment.

Both these patients were similar in presentation. Had they shown certain additional risk factors, one might have leaned away from home treatment and towards hospital. We look for such signs as history of impulsive behavior, especially related to previous suicide attempts, past potentially lethal suicide attempts, secretiveness, unwillingness to participate in a suicide safety plan, current substance abuse, psychotic symptoms and signs, or even what clinicians call "a psychotic feel" about the patient. Other considerations are: what has prevented them for committing suicide so far—what are the barriers? How open are they with their family—what is the quality of the relationship? The interaction with the case managers is important—do they experience them as helpful? Do you see their hopes rise during the interview? Are they cooperative with the suicide safety plan? For example, one man resented our wishes to remove a large supply of old toxic medications from his home and to involve his common-law wife, accusing us of being controlling, so we did not accept him for MCHT.

It is not enough to have a willing family member to share the responsibility; we have to make sure they can do the job. Are they exhausted, lacking the wits, or unable to influence the patient? Can other family members help? Sometimes we help them develop a roster of helpers to be in attendance. Of course, the significant family member may be part of the patient's problem—there is no point in relying on an abusive spouse.

The decision about suicidal risk is not once and for all. After a night in the hospital and a good sleep, many patients will be able to transfer to MCHT. Conversely, a family may try to manage the patient at home only to discover that it's an intolerable risk, and then want them in hospital. Some patients respond to contracts, although they are seen as only an adjunct, not binding, and not a foundation of suicide risk management.

Suicidal patients work with their case manager to reduce the risk. Getting rid of aids to suicide is an obvious place to start. These can include guns and ammunition, medicines, hoses, and access to vehicles. Suicide can be associated with intense bursts of affect. These can be controlled with anxiolytics for panic and anxiety and anti-psychotics, such as olanzapine for self-hatred, agitation, and intense self-critical rumination. Severe psychosocial stressors such as rejection by a loved one, threats of or actual financial loss, and other losses, such as a job, can lead to suicide attempts; a case manager can often predict likely triggers and can coach the patient and family about these risks and how to cope. They catch deterioration quickly by proactive phone calls in the evening or on the weekend; e.g., "How did the court case go today?" A suicide safety plan is developed and written out for patients, including who to call in an emergency, how to calm themselves down, what to tell themselves if they get certain feelings and thoughts or predicted stressors occur. Offering to call the patient in the evening or at the weekend is a powerful reassuring tool—"you're calling me at home?"—there is a lot of therapeutic mileage when the patient perceives staff as going beyond the call of duty.

After Hours Emergency Coverage

While essential to an MCHT service, the after hours provision is likely to be less arduous than one would expect. Emergencies in MCHT are usually predictable-if you know the patient well enough. The case manager quickly engages the patient and family and becomes so thoroughly familiar with their problems and possible outcomes that they can anticipate and forestall most emergencies. They are coached regularly regarding what to do if symptoms worsen or stressful events occur; as-needed medication is arranged in advance. Patients reach the emergency on call person at Hazelglen by phoning a special number that pages the staff.

Almost all emergency calls can be dealt with by phone; staff very rarely meets with the patient after hours. If face-to-face contact is required in the evening or at weekends, the hospital crisis clinic nurse takes over; patients can go there by taxi provided by Hazelglen. Other services, e.g., Edmonton and Victoria, use the psychiatrist on call for emergency contacts. Common reasons why patients call include they cannot sleep; something new in their life, such as a new relationship difficulty; social emergencies, such as a cheque has not arrived; anxiety and worry; questions about medication; and concurrent medical problems. Common interventions include: asking what has helped before; what they can do to help, e.g., hot bath, rosary, walk, extra medication; suggesting that they go and stay with someone or that someone stay with them. The promise of a call back in an hour or two to see if they have improved is very reassuring.

Role of Program Psychiatrist

The role of psychiatrists in MCHT is the same as in other settings, but their approach to the job may be different to that in a hospital or mental health clinic, and their practice activities will certainly be different.

In a hospital it is easy to fall into a traditional medical hierarchical role, in which they give "orders" to the nurse, the patient is a passive participant in their treatment, and the family deals chiefly with the social worker. Home treatment works best, if the psychiatrist's attitude and modus operandi are in harmony with the key elements and principles described in Chapter 4.

In MCHT, the responsibility for care and decision making is spread more evenly: the case manager has to be able to work independently with the patient and family in an unstructured home and community setting, patients take more responsibility for their care, and the family have some say in decision making and a role in care functions. A collaborative, consultative approach is therefore suggested. Psychiatrists' opinions and decisions about diagnosis and treatment should, whenever possible, be developed in concert with the case manager, who has a lot of useful clinical information, having spent many hours with the patient and family.

Practice activities will include home visits, alone or with the case manager; interviews, which include the family and caregivers; and informal, on-the-fly consultations. The case manager should be prepared to see patients in the street and in coffee shops and should make themselves readily accessible by phone or pager.

It is helpful, too, if they can involve themselves in the day-to-day running of the service and development of policies. The ability to perceive how the service fits into the local community and mental health system is useful, as well as knowledge of local agencies and politics.

Preferably, the psychiatrist will spend 40–50% of their time with the program and make themselves available by phone after hours (e.g., the Hazelglen psychiatrist is available 8 a.m.–10 p.m. 7 days a week; usually, they will get few calls).

Team Functioning

To respond to patients' needs rapidly, other case managers need to be aware of their clinical situation; often, particularly in larger teams, care is shared between two or three other workers. Daily morning team meetings and handover meetings are useful to keep everyone up to date with the patients, and are essential for teams with larger services, extended hours, and two shifts. Other forms of inter-team communication are the patient's chart, a summary sheet of all the patients, their medication, key family members, and clinical issues, which is updated at the weekly team meeting or on a large white board. What is most important in MCHT is that, by whatever means, staff constantly communicate with each other—there is no room for staff who "do their own thing" with their patients.

At Hazelglen, staff operate as generic mental health workers—in other words, they all take responsibility for their patients' treatment, do assessments, contribute to diagnosis, make a treatment plan, conduct psychotherapy, and monitor medications. The social worker and the occupational therapist on the team may be asked to consult in their area of special expertise, such as assessing the functioning at home of an elderly patient or helping with a complex family conflict; the nurse may be asked to assess a patient for a physical medical problem.

At the weekly team meeting each patient is discussed in depth, and issues are discussed in a safe, non-threatening manner in which staff receives supervision from the psychiatrist and from each other. Patients' progress is discussed and modifications to treatment plans are planned as necessary.

Safety

Practical experience in all MCHT programs indicates that safety of staff and patients is usually not a major issue; some of the reasons for this were outlined in Chapter 4.

As usual, prevention and preparedness are best. Part of the intake procedure is always aimed at assessing safety risk. One reason for the relative safety of MCHT is that patients are usually willing to receive help, so one needs to exercise care regarding patients who are reluctant to receive help, especially if you sense they are being coerced by the family or others. One of the few dangerous situations we had at Hazelglen was when a well-meaning member of the local parent support group, with the patient's mother, brought a young manic man, against his wishes and against our advice, to our office. He got quite wild and the police had to be called.

Obvious red flags for risk are current substance abuse, previous history of violence; antisocial activities; suspiciousness regarding others, especially if directed at health care providers; certain symptoms of psychosis, which cause the patient to feel threatened by or compelled to hurt others; and current problems with anger control.

The environment needs to be assessed, especially whether weapons are available; prior knowledge of unsafe neighborhoods and apartment buildings is useful. These considerations are much more crucial in impoverished inner-city areas than in rural and suburban areas. Some programs, such as in Victoria, B.C., conduct a mandatory safety check of the home before the patient is accepted. Concerns include weapons, vicious pets, and dodgy family members or roommates.

If there are safety concerns, then the usual procedures have to be modified, such as going in pairs or meeting at the office or in a coffee shop. Protocols regarding informing others of your intended time of visit and expected return need to be developed. These and other more detailed safety precautions, such as where to sit, where to park, and when to leave in a hurry, are taught to new staff members.

Treatment Plan

After the initial visit, the treatment plan is discussed and outlined with the patient and their family. They are given a written copy, and a copy goes on the chart. As mentioned in the principle of time-limited interventions in Chapter 4, this plan should be tightly focused and may include target symptoms. This may have required considerable discussion with the patient and his family, whose expectations may be quite unrealistic about what home treatment can accomplish. It can be quite overwhelming when we first encounter some patients and their story unfolds. Issues that are contributing to the current crisis include immediate and extended family conflicts and loss such as separation, divorce, bereavement, pathological interactions, and abuse, and practical problems, such as poverty, no rent money, eviction, job loss, job stress, custody and access battles, and legal problems.

The treatment plan describes what the patient's goals are, what treatment is suggested, and who is responsible for what.

Working with Family and Caregivers

The family is usually essential to home treatment for many reasons. Often, it is they who seek help for the patient in the first place; for example, by taking him to the emergency room and requesting admission to hospital, maybe because they cannot cope any longer and the situation has become a crisis for them. Whether they can cope with the assistance of the MCHT team or whether they will demand hospital admission is vital to the success of MCHT. If they do agree to MCHT, they can be of great help with the assessment and be useful partners in the treatment.

Often, it is simple to involve the family, but sometimes there are barriers. It is not unusual for everybody to work outside the home, for long hours and on shifts. This may preclude them from the initial interview, and the case manager may have to make an effort to accommodate their schedule and go back in the evening. They may be part of the patient's problem, and it is impossible or even counter-therapeutic to involve them; for example, adolescents having major problems with their parents may insist on keeping their parents out of it.

Some patients just don't want their families involved, for no good reason that you can see. There have been occasions when we could not envision caring for a very sick individual without some help from other persons in their lives and had to conclude that MCHT was not workable unless they allowed that. The family may decline to be involved because they are burned out or because of long-standing conflict or emotional distance. A standard principle of mobile crisis home treatment is to assess the degree of family burden. In general, family burden has not been greater with home treatment; it allows the patient to continue to have a functional role in the family, and this appears to offset any increase in burden caused by the avoidance of hospital. Families appreciate that the patient can still play an important, albeit diminished role; for example, a depressed woman may still be able to provide basic child care for parts of the day, whereas if she were in hospital, major and inconvenient provisions may have been necessary. There may be much conflict in the family about the patient's present breakdown some insisting on hospital or some not agreeing that there is a psychiatric problem at all. Members of some cultures don't "believe" in mental illness, or are deeply ashamed at the idea and can't bring themselves to acknowledge it.

The case manager has to quickly assess all this, starting at the intake procedure, deciding who are the key family members and caregivers for the practical purpose of home treatment. Family need not live with the patient, but be close enough to be involved, and the case manager needs to negotiate with the patient, if necessary, who is going to be involved with his care, and how. Release of information forms are completed as necessary.

At the initial interview, or as soon as possible, the family's opinion about the crisis is obtained and their attitude to home treatment and their expectations are assessed. Do they have the resources to help—the time, energy, and ability? The process of home treatment is explained, and they are introduced to the idea of helping with the treatment. What the patient can still do in the home is also discussed; for example, could they drive and pick up children from school or take them to swimming lessons?

An important concept in home treatment is that the family is part of the treatment; they substitute, to a degree, for the help that the patient would have received in hospital. From the list of the components of in-patient care, outlined in Chapter 2, the following lend themselves to family involvement: interpersonal contact, on-going assessment, hostel services, helping with self-care, drug therapy, assessing competence in daily living activities, and liaison with the outside world.

SIDEBAR

Is the Service Caring for the Caregivers?
A Snapshot of One Team and Their Patients' Families

Qualitative research on the Intensive Home Treatment Team of South Leeds, Britain (Godfrey and Townsend, 1995), revealed the following concerns of caregivers. (11 caregivers were interviewed).

The main thrust of IHTT involvement was in relation to the person who was ill. Most caregivers acknowledged the value of the service for the patient and recognized significant advances from their past experiences with specialist mental health services. They valued the professional support, both to prevent admission and to enable discharge. Many also had a good relationship with the workers.

> *"At least I could sit and talk and didn't feel as though it was all my burden any more. The 24-hour phone number from them was brilliant . . ." made me settle and sleep, because before I had that, there was just no chance. I was on edge all the time listening for him, thinking "God how do I get him to hospital with four kids at night. But with these . . . they could have arranged all that for me, and I would not have had to go with him."*
> —Elinor Harvey, sister

However, whilst some caregivers felt supported by the fact that the team was working with the ill person, caregivers generally were critical of the unresponsiveness of the service to their needs or even an acknowledgement that they might have needs arising from the impact of the illness.

Unmet needs identified by caregivers included counseling/ support in their own right, as well as help with practical tasks around child care, and home care and a need for couple of hours' break. There were also unmet needs in relation to the children of service users, on whom the illness had an impact. They needed advice on how to explain what was happening to the children, some of whom might need support in their own right.

Their experience with acute mental health services was one of being made "invisible" as far as their own needs were concerned.

> *"No-one came to see me if I had any problems. No-one has ever asked anything about me. But I'm here as well. I'm just left to cope. There are times when I could do with going to see a psychiatrist myself. What I need is just someone to call and talk to me now and again. Or even someone who called me to ask if they're any problems. To help you release your feelings."*
> —Theresa Cartwright, mother

It was notable that a number of people suffering severe and chronic depressive illnesses related their problems to a childhood history of family breakdown and sexual abuse. Dealing with these issues posed difficult problems for partners of the ill person. Firstly, there was the impact on current marital and family relationships. Secondly, there was the issue of how partners were perceived by professionals.

> *"When the abuse was first revealed, there did not seem to be an acceptance that a partner—and a man could be supportive. But I do want information so that I can cope and work out what is best for our family" "It was devastating when the abuse first came out, but no-one was available to talk to me as her husband about it. I needed to understand what it did to her. But there was nothing."*

Two factors appeared crucial in enabling caregivers to cope. One related to the nature of the relationship with the patient and the extent to which it involved a mutual sense of support and obligation and, in the case of partners, a past and current pervasive sense of marital closeness. However, there were also examples where the impact of the illness had strained and disrupted the relationship. One person described her current marital status as "separated by illness."

The other factor concerned the resources available to or accessible by the carer. People had different access to support systems, both formal and informal; hence the need for workers to carry out a sensitive and thorough assessment of needs, not only of the patient but of the significant others within their social milieu. This involves an understanding of the dynamics of the relationship, as well as the ambivalence expressed by some caregivers in seeking help in their own right.

> *"I'm not very good at asking for help. I prefer to try and sort things out myself which isn't always the best way. You get on with the job and you don't see yourself in the role of carer and you don't see yourself in need of support and you do. And it's also working out what is acceptable for my wife. It's keeping the balance and not making her bad as well."*
> —Brian Jones, partner

The inadequacy of the response of the acute mental health service to the needs of caregivers is not simply an issue that has emerged with the Intensive Home Treatment Team. Rather, the provision of an acute service within the person's own home, has highlighted the manner in which mental health services have traditionally either ignored or blamed close relatives for the illness.

How Families Can Help Provide Some Components of Hospital Treatment

Interpersonal Contact

Many acute patients find it difficult to tolerate being alone for very long, and sometimes not at all. The reasons are not always clear; it is usually associated with severe anxiety and agitation. Sometimes, the reason is clearer and more specific, such as fear of harming themselves, or frightening hallucinations or delusions. Families can help a lot, by offering to stay with the patient or having the patient stay with them, or visiting them frequently, or a combination of all three, the tasks being distributed among all the family and caregivers. A lesser degree of support may suffice, such as agreeing to be easily accessible all the time by telephone and agreeing to come over quickly if necessary.

On-Going Assessment

This is important if the patient's symptoms and/or behavior may change rapidly for the worse, or if their ability to function alone is shaky. Or, it may be required because you don't know what is going on; the patient is quite ill, but the diagnosis in unclear; you may be worried that they may be in danger of rapidly becoming psychotic or descending into severe, comorbid substance abuse. The family are educated about the likely causes and nature of the illness, possible course of events in the next 24–48 hours, what to watch out for and how to respond, and how to reach the case manager quickly or the after hours service.

Hostel Services

This may be the easiest part of treatment for the family to help with. They may not need to stay with the patient, but visit frequently to help clean up, do laundry, provide food, and shop. These activities are closely linked to the following two other components:

Help with Self-Care and Assessment of Competence in Daily Living Activities

The family is taught how to assess the patient's functioning and to report their findings and concerns. The case manager may need to use some diplomacy in getting the patient to accept the sick role—some don't accept it without a struggle, battling valiantly in the face of severe psychomotor retardation and paralyzing lethargy, for example. On the other hand, they may have to protect the patient from patronizing or domineering behavior by the family. As the patient gets better, the family may need some encouragement to back off; for example, allowing the patient to drive short distances when, two weeks before, the family had to chauffeur them everywhere because they were not considered safe on the road. The patient can still contribute to family life, and their activities will gradually change as they improve.

Drug Therapy

Family can be taught to do some of the fairly simple nursing activities involved in drug therapy. They can take control of the bottles of medicine and give tablets as required, or monitor the patient's use of a daily dosette box. They are alerted to possible side effects; patients sometimes need repeated reassurance about these.

Activities

Patients find it hard to manage their day. They can't decide what to do next, can't initiate even simple activities, and find time heavy on their hands. Families can help here by developing a structured plan of activities for the day and doing some of them with the patient, such as taking them for a walk or for a coffee.

Liaison with the Outside World

Patients in a crisis sometimes have many stresses impinging on them from the wider community, such as problems with police, government agencies, debt collectors, landlords. The family can help by helping the case manager understand these problems, what has already been tried, and what may be of help. Families can be encouraged to intervene on behalf of the patient with the case managers guidance.

A Summary of the Process of Mobile Crisis Home Treatment from Start to Finish: Two Schemes

Hoult (personal communication, April 23, 2002)

Assume That the Problem can be Managed in the Community

1. At the time of receiving the referral:

   • Get as much information as possible from the referrer; especially what the person is doing (but be aware of second- or third-hand information). Who are the other people involved (the social system)? Find out the referrer's expectations.
   • Negotiate a time for the initial assessment. This is best done in the home and in the presence of key elements of the social system; however, it may be difficult to get all players together at the beginning, and may be done later as people become available.
   • Obtain as much information as possible from clinical records, current mental health worker, family and social network.

- Ask that key elements of the social system be present at the time of the assessment.
- Prepare what you think you will need; e.g., medication.

2. Initial assessment

- Let them talk about

  What the problem is and who has it
  History of present episode
  Clinical signs and symptoms
  Previous history
  Interpersonal relationships
  Disturbed behavior
  Risk
  Willingness to cooperate

- Tolerate the drama and anger
- Involve the social network if possible
- Form a relationship

3. Plan

- Explain what the team can do it's availability
- Formulate options, consequences of options
- Decide what resources are needed and what is available
- Involve the social network
- Wait for an opening

4. Implementation (immediate)

- Explain the plan
- Reconfirm team's potential to visit
- Address accommodation, money, or other practical problems
- Remove or reduce stressors
- Administer medication
- Try to ensure that the patient sleeps if this has been a problem
- Give advice, guidance, and directions
- Tell everyone how to contact the team
- Make sure everyone understands the plan
- Promise help if trouble arises
- Arrange time of next visit

5. Implementation (medium term)

- Frequent visiting (twice daily, or more if required)
- Monitor mental state
- Monitor (maybe supervise) medication
- Address practical problems
- Address family, social network problems
- Counsel
- Provide education for patient and social network
- Continue to build the relationship with patient and social network
- Titrate level of service, dependence

6. Implementation (the final stage)

- Less frequent visits
- Maximise patient's independence, control
- Arrange adequate follow-up and ensure seamless transfer
- Stay involved until crisis is over

The Process of Mobile Crisis Home Treatment from Start to Finish

McGlynn & Smith (1998)

1. Assessment

- Rapid response
- Home assessment
- Multi-disciplinary assessment
- Focus on "here and now"
- Involve relevant others, caregivers and family using problem solving approach
- Risk assessment

2. Planning

- Team approach and team decision making
- Focused crisis plan with short-term goals based on negotiation with patient
- Decide number of visits and level of input based on available options
- Focus on discharge planning at an early stage

3. Intervention

   - Engagement and therapeutic alliance
   - Allocate named worker in team
   - Commence medication
   - Family work
   - Frequent monitoring and continual assessment
   - Explanation as to why crisis has happened
   - Practical interventions; e.g., benefits
   - Give contact number of team in case crisis occurs during treatment

4. Resolution

   - Linkage with on-going care
   - Maintain contact until the above is well in place
   - Learning opportunity—why did the crisis happen? Relapse prevention strategies, and coping strategies
   - Joint visits with patients and regular worker prior to discharge
   - Develop longer-term community care plan; involve family/caregiver
   - Liaise with relevant others; e.g., primary care physician
   - Request feedback from patient

The next two chapters describe how MCHT is applied to the treatment of depression, schizophrenia, first episode psychosis, mania, borderline personality disorder, and postpartum disorders.

Chapter Seven

Mobile Crisis Home Treatment of Mental Disorders: Part I

"Setting is where the treatment occurs . . . the choice of setting does not necessarily depend on the severity of the patient's illness. Many patients who are severely disturbed can be and should be treated on an outpatient basis . . . choice of setting will inevitably influence . . . components of treatment . . . the setting does not preclude their consideration."

(Perry, Frances, & Clarkin, 1990)

In their book on treatment selection, Perry, et al., (1990) recommend a more discerning approach to treatment selection and add support to the notion that intensity and type of treatment can be uncoupled from location; the most intensive level of service does not necessarily have to take place in the most restrictive setting; i.e., hospital. Before clinicians arrange hospital admission for their patients in a crisis, they should consider what *specific* components of in-patient treatment are needed, and with what degree of intensity. What is the specific "insufficiency" that the patient is showing (see Chapter 2).

All functional mental disorders can be treated by MCHT if the right conditions prevail. MCHT may be able to provide whatever components of in-patient treatment the patient needs, using their current supports. Using the components of in-patient treatment list in Chapter 2, and the key elements and principles described in Chapter 4, the following two chapters describe how six acute mental disorders are treated: depression, schizophrenia, borderline personality disorder, mania, first episode psychosis, and postpartum disorders. Only those aspects germane to home treatment are included; it is assumed that staff are experienced enough to be familiar with the general principles of managing these conditions. This account is supplemented by numerous case histories.

MOBILE CRISIS HOME TREATMENT OF DEPRESSION

This discussion of the home treatment of major depression will be anchored by the Practice Guidelines of the American Psychiatric Association (American Psychiatric Association, 2000) and the Clinical Guidelines for the Treatment of Depressive Disorders (Canadian Psychiatric Association and the Canadian Network for Mood and Anxiety Treatments (2001), plus the list of components of in-patient treatment outlined in Chapter 2, and the key elements and principles in Chapter 5.

What clinicians are concerned about, and what they do with patients and their families in treating a specific mental disorder, will frequently apply to the treatment of other disorders, so the next two chapters should be read as a whole.

Choosing the right setting for the treatment of severe acute depression depends upon symptom severity, comorbidity, suicidality, danger to others, level of functioning, and available support system. Other important considerations are the patient's ability to adequately care for himself, provide reliable feedback to the clinician, and cooperate with treatment.

MCHT can substitute for in-patient treatment of depression or shorten its duration dramatically. Its flexibility, intensity, and 24-hour availability enable it to tackle many of the above clinical issues. There is a certain degree of suicidality, illness severity, dysfunction, and social support breakdown that is beyond out-patient management, but for which, MCHT can adequately provide many of the 20 components of in-patient care

Table 7.1

Indications for Hospital Admission of Depressed Patients

- Serious threat of harm to self or others
- Severely ill patients who lack adequate social support
- Complicating psychiatric or medical conditions
- Unlikely to cooperate, or not responding adequately to out-patient treatment
- Diagnostic evaluation (especially with comorbid medical or psychiatric conditions
- Rapid deterioration or marked severity of depression (including hopelessness, suicidal ideation, or psychotic features)
- Inability to function at home
- Breakdown of social supports

described in Chapter 2. Apart from suicidal ideas and behavior, the array of problems that can tip the balance towards hospitalization of a depressed patient—the reason for the insufficiency—include intolerable symptoms and behavior such as severe agitation, constant pacing, importuning, severe irritability, inability to eat, staying in bed all day, not washing for days, extremely poor adherence to medicine because of preoccupation with side effects, failure to attend to medical conditions such as diabetes, excessive drinking, odd, psychotic behavior, and refusal or inability to come to outpatient appointments.

What kinds of patients would not be suitable for home treatment? Obviously, patients who refuse treatment, although there are degrees of refusal. Some patients are adamant, and have absolutely no insight and no family capable of cajoling them into treatment, but there are others who, with strong encouragement from the family and a gentle, winning approach from the case manager, can be drawn into treatment. MCHT probably has an advantage over in-patient treatment in this aspect—it may be easier to persuade the reluctant patient to accept treatment at home than in the hospital. Where a patient's needs and severity are not balanced by the family's strength, willingness, and wish to avoid hospital, MCHT is unlikely to work. A patient who is suicidal, impulsive, abusing alcohol, thinking in a distorted fashion, and without any supportive family is clearly unsuitable; similarly, a frail, elderly, medically unwell person with only an equally frail spouse for support.

Components of psychiatric management of depression include diagnostic evaluation, evaluation of safety of patient and others, evaluation and addressing of functional impairments, establishing and maintaining a therapeutic alliance, monitoring the patient's mental status and safety, providing education for patient and family, enhancing treatment adherence, working with patient to address early signs of relapse, and providing medication and psychotherapy.

Initial Assessment

Assessment, as always, focuses on the reason for the insufficiency—just what exactly has tipped the balance, creating the need for admission to hospital or an alternative such as home treatment. The reason may lie with the patient, the family, or both. It is important to nail down, as specifically as possible, who brought the patient to the emergency room or who called the family doctor. Why at this time—what was different today, compared to yesterday? Was it the patient, who suddenly became frightened by the intensity of their suicidal thoughts? Was it the adult daughter, visiting from out of town, who discovered that mom hadn't eaten for two days, had no food in the fridge, and had lost thirty pounds? Or, maybe it was the family doctor, who became alarmed at the rapid deterioration of the patient and discovered they were not taking their medicine and putting themselves to sleep with large doses of whisky. Suicide risk assessment and management is dealt with in Chapter 6.

It is useful to find out what treatment and coping techniques have been tried already, and why they may have been ineffective; what was the experience in previous episodes of depression: what helped, and what are they afraid of happening again? Assess the level of anxiety and agitation, insomnia, and psychotic symptoms; if these are severe, they can "sink the home treatment ship" quickly, by losing family trust in the service and fueling demand for hospital admission. Psychotic thinking, or even quasi-psychotic distorted thinking, intense self-hate can cause the situation to quickly get out of control. Practical help may be needed quickly, with nutrition, childcare, and social stressors that may have helped trigger the crisis.

Support for the Social Network and Work with Families

The role of the family will vary with age and circumstances. For example, in the case of depressed adolescents, they may insist that their family is not included, which can present ethical and clinical dilemmas; but, if the parents are regarded by the patient as part of the problem, you may have no choice. However, sometimes if you cannot negotiate an adequate support network, and they are thought to be in some danger of hurting themselves or suffering severe dysfunction, you may have to refuse to admit them to the MCHT service and insist on hospital admission. School guidance counsellors, parents of friends that they may be staying with, and their peer group can sometimes provide support. Usually, though, it's the parents who have initiated the request for help. One of the first tasks may be to find out who is in the patient's social network. They cannot always be relied upon to identify who their supports are. They may be ashamed, demoralized, fearful of burdening others, and feeling undeserving, so they don't reach out for help, which contributes to their having a crisis. We don't want to trample on their autonomy and be paternalistic by going over their heads, but sometimes we have to tread a fine line to set up the supports needed for home treatment to work. Most times, though, the family is already involved and willing to arrange all the supports needed.

Families sometimes can have unhelpful and inaccurate ideas about depression: that the patient is lazy, attention seeking, needs to "smarten up," or have more faith in Jesus. They cannot believe it is a mental problem—the physical devastation that depression can cause makes them convinced that it's a medical problem that you have missed. They may not realize how sick and impaired the family member is or, may in some cultures, may have difficulty believing in the concept of depression at all, or be deeply ashamed.

A severely depressed person in the home can be exhausting and frustrating; whether it's the irritable acting-out of the adolescent, the constant hand-wringing rumination of the middle aged, or the whining importuning of the elderly. The degree of family burden needs to be assessed as soon as possible. Other common concerns of families are restless, sleepless nights, worry about suicidal risk, and having to take over much of the patient's regular duties. Their response to all this may vacillate between imploring patients to "pull themselves together," and mollycoddling. Or, the family as a whole may be split between these two poles.

One of the key components of psychiatric management of depression is education (Brent, 2001; Rush, 2001).

Rush states that patient education markedly improves medication adherence and clinical outcomes, "The principles underlying patient and family education are 1) reiterate key points, 2) deliver less complex information early and more complex messages when patients are more stable, and 3). emphasizing patients' participation in their own treatment." Initial education consists of explicit information about the symptoms of the illness and the medication prescribed. Patients and families learn how to monitor symptoms and medication side effects. They often comment on how much more they have learned about their illness and treatment in MCHT compared to previous experiences in hospital. The responsibility given to them and their families stimulates them to learn, in their natural surroundings; the education has an immediate practical impact and staff are committed to constantly making sure everyone understands enough so that home treatment is proceeding safely. Some hospital procedures of giving medication, such as patients lining up at a window, don't lend themselves to private, lengthy educational talks about pills.

Drug Therapy

Antidepressant medicines are usually required for the severe level of depression treated in MCHT. Some patients are unwilling to take these drugs, fearing dependence, side effects, or wanting to do it on their own, and get to the real root of the problem. Outside the controlled setting of a hospital, with a passive patient often lining up with other patients to be given their pills, considerable effort may need to be expended to start and keep a patient on these medicines; treatment adherence can be poor. Much education and reassurance may be needed. Depressive illness can present as a crisis, partly because of severe agitation, restlessness, and insomnia, so rapid control of these symptoms is recommended. Benzodiazepine anti-anxiety medicines are useful, but some patients do better with the newer anti-psychotic drugs, such as olanzopine, especially if thinking is distorted, frank psychotic symptoms are evident, or there is intense self-hatred. Decreasing agitation and insomnia can decrease suicidal risk. Patients and family may need a lot of guidance as to when and under what circumstances to take PRN or as-needed drugs. For safety, it may be necessary for the family to have control of the medicines. Written instructions, "post it "notes stuck on the fridge or bathroom mirror are helpful.

Psychotherapy

Psychotherapy is mainly supportive at first, with an emphasis on maintaining hope, helping them tolerate the pain and disability of depression, and guiding them about what to expect and how to cope with symptoms. Relaxation exercises and tapes are helpful. Cognitive, behavioral, and interpersonal psychotherapy have the best-documented effectiveness in the literature on specific treatment of major depression, and elements of these are used particularly when the very acute phase of the illness is diminished. Patients are given chapters of *Mind over Mood* (Greenberger & Padesky, 1995) to read and complete exercises. Problem solving, help with decision making, activity monitoring and scheduling, coping cards, graded exposure, and role playing are common interventions. Many are struggling with interpersonal problems that may have precipitated the acute depression: breakup of a relationship, marital separation, family conflict, and job stressors are common examples. Interpersonal psychotherapy is helpful, which involves explaining depression, linking it to the relationship issues, and focusing on how to cope with loss, grief, and conflict. Short term, crisis-based family and couple therapy is helpful.

Management of Problems in Activities of Daily Living

The most important deficits are focused on, which may be as basic as not getting out of bed all day. The therapeutic relationship, appropriately laced with humor, is used; for example, deliberately making a home visit first thing in the morning, phoning shortly before you arrive and gently creating expectations to be up and dressed. The case manager may need to be very actively involved at first and personally deal with practical matters. Sorting through unpaid bills to decide what is absolutely necessary to pay first may avoid power and phones being cut off. External agencies may need to be recruited for some functions in the early stages; for example, home care nursing or home making, meals on wheels, taking a patient to a food bank, and local churches are very helpful.

Providing guidance about daily functioning can sometimes be quite tricky. It's not unusual for guilt-ridden patients in MCHT to insist on trying to keep up their premorbid level of functioning; the resultant failure exacerbates their sense of worthlessness and increases their anxiety. This can be so problematic that hospital treatment may be preferred, where they are forced to accept the patient role and to rest and wait for the treatment to work. Education plus rearranging the roles of other family members is helpful in these cases. Very specific instructions about what activities and responsibilities they can handle may be required and need to be written out, a kind of activities schedule in reverse, intended to slow them down.

Driving ability is another difficult topic. It's not easy to determine when, and whether, a depressed patient taking sedative drugs can drive. This function is so necessary to be able to perform other functions, like shopping and child care; patients may not be cooperative or may overestimate their abilities. Again, family members can be helpful with these decisions.

On-Going Assessment

Using the family as an additional eye, the case manager continuously monitors progress, relapse, complications, functioning, and safety. They are coached as to the likely course of events, what can go wrong, and how to observe and record. Rating scales such as the Beck Depression Inventory and daily mood graphs are used. Patients often see no progress from week to week and easily get discouraged, as they may have unreasonable expectations of a rapid recovery. It is useful to chart their progress quantitatively to demonstrate progress. Suicidal thinking, side effects of medicines, crucial areas of functioning, and expectations are all important.

Electroconvulsive Therapy

This can often be provided by MCHT; contraindications would include the elderly, physically frail patients, those with significant active medical complications, and those without enough support for someone to stay with them on the day of treatment. It may be desirable for the case manager to accompany the patient to and from the hospital, or the family can do this. Headache, confusion, and degree of improvement are monitored. Clinical guidelines for ambulatory ECT are described in a report of the Association for Convulsive Therapy (Fink, Abrams, Bailine, & Jaffe, 1996).

Help with Self-Care

Very depressed patients often neglect this by not bathing for days, wearing unwashed clothes, not attending to medical problems such as diabetes, and eating poorly. In MCHT the case manager assesses this, and if the patient cannot be coaxed or convinced to attend to these, the family or home care nurse may have to step in. Some larger MCHT programs employ practical aids to help.

Activities/Structure

One reason that depressed patients improve in hospital is that they have a structured day, with expectations that daily living activities will be completed and provision of simple activities. Time passes slowly for seriously depressed patients at home, and even the simplest decision is hard; consequently, at the end of the day, they look back, demoralized, and feel that yet again they have done nothing. The case manager can help them and their families arrange a schedule of activities and, if necessary, take them out; for example, going for a walk to a local coffee shop. These are sometimes productive sessions, psychotherapeutically—patients feeling more able to bring up issues in this relaxed time, with no expectations to talk about their problems.

Activities with pets are one of the least threatening—pets don't judge, and one reason patients don't want to go to hospital is worry about care of their dog or cat. Pet care such as grooming and walking can be incorporated into a schedule. Physical activity is very helpful and, in the case of the elderly, vital, to prevent the deconditioning that can contribute to the vicious cycle of: depression, inactivity, deconditioning, social isolation, depression. Elderly patients are encouraged to walk up and down their apartment corridor or do simple calisthenics with the case manager.

CASE HISTORIES OF MOBILE CRISIS HOME TREATMENT OF DEPRESSION FROM THE HAZELGLEN SERVICE

A 34-Year-Old Female with Major Depression with Psychosis

Donna is a 34-year-old factory worker, who has lived with her common-law husband Bob for the past year, and her two children, a boy, 6, and a girl, 9. She was referred by her family doctor because of severe depression associated with psychotic symptoms and poor adherence to medicine.

This was her third major illness, and two years previously, she had been admitted to hospital in another city for 25 days with a similar condition that had been diagnosed as schizoaffective disorder. At that time, she had been a single mother, living on social assistance, and worked part-time as a dishwasher.

Her family doctor had been trying to treat her with anti-depressants and anti-psychotics, but her adherence was so poor that she had given her an injection of flupenthixol decanoate, a long-acting, depot anti-psychotic, shortly before the referral.

June 11, 1600 hours initial interview at home by case manager

Donna complained of being restless, uptight, having insomnia, having a poor appetite, being indecisive, being unable to concentrate, and being forgetful. She had walked off her last job a week previously without telling anyone, and was keeping her 9-year-old daughter home from school to be at home with her for "companionship." She appeared depressed, fearful, slow, and markedly indecisive; she denied suicidal thoughts, but at times wished she were dead.

June 13, first office visit with psychiatrist

She had been very reluctant to come in and had to be coaxed by the case manager. Her past history indicated that this was her third breakdown in four years. Two years before she had heard voices, thought someone was in the basement, had strange thoughts that she had been fired from work for "screwing up," and would phone co-workers at home late at night. Suicidal thoughts had prompted her sister to take her to the hospital for admission.

On examination, she appeared very suspicious and was secretive, admitting to strange thoughts, but not divulging them, and denying hearing voices; but, at a subsequent interview, admitted that she had heard them before she got the first injection from the family doctor. She thought life was not worth living, but it was the children that stopped her doing anything to herself.

She was functioning poorly at home; Bob had to do the shopping and she was not cooking. She alluded to problems with Bob; they had been together one year, he hit her occasionally, and she seemed perplexed and vague and very unsure. It was not clear to what degree her concerns were delusional: she had her bags packed by the door, ready to leave with the children and "drive around."

Family history revealed that her mother had been hospitalized with depression and her father had been an alcoholic.

Her diagnosis was thought to be major depression with psychosis; her GAF score, 40.

Because of intense anxiety, she was prescribed lorazepam 0.5 mg 2–3 times daily. Her family doctor had attempted unsuccessfully to start her on a previously effective anti-depressant, nortryptiline; this was started at a dose of 25 mg daily, and she was given a dosette box to help with adherence.

Problems highlighted were her relationship with Bob—he "drank too much at times"—and she also drank excessively at the weekends, causing her to stop her tablets then. Her understanding of depression and medicine was very poor.

June 15, home visit by case manager

Feeling better until she had an argument with Bob. Keeps bags packed at the door, in case she wants to leave. Educated about depression, and counseled against sudden major decisions.

June 18, office visit with psychiatrist

Improving—adherence still poor—did not take nortryptiline last night because it made her "tired and spacey"—Bob, also present, said she was "more spacey without the drug." Reluctant to take medicine—dysfunctional attitude to illness—"I need to get to the root of it—I should not be dependent on pills." Admitted, for the first time, to having heard voices in this currrent episode of her illness—before the first injection of flupenthixol.

June 22, office visit with case manager

Less anxious, more secure about relationship with Bob. Adherence still shaky—misses medications because of drinking or forgetting. Given teaching video on depression, encouraged to watch it with Bob. Education provided about medicines, alcohol, and depression. Dosette box filled. Encouraged to attend a support group on women's issues put on by Family Crisis Shelter when she was feeling more stable.

June 22, office visit with psychiatrist

Weepy, labile, reluctant to talk, still uneasy about Bob's fidelity, which seemed to be an irrational fear. Advised to stick to two drinks only at weekend.

June 26, home visit with case manager, Bob, and children present

Injection of flupenthixol given. Mood better, less labile, Bob sees improvement, and attributes it to medication, which she is now taking as prescribed. Plans made to soon join local self-help group on depression.

June 30, phone call to case manager

Upset, weepy, had fight with Bob; left with daughters, to stay with sister.

Home visit, later that day

Bob present (with beer in hand), got irritated when Donna became weepy and accused him of not being demonstrative enough. Role of alcohol becoming clearer—situation had deteriorated over the weekend, with Bob drinking heavily, and pressuring Donna to "party" with him. An argument ensued, with Bob pushing and shoving her. She is very uncertain as to what she should do. Case manager reviewed options with her: call police when being abused physically, family crisis shelter, Al-Anon, temporary separation. More education provided about depression, drinking, and medications.

July 3, home visit with case manager

Bob joined in for part of visit. Some improvement; had outing yesterday with female friend and children.

July 6, office visit with psychiatrist

Weepy, discouraged, thoughts of wanting to die, troubled by lack of motivation, relationship with sister, "bored." Nortryptiline dose increased to 75 mg, activity schedule suggested, encouraged to come to group at the office.

July 10, office visit with case manager

Weepy, continuing to be upset at Bob's lack of communication, expressing much self-criticism, thinking that her friends "hate" her, concerned that sister (who lives next door) is distancing herself. Donna had, until now, refused us permission to interview her sister—encouraged to allow this. Simple education about depression, provided to her two children, who accompanied her—because their lives have been much affected by their mother's illness.

July 16, home visit with case manager

Due to insufficient response to nortryptiline, sertraline 25 mg added; previously discussed with psychiatrist.

July 20, office visit with psychiatrist

Significant improvement on all fronts—increased energy, activity, concentration, mood, sleep—no signs of distorted thinking.

July 22, office visit with case manager

Maintaining improvement—attributes this to addition of sertraline. Feels "less emotional," more relaxed—planning holiday with Bob.

Donna continued to improve, up to her discharge on September 9. Her relationship with Bob continued to be stormy, and she spent two nights in the Family Crisis shelter because he had slapped and shoved her. She continued to attend the women's issues group, Mutual Aid, and the children also attended a support group.

Gradually, she developed more confidence, got a new job in food services that pleased her, and her relationship with Bob became more stable at the point of discharge. At discharge, she had gone four weeks without flupenthixol, with no psychotic symptoms. Long-term maintenance with antidepressants, symptoms and signs of relapse, and subsequent interventions, such as restarting anti-psychotic medications were reviewed.

Total number of interviews: 17 (8 in the home)
Total direct hours of care: 18.5
Total indirect hours: 5.5

Points Illustrated in this Case History

Almost certainly, Donna would have been admitted: she was psychotic, in danger of impulsive actions with her children such as taking off, with no rational plan (she had already kept the 9-year-old home from school for a week). This episode was a similar illness to the breakdown two years previously that had resulted in hospital admission for 25 days. Adherence to medication treatment was almost nil; she was abusing alcohol, and often stated that she wanted to die. Her home situation with her partner was very stressful.

The case manager had to provide large doses of education at every visit, to both the patient and her partner, mainly verbal, plus the use of a video. Her lack of adherence to medication was complex, and treatment in the home setting undoubtedly helped to reveal the damaging pattern of interaction, in which she abused alcohol at the weekend, causing her to stop her medicine, and leading to domestic fights, followed by an increase in depression and feeling of being in a crisis. Guidance about alcohol, use of dosette box (filled by the case manager), and education helped adherence, as did the gradual improvement that enabled them to see improvement connected with taking medicine. Other key elements of MCHT were rapid control of anxiety and psychotic symptoms with anti-anxiety medicine and anti-psychotic medicine (in depot form); referral to agencies, such as the Family Crisis Center and the support group; rapid response of case manager to crisis call (home visit later that day); working with the family (Bob, and the children); supportive and problem solving psychotherapy, and the role of the psychiatrist in adjusting her medicine (adding sertraline), which enabled a complete remission of symptoms.

A 48-Year-Old Woman with Major Depression with Psychosis

Alison is a 48-year-old single woman, who lives alone in a home owned by her parents and works in an office.

She was referred by her psychiatrist because of suicidal thoughts, severe depression and agitation, and psychosis, which had become much worse since her boss had told her on January 10 that, as she was unable to function at work, she would have to go on sick leave. Her psychiatrist had been seeing her since the past September for depression following the break up of a 10-year relationship with her boyfriend. At his first consultation, he noted that she had been admitted 12 years prior for a what sounded like a manic psychosis at the time of her divorce; she had been experiencing auditory hallucinations for the past five years, which referred to her marriage, but had been able to work. His treatment with anti-psychotic medicine had been unsuccessful because of side effects, and she had steadily become worse.

February 7, first visit with case manager, at her home

Very agitated, restless, rubbing her legs. Staying at her parents' house during the day because she is unable to stay alone. Hearing voices telling her what food to eat, to do the laundry, and hearing neighbors talking about her divorce. Suicidal thoughts of carbon monoxide poisoning since sent home from work on January 10, denies intent: "I don't have the guts." Feels very hopeless "I don't know what to do, to get out of this mess." Current medication: chlorpromazine 25 mg, an anti-psychotic medicine (for sleep and hallucinations), paroxitene 20 mg (prescribed six days prior), lorazepam 1 mg twice daily. Agreed to not commit suicide and to allow the case manager to try to help her.

February 8, home visit cancelled due to snowstorm

February 9, home visit, parents present

Her parents are finding her dependence on them very stressful. Alison was given an anti-psychotic drug, 2.5 mg, olanzapine, prescribed by her psychiatrist following phone consultation; she was reluctant to take more medicine, at first, but finally accepted it, with urging from her parents. She had no drug benefit plan and could not afford to buy her medicine, so the case manager provided her with free samples. A seven-day supply of medicines was provided in a dosette box.

She was encouraged to get additional support from her brother, friends, and church, but was reluctant; she had lost most of her friends in the breakup with her boyfriend the previous August. The case manager provided her with a schedule of daily activities to provide some structure and promised to phone her daily over the weekend.

February 10, phone contact

Able to delay going to parents until 3:30 p.m., did some housekeeping and made lunch. Not using daily activity schedule. Auditory hallucinations have almost disappeared; hears only a high-pitched noise "like crickets or birds."

February 12, phone contact at parents' house

"Not too bad"—spent most of weekend at parents' house, sleeping better, went for walk with father.

February 13, first interview with Hazelglen psychiatrist at the office, accompanied by her brother

Alison was very agitated, such that a full interview was not possible. Her hallucinations had ceased and the main symptoms were extreme agitation, fear of being alone, irrational hopeless thoughts, and suicidal ideas. The suicidal risk and heavy burden on their parents was discussed with her brother Bob, who agreed to try to establish a network of family and friends with whom she could stay with, either at their house or at her own. He confirmed the family's willingness to share some responsibility for suicide prevention by staying with her.

February 16, home visit by case manager

Having severe migraine with vomiting.

February 17, phone contact

"Not bad."

February 19, home visit by case manager

Still feels that she cannot do anything, but then reported she had cooked her dinner at the weekend, something that she had not done for a long time. Discussion regarding activity schedule—able to think of things to do the next day, but on waking she is too anxious. Urged to contact friend in nearby town; case manager will contact Bob and ask him to contact her church on her behalf.

Alison was stressed by weekly calls from her boss, enquiring about when she would be returning to work. She had begun to ruminate obsessively about adjusting to her new bifocal glasses, thinking she could never adapt to them. Case manager intervened at work—called the boss, who seemed supportive, and asked her to call only monthly.

February 20, office visit with psychiatrist

Denied suicidal thoughts, no hallucinations, calmer, but still obsessing about bifocals—very pessimistic.

February 21, home visit with case manager

Case manager phoned brother to try to arrange more support from friend and a cousin. Still obsessing about glasses; says she will never be able to work again because of inability to adjust to them.

February 23, home visit with case manager

Less agitated. She was reluctant to increase dose of paroxitene to 30 mg as suggested by psychiatrist, but willing to try. Alison slowly continued to improve during a further nine visits, five of which were in her home, four of which were phone contacts. She gradually did more, including hiking with a group she belonged to, playing cards, working on the computer, needlework, and reciprocating her parents' help, by cooking dinner for them. She was eventually able to resume living alone. She continued to need a lot of reassurance about side effects, such as sweating and weight gain. By March 26 she had returned to work part-time, and she was discharged on April 11.

Total number of visits: 16 (11 in the home)
Total hours of direct care: 21
Total hours of indirect care: 3.5

Points Illustrated in this Case History

This patient would likely have needed admission if home treatment had not been available. She had been experiencing psychotic symptoms—auditory hallucinations—for five years, and, after her breakup with her boyfriend of ten years, had become severely agitated, helpless, hopeless, isolated, and unable to stay alone during the day. She had suicidal thoughts of using carbon monoxide. She had ceased to do many of her activities, including food preparation, and her elderly parents were feeling very burdened at the time of the referral. She was reluctant to take adequate psychotropic medicine, and likely would not have adhered to conventional out-patient drug treatment.

The case manager worked very closely with her parents and brother, supporting them and enlisting their help in getting her to take medicine, watching her closely, providing much-needed interpersonal contact, and willing to accept some responsibility regarding suicidal risk. Attempts to get Alison to connect with anyone other than her immediate family were not successful, and so family burden was managed mainly by providing support and reassurance of eventual recovery.

Rapid control of hallucinations, agitation, and insomnia were accomplished by provision of an anti-psychotic drug, prescribed readily by her psychiatrist. She could not afford to buy her medication, so free samples were provided in a dosette box. Phone contact was used six times, most of the 3.5 hours of indirect care.

Focus on daily activities, structure, intervention with employer, and practical problem solving concerning such things as her bifocal glasses were features of her treatment.

Mobile Crisis Home Treatment of Schizophrenia

Indications for hospital treatment of patients with schizophrenia are quite broad (American Psychiatric Association, 1997; McEvoy, Schleifler, & Frances, 1999):

Table 7.2

Schizophrenia: Indications for Hospital Admission
• Risk of harm to others
• Risk of suicide
• Severe disorganization
• Acute psychotic symptoms
• Risk of accidental injury
• Unable to care for self and need constant supervision
• General medical or psychiatric problems where out-patient treatment would be unsafe or ineffective

This leaves a lot of scope for the use of MCHT as an alternative to hospital admission. Any one of the above clinical situations may be too acute for out-patient management, but, because of the flexibility, intensity, extended hours service, and 24-hour availability of MCHT, may be managed without admission. The American Psychiatric Association (APA, 1997) guidelines recommend that the least restrictive treatment setting be used, depending on the need for particular treatments, family functioning, social supports, and the preferences of the patient and the family.

Common clinical situations that can lead to requests for hospital admission include acute severe exacerbations or recurrences of psychotic symptoms and ensuing disturbing behavior; failure of out-patient/day hospital treatment because of poor adherence to treatment, not showing up for appointments, or medication proving ineffective; tricky switches in medication in an already fragile patient; inability to care for self; caregiver burden and distress; and comorbidity, e.g., poorly controlled diabetes, substance abuse, and psychotic symptoms. As well as enabling the patient to bypass the hospital completely, MCHT can facilitate early discharge from hospital.

The success of MCHT in treating schizophrenia depends a lot on the relationship between the caregivers and the patient, who may be distrustful of mental health professionals, have little insight into his own illness, and not want treatment. But, if there is at least one person whose advice they will follow, such as a parent, sibling, or community case manager, it can make all the difference; the effectiveness of MCHT may hinge on that relationship. For example, in the case history that follows, Ken, a severely ill, homeless, chronic paranoid schizophrenic man, the role of a trusted police officer in getting him to take his first injection was crucial.

Some very ill patients can still have a positive attitude to home treatment; there is sometimes a surprising lack of correlation between the severity of psychotic symptoms and behavior, and the ability to cooperate sufficiently with treatment. Some MCHT programs, such as in Victoria, B.C. (Chapter 3), have found that patients with schizophrenia are more willing to present themselves for treatment, and disclose their psychotic relapse earlier to their therapist because home treatment is available, and it does not mean an automatic trip to the hospital.

The goals of psychiatric management in the acute phase of schizophrenia are prevent harm, control disturbed behavior, suppress symptoms, effect a rapid return to the best level of functioning, develop an alliance with the patient and the family, formulate short- and long-term treatment plans, and connect with maintenance and follow-up care (APA, 1997). Developing an alliance with the family is often the first priority, because patients with schizophrenia usually have very limited insight into their illness and its treatment. But families may not be up to the job: they may be burned out if the illness is chronic and severe, or MCHT is offered too late in the current episode; some may be willing, but lack the capacity to cope. Some families have developed harmful, unhelpful patterns of relating to the patient, the illness, and each other, which may help trigger a relapse. Other, non-family supports need to be assessed too. Most chronic patients have other care-givers, such a community case manager, and one job of the MCHT staff is to orchestrate the efforts of everyone involved.

Initial Assessment

Family members and/or a community support person should be present to aid in getting an accurate history of the presenting problem. Also, one needs to estimate how much help will be forthcoming from caregivers, and ensure their commitment to being part of the treatment. It is important, though, to give the patient a chance to speak privately; they may be reluctant to reveal their psychotic symptoms in front of the family, and they need to be free to talk about family problems. What are the triggers of this acute episode? A common cause can be a change in the environment, such as a move to an-other apartment, new neighbors, or change in caseworker. Frequent stres-sors are landlord/rent problems, having the phone cut off, and conflict with friends. Stopping their medication may have set the ball rolling.

The presenting problem may not be psychosis; their schizophrenia may be under reasonable control, but a comorbid disorder such as depression, anx-iety, or substance abuse may have reached crisis proportions. A history of their recent physical health needs to be obtained; physical illness can exacerbate psy-chosis, and patients don't always know how to describe health problems. They should be given a physical exam soon after admission to the service.

Due to the nature of schizophrenia, you cannot always rely on what patients report about their illness; they often deny psychotic symptoms. You do not have the luxury of observing them in a controlled setting for the next eight hours, as in hospital, and so a direct approach may be needed in ques-tioning about symptoms. You may have to be a "detective"—-making de-ductions about their mental state and functioning from the appearance of their dwelling places, such as bizarre foods and costumes. Casual wandering around their homes, chatting informally about family pictures, looking at evidence of recent activity, such as writings, newspaper clippings, or odd ob-jects, can reveal a lot.

You may need a strong stomach to cope with some patients' sur-roundings, which may stink of smoke and show evidence of dog dirt and urine. Most important is not to react—you have to be a good actor—and avoid doing anything that would offend the patient or lose their trust. It is important to whom, and how you speak during the visit; for example, talk-ing to a neighbor outside without permission from the patient may arouse suspicion, jeopardizing the whole visit.

At the end of the assessment, you have to make sure the patient will be safe and has the basic necessities of life until the next day. Are they not drinking and dehydrated, is there food in the fridge, are the utilities functioning? Don't assume anything; e.g., the delivery person from the pharmacy may need a $2 prescription fee to be paid, which the patient may not have; one has to think like a parent in some respects.

Working with Families

Family education needs to start right away. Often, they have to take control of and monitor the medication. They need to be taught what to watch for regarding psychotic symptoms and how to respond; e.g., visual clues to hallucinations such as looking distracted, moving of the lips, and whispering. They are taught to recognize extra pyramidal side effects and what to do. The patient's odd behavior needs to be discussed fully and freely; family intolerance can scuttle a home treatment plan. They need to learn to not get into power battles about such things as getting up in the middle of the night, wandering around, and watching TV or smoking; their limits of tolerance have to be assessed. The role of excessive expressed emotion needs to be explained. The family's emotional distress often needs active intervention, with supportive psychotherapy, reassurance, and a chance to blow off steam. In MCHT, a patient has more say in his treatment—he is less likely to assume the passive role so automatically assumed in a hospital. And yet, in a relapse, not well enough to always have the last word he is needing help from their family or other supports, who have to adopt a caregiver, parental role, if only for a brief time. Negotiating all this in order to put together a home treatment plan is one of the more challenging, but rewarding, tasks; it can be impressive to see how hard patients and families work at this, motivated by love and wish to relieve suffering, and to avoid hospital admission.

Drug Therapy

Rapid control of symptoms and disturbing behavior carries the day. For credibility of the MCHT service and relief of anxiety in the patient and family, early signs of progress are important. Patients may fear loss of control in the middle of a psychotic break while free in the community; such loss can mean jeopardizing their job or apartment. Short-acting depot intramuscular preparations of anti-psychotics, such as zuclopenthixol acetate (Clopixol-Accuphase) are useful, both for speed of action and adherence problems; similarly, medications in liquid form or as a rapidly dissolving tablet (Zydis form of olanzapine). Sometimes, simply reintroducing a recently discontinued medicine or increasing the dose of an existing medicine is sufficient.

Non-psychotic symptoms and behavior, such as severe insomnia, or agitation, may be more of a priority, when a benzodiazepine preparation is useful.

On-Going Assessment

One of the reasons why patients with acute schizophrenia get admitted is to keep an eye on them—their mental state can change unpredictably, and psychotic symptoms and behavior can emerge with alarming rapidity. They cannot be relied upon to monitor their symptoms and call for help.

MCHT can carry out this function adequately for many patients. Frequent home visiting, liberal use of phone check-in, reliance on coached family members and other supports, and regular training and reminding of patients to help them monitor themselves are the keys. It is important to focus on previously agreed-upon target symptoms and behaviors; specific areas of dysfunction, such as grooming and eating; and safety, of self and others. By now, specific psychosocial triggers will have been identified, although on-going assessment may reveal more. Progress in handling these stressors is monitored, and the patient's ability to cope is measured, so the degree of support can be titrated accurately.

In home treatment, psychotic symptoms may be more visible; the illness is in its more raw form—patients are less sedated than in hospital, because they have to carry on their normal life (you cannot "knock them out" with large doses). How they respond to the phone, answer the door, and deal with neighbors are all clues to psychotic thinking. While they may appear stable at home, accompanying them to a stimulating shopping centre, for example, may stimulate symptoms unexpectedly.

Although frequent often daily, visiting is desirable, patients may not allow that—they cannot tolerate that degree of contact, and you may have to compromise (see case that follows, Ken; and case Chapter 8, David, in section on first episode psychosis. Readers may be surprised at the length of time between visits, but that's all he would allow; we had to rely on his friend to alert us if there was a problem.) We have to bear in mind that our patients may cope better than we expect; some have lived with psychosis for many years.

Practical Help

Staff may have to turn their hand to a wide variety of problems that can aggravate the patient's clinical state. It is important to actively scan for problems; because of cognitive impairment, long-term resignation, demoralization, and psychotic preoccupation, patients may be unable to identify what they need help with. Common issues are landlord/housing/neighbor problems, interpersonal, family conflict, money problems (check not arrived, can't pay rent), and forced change in routine; e.g., some supportive comforting activity is no longer available.

The case manager's response will vary, but, if possible, the patient is given the degree of responsibility that they can handle; for example, a patient may be accompanied to a government office but, encouraged to do the talking for himself.

Psychotherapy

In the acute phase of the illness, psychotherapy is geared to reassurance, helping patients counteract psychotic thinking, and explaining symptoms. They need guidance to avoid overstimulation, stressful relationships, and help to avoid exposing themselves to situations where they may fail and embarrass themselves; unlike in hospital treatment, it can be hard to protect them. A young patient may insist on going to his college classes or part-time job, even though this is beyond his ability, and may cause him to behave strangely, drawing unwelcome attention. You have to help them face up to their denial and their desperate urge to carry on leading a normal life. A common problem is exposure to recreational drugs and heavy alcohol use that may have been part of their previous social life. They may bridle at proscriptions regarding not smoking marijuana and restricting alcohol use. All this falls under the treatment guideline of helping them understand and adapt to the psychosocial effects of the illness.

Brief Hospitalisation

Frequently, home treatment services and the local hospital need to work as willing, flexible partners in the care of these patients. The course of MCHT for a patient with schizophrenia may be marked by series of very brief hospital stays when the situation gets out of control; the respite from stress, and being provided with nursing care for a few days can get them on their feet again. They may be more willing to go to hospital voluntarily if they know they can be discharged soon, back to home treatment. This recurrent use of very brief hospital stays makes the most economical use of beds. The point to be made here, is that home treatment should not be seen as success, and hospital as failure; the optimal treatment is often: a smooth mixture of both predominantly home treatment, with a judicious sprinkling of hospital.

Sometimes, MCHT can serve paradoxically as a more gentle mechanism to admit a patient who is on the verge of being admitted involuntarily, which can be coercive and traumatic, with use of police and restraints. MCHT can "soften" a patient's resistance—sometimes enough so they will reluctantly agree to try it for a few days.

Link Patient with Other Agencies

MCHT case managers should be very familiar with the local agencies that serve these patients, knowing the culture, personalities, and characteristics of their patients. It is important to get the fit and the timing right to link these fragile patients with the support they need. Of course, there may not be a lot of choice; a good MCHT program is constantly on the lookout for what may be small organizations, such as supportive church groups, that can help their patients.

A Mobile Crisis Home Treatment Service for Schizophrenia

The Home Treatment Program for Acute Psychosis, Toronto, Canada

This report (Wasylenki, et al., 1997) is of interest for a number of reasons. First, the target population was confined to a group of 400 severely ill, difficult to treat, and often treatment-resistant patients; approximately 80% have a diagnosis of schizophrenia, schizoaffective, or paranoid disorders, and 40% have a co-existing substance abuse disorder. Second, continuing the tradition of Fenton and Pasamanick (see studies in Chapter 1), the home treatment was provided by general, not specialist, psychiatric nurses and social workers—staff affiliated with the Home Care Program for Metro Toronto. Thirdly, and most importantly, it was a collaboration between a mental health program and a general home care program; as these or similar organizations are in place across Canada and the U.S., the model has wide applicability.

The home treatment program for acute psychosis is a partnership between the Continuing Care Division (CCD) at the Clarke Institute of Psychiatry (now the Centre for Addiction and Mental Health) and the Home Care Program for Metropolitan Toronto (HCPMT). The Continuing Care Division provides psychiatric treatment and clinical case management for approximately 400 severely ill patients. The Home Care Program for Metropolitan Toronto coordinates the provision of in-home services for approximately 14,000 patients each day. Services are provided by such agencies as St. Elizabeth's Visiting Nurses Association and the Visiting Homemakers Association.

To start the program, staff from CCD organized a week-long training experience for nurses, homemakers, social workers, and coordinators. Topics covered included major mental disorders, psychiatric medication, principles of crisis intervention, and working with families and caregivers. When a CCD patient was in need of admission to hospital, the patient was offered home treatment as an alternative. Within 48 hours, visiting nurses, homemakers and social workers began to provide intensive support; in urgent situations, services were provided in the home immediately. But, in most cases, the decision to offer home treatment had a settling effect upon both the patient and others, so intensification of the existing case management support from CCD was sufficient to tide the patient over for 48 hours.

The visiting nurse was available 24 hours per day and a CCD psychiatrist provided back up 24 hours a day. Services provided included medication management, interpersonal support for patients and caregivers, behavior management, maintenance of housing and/or entitlements, assistance with activities of daily living, maintenance of linkages with other programs and services, reality orientation, and social/recreational activities. Once the patient had stabilized, on-going care reverted to the psychiatrist-case manager team in the CCD.

This report describes the impact and comparative cost of this MCHT program and also describes the processes necessary to establish the program. During the project period of eighteen months, 34 episodes of home treatment were completed involving 27 different patients. To be eligible for home treatment, patients had to be in need of immediate admission to hospital by the attending psychiatrist. The only patients excluded from the program were those judged to be imminent dangers to themselves or others. Unfortunately, the number of patients excluded was not provided.

No patient offered home treatment chose to be admitted. For over half of the patients, no family member or caregiver was involved; 92% were single. Although approximately 80% of all CCD patients had a diagnosis of schizophrenia, schizoaffective disorder, or paranoid disorder, and 40% had a co-existing substance abuse disorder, fewer patients in the home treatment program had a diagnosis of schizophrenia, schizoaffective, and paranoid disorder (60%), and only 7% had a diagnosis of substance abuse disorder. These figures perhaps indicate the difficulty in treating substance-abusing patients in home treatment.

The 18-item Brief Psychiatric Rating Scale (BPRS) mean score at admission was 41. The BPRS scores diminished significantly to a mean of 35.

The authors developed two interesting scales designed to measure opinions about home treatment compared to hospital treatment. The Attitude Questionnaire consisted of items designed to elicit respondents' general preferences for home treatment over hospital treatment, with 1 indicating the most negative and 10 the most positive. Patients, families, and providers all showed positive attitudes. Hospital providers were less positive than community providers (4.9–5.0 compared to 6.5–9.1).

Patients and caregivers showed a clear preference for MCHT on the Treatment Comparison Questionnaire, which compared respondent's experiences in the home treatment program with previous experiences in hospital along 11 different dimensions:

Table 7.3

Treatment Comparison Questionnaire

Advantages for home treatment
- More communication with staff
- Provided help more readily
- Opportunity to plan and make decisions
- Less anxious and stressed
- Relationships less disrupted
- Daily routine less disrupted
- People expressed fewer negative attitudes
- Treated with more dignity and respect
- Provided more support

Advantages for hospital treatment
- Felt more safe
- Less difficult to separate emotionally

Average length of stay in home treatment—26 days
Average number of nursing care visits—48

Table 7.4

Cost Analysis of Home Treatment Program

- Home treatment program per diem—$139.78
- Hospital per diem—$637.00
- Average cost per episode, home treatment—$3,634.28 (26 days × $139.78)
- Average cost hospital—$17,836.00 (28 days ×$637.00)
- Daily nursing hours, hospital—8 ($205.68)
- Daily nursing hours, home treatments—2 ($123.29)

Case history of mobile crisis home treatment of chronic schizophrenia—Ken, aged 42

Ken is 42, single, and homeless, literally living on a bench in downtown Kitchener, Ontario, for the past year.

He refuses all help, including social assistance, and believes he has no need for money. From time to time he is persuaded to stay at a nearby hostel for homeless men, but he refuses to bathe or change his clothes, so eventually they have to ask him to leave. He was recently re-admitted to the hostel because of growing community concern about his living on a bench in the cold weather; local people give him food and offer him money, which he declines, telling them to give it to somebody who needs it more. Staff at the hostel, the House of Friendship, referred him to Hazelglen, the MCHT service.

April 11, psychiatrist visit to hostel

History obtained from Ken and staff members. He is single, has always been a loner, and worked in a factory until 13 years ago when he became mentally ill. He said he had been fired "for setting up the wrong chemical," had physically assaulted his mother, spent a night in jail, and then ended up at the hostel showing signs of psychosis. He has been homeless for 13 years, has resisted all attempts to get him treated, and has never fit in to various group homes and hostels.

He appeared very unkempt and filthy, with a long, straggly beard, and an old woolen hat, covering up a prominent sebaceous cyst protruding from his forehead. He was very thought disordered and delusional.

Regarding his father, he said: "I go and see my father—he's a doctor—he's military and government and so forth, and all this type of thing . . . he doesn't put out his name—he has an attorney behind him—he just uses a short form—that's why I don't know his name." Regarding his mother, "she had something to do with inventing journalism—government secretaries and all that" He did not want any money, saying he does not need it. He did not know the year, month, or day.

A diagnosis of chronic schizophrenia was made; his GAF score was 25. The only people he would take notice of were the police, who had taken a kindly interest in him over the years. Because he followed no one's direction or advice except police officers', the treatment plan was to ask the police to "tell him to take injections of medicine" (not in any coercive "law enforcement fashion"); otherwise, he likely would have to be admitted involuntarily to hospital.

April 19, hostel visit by case manager

Although at first reluctant to take this role, a police officer told Ken he should take an injection of medicine; 25 mg of pipotiazine (a depot injectable antipsychotic) was injected intramuscularly.

April 21, 24; phone call to staff
No side effects, no improvement.

May 8, staff phone call from
Ken drooling and stiff (extrapyramidal side effects)—he accepted 2 mg of benztropine (anti-parkinson drug).

May 9, hostel visit by case manager
More lucid, oriented in time, staff report he is more sociable.

May 17
Ken taken to the hospital out-patient clinic for an antipsychotic injection, in order to get him used to going there; still drooling. Gave permission for us to speak with his mother, who had shown a recent interest in him after hearing about his improvement.

May 19, psychiatrist visit to hostel
Staff reports more compliant with grooming, more aware of time, accepted money from social services, more interaction with staff. Drooling still, but not taking benztropine consistently. Less psychotic talk, willing to continue taking medicine, better eye contact.

May 31, interviewed on street corner downtown
Still delusional—more focused.

June 6
Mother located—gave history. Staff report Ken stable.

June 7, hostel visit by case manager
Ken could not be found. Staff says he refuses to visit his mother.

June 14
Taken to clinic for injection, more clear conversation.

June 15, phone contact with staff
Very difficult to engage Ken in any activities.

June 19, phone contact
Ken initiates conversation, is clear and logical, and has purchased a pair of shoes (major step—he had clung on to his filthy dilapidated shoes until now).

June 28, phone contact

Decreased delusions.

July 20, hostel visit by case manager

Ken not available. Staff reports he still denies any need for material items; one staff member has become his trustee.

July 26

Given tour of Achievement in Motion, a rehabilitation facility. Showed little interest in attending. Delusions increase when one talks about his family.

August 15

Two unsuccessful attempts made to meet with Ken. Staff reports he is resistant to any attempts to involve him in any activities. Discharge from home treatment to team at the clinic. Now taking pipotiazine 100 mg every three weeks. Ken was successfully placed in a group home and remains there to this day, attending the clinic regularly.

Total interviews attended: 5
Total direct hours: 11
Total indirect hours: 3

Points Illustrated in this Case History

The successful outcome of Ken's treatment hinged upon the unorthodox use of the police, who took some persuading, to get him to take anti-psychotic medicine—an example of "thinking outside the box" which is sometimes necessary in MCHT.

Ken's need for interpersonal distance was respected; often he would not be there when prearranged visits were made. We got around that by working with two very dedicated hostel staff, coaching them about what was needed to treat Ken, and by a willingness to meet with him on the street, which he preferred. Attention was given to practical problems, such as social service money, shoes, and clothes.

Case History of Chronic Schizophrenia—Mary, Aged 49

Mary is 49 years old, has chronic schizophrenia, and has had numerous involuntary mental hospital admissions, usually because she is hearing voices and behaves violently towards her family. When she is well, she does simple work in her sister-in-law's cleaning business; her husband is on social assistance. She usually refuses to attend psychiatric out-patient clinics and is non-compliant taking medication; a worker visits her from the local mental health association.

It was this worker who called a mobile crisis assessment service, who, in turn referred her to Hazelglen Mobile Crisis Home Treatment on December 16. She had been discharged from the local mental hospital in October to the care of her elderly aunt, with whom she was living. Her aunt Lily had become alarmed by her behavior; in particular, she had been "waving scissors around" and was up most of the night, screaming at voices.

December 17, home visit by case manager and psychiatrist

When phoned, she declined home treatment; we decided to make a home visit anyway. Mary, who did not object to our visit, smoked constantly, was vague and evasive, and could not provide any useful history.

Aunt Lily gave the following history: she had been admitted to the mental hospital in October because she was hearing voices and had been threatening to kill her husband. Since discharge, she had been hearing voices and talking at night, pounding on the floor, screaming, "You're going to get it." She laughed uncontrollably, neglected her self-care, smoked constantly, and stored her cigarette butts in the freezer.

Lily's husband was said to have Alzheimer's Disease. Lily could not breathe properly because of the smoke and had given Mary an ultimatum—that she must take medicine or she would have to go back to the hospital. The family were concerned that "she is now acting the same way as before they took her away."

It was clear that Mary was perilously close to being admitted to the hospital involuntarily again. She was not likely to take oral medicine, so she was offered an injection. She said she would take it "just this once." Twenty-five mg of zuclopenthixol acetate (a depot injection that lasts 24–48 hours) was given, the aunt was given instructions about what to expect, and some tablets of trihexyphenidyl (an anti-parkinson medicine) were left in case of extrapyramidal side effects.

December 19, telephone contact with aunt

Mary was resting more, and had not shown any threatening behavior.

December 21, home visit by case manager

Lily said Mary was "more like herself" less restless, less talking to self. Mary allowed the case manager to give an injection of zuclopenthixol decanoate, 50 mg (a longer-acting depot antipsychotic). Mary was dismissive of the case manager, refused to be engaged, and said "no more needles."

December 27, telephone contact

No side effects, doing much better.

December 30, home visit by case manager

Aunt reports Mary is becoming louder, more restless, she feels the effect of the medicine is wearing off; however, Mary is more receptive to the visit.

December 31, home visit by case manager

Injection of zuclopenthixol, 50 mg.

January 2, telephone contact

More settled.

January 7, home visit

Talking incessantly, sleeps at night. House very cold, furnace not working. Case manager will refer aunt Lily's husband for placement and respite care.

January 8, home visit

Zuclopenthixol 100 mg given. Mary is starting to show stereotypical arm movements—strange gestures.

January 12

Case manager accompanied her to lab for blood tests.

January 19, telephone contact

Mary returned to her husband last night—still has some preoccupation with voices, but is not doing the hand gestures.

Mary had 10 more visits, and by May 6 was much more stable, was working at cleaning, and was able to go for injections to her family doctor's office. She rejected any other psychiatric care, but was still being visited by her worker from the mental health association.

Total home visits: 18
Phone contacts: 5

Points Illustrated in this Case History:

This patient would certainly have been admitted if home treatment were not available. An assertive approach was taken, going to the home in spite of the patient declining treatment on the phone. Rapid control of psychotic symptoms using short-acting depot antipsychotic medicine was achieved. The family was very tolerant and supportive.

The patient, although psychotic, non-compliant, and lacking insight, was passively accepting of help, allowing an injection on the first visit. Most of the treatment was done through the aunt; the patient never gave much information about herself and could not be engaged in any discussion. Practical help was provided for family, referring the demented uncle for respite care in an attempt to decrease caregiver burden.

The Home Treatment team stayed on until she could be stable enough with care from her worker and family doctor.

TREATMENT OF BORDERLINE PERSONALITY DISORDER

> *"Do not hospitalize a patient with borderline personality disorder for any more than 48 hours. My self-destructive episodes—one leading right into another—came only after my first and subsequent hospitalizations, after I learned the system was usually obligated to respond."*

> A recovered patient (Williams, 1998)

Not enough is known about mobile crisis home treatment of patients with borderline personality disorder (BPD) to provide much clinical guidance; this section is therefore more of a discussion.

The literature suggest that MCHT may have a role, and are full of warnings and cautions about hospital admission. These range from always avoid hospitalization, to admit for no more than one or two weeks. Hospital treatment is almost universally regarded as having major side effects: fostering regression, increasing behavior problems, and encouraging dependence and repeated admissions.

Gunderson (2001) describes four levels of care for BPD level IV (hospital), III (Residential/Partial Hospitalization), II (Intensive Out-patient), and I (Out-patient). Most patients use brief hospitalization (Level IV) for crises, but otherwise remain in (Level I) out-patient care. Treatment delivery models between these two levels should be available in order to avoid admissions and keep them short. Gunderson recommends greater development and use of Level II, intensive outpatient care, including that which is modeled on assertive community treatment, which shares some components with MCHT. This level of care can also reduce the need for residential and partial hospitalization (Level III). Hospital admissions longer than 1–2 weeks encourage regression and idealized or dependent attachment; when longer hospital stays do occur, it's not usually because they are therapeutically necessary, but because appropriate step down services are unavailable (Levels II or III). Health care systems that do not have all the levels available will be cost ineffective. The importance of graduated and careful discharge planning is brought home by the observation that many suicides occur just after discharge or just before a mandatory discharge.

Gunderson's model of intensive out-patient care recommends the use of self-assessment groups and case management. Such groups can be effective with as few as three members, with flexible attendance requirements, and can easily be incorporated into an MCHT team; the Manchester Home Option Service described in Chapter 3 combines MCHT with a group therapy approach (although not specifically for patients with borderline personality disorder). The success of these programs depends on their ability to "offer sufficient holding to counter regressive flights and to support sustained community living" (Gunderson, 2001).

American Psychiatric Association Practice Guidelines (APA, 2001) only mention partial hospitalization as an alternative to "brief hospitalization." Indications for one or another of these are included in: Table 7.5 and Table 7.6.

Hospital admission for several of these indications may possibly be avoided by MCHT, using the 20 components of in-patient care that can be delivered to a patient at home, provided that caregiver support was commensurate with acuity. For example, from Table 7.5: non-adherence with out-patient treatment, complex comorbidity, and symptoms of sufficient severity, could be managed by such elements as intensive home visiting, extended hours, working closely with caregivers and families, and 24-hour emergency availability.

MCHT could also manage some patients showing transient psychotic episodes and symptoms of sufficient severity (see Table 7.6).

Table 7.5

Borderline Personality Disorder: Indications for Partial Hospitalization
(or Brief Hospitalization if Partial Not Available)

- Dangerous impulsive behavior unable to be managed with out-patient treatment
- Non-adherence with out-patient treatment and a deteriorating clinical picture
- Complex comorbidity that requires more intensive clinical assessment of response to treatment
- Symptoms of sufficient severity to interfere with functioning, work, or family life that are unresponsive to out-patient treatment

Table 7.6

Borderline Personality Disorder: Indications for Brief Hospitalization

---

- Imminent danger to others
- Loss of control of suicidal impulses or serious suicide attempt
- Transient psychotic episodes associated with loss of impulse control or impaired judgment
- Symptoms of sufficient severity to interfere with functioning, work, or family life that are unresponsive to out-patient treatment and partial hospitalization

---

Paris (2002) is very clear about the need to avoid hospital admission. He states that it makes sense to admit patients for treatment of brief psychosis and life-threatening suicide attempts to assess precipitating factors and review treatment plans. The value of hospital treatment is much less clear for suicidal threats, minor overdoses, or self-mutilation. Once hospitalization is introduced, admission can become repetitive, because the patient becomes suicidal again shortly after discharge. Hospitalization is a two-edged sword, because the psychiatric ward can reinforce the very behaviors that therapy is trying to extinguish. Borderline patients self-mutilate more in hospital since patients who cut themselves or overdose receive more, not less nursing care, and for patients with poor social support, hospital can provide a reinforcing level of social contact.

Paris discusses litigation, and the fear of it, that causes clinicians to admit BPD patients against their better clinical judgment. The issues he raises are particularly relevant to clinicians working in community mental health services, like mobile crisis home treatment, that try to keep these patients out of hospital. Only a very small fraction of completed suicides leads to litigation, and the majority, 80%, end with a decision for the clinician. The vast majority involve patients treated for major Axis I disorders, usually focusing on whether the patients were discharged too early, not whether they should have been admitted in the first place. Litigation after completed suicide of a chronically suicidal patient (often the case with BPD patients) is rare. When the clinician is found liable, it is usually not just because of the suicide—most courts know that suicide cannot always be prevented and do not routinely hold clinicians responsible when it happens. Liability depends on other issues, such as gross clinical misjudgments, the failure to assess patients carefully, and the absence of adequate records documenting the management plan. Involving the family in the treatment of chronic suicidal patients makes litigation less likely. The goals of meeting with family members are the same as with all MCHT patients: to inform them of the rationale behind treatment, to educate them about the management plan, and to obtain cooperation with therapy. Family members, who themselves have had to endure a patient's suicidality, will feel supported by being brought into such an alliance. If there is an unfavorable outcome, they will have less reason to feel angry and excluded.

Hospitalization is of unproven value in preventing suicide by these patients, and fear of potential litigation should not be the basis for admission. Empirical evidence that clinical interventions have any systematic effect on suicide completion is notably lacking. Chronic suicidal behavior in BPD patients can best be understood as a way of communicating distress. If an alternative to hospital is required, Paris suggests the use of partial hospitalization, which is effective because of its highly structured program.

Dawson and MacMillan (1993) believe the worst and most damaging behavior of borderline patients are products of their unfortunate relationships with health care professionals and institutions. In the interpersonal relations between the patients and the health care organization, the "currency" of the transaction includes suicidal threats and behavior, self-harm, symptoms of illness, loss of control, conflict over medications, and helplessness. They advocate "relationship management," a method of dealing with borderline patients that avoids or undoes these transactions and is based on four principles, one of which is to avoid hospitalization. The "currency" of the transaction between patient and clinician is vastly expanded in hospital to include seclusion rooms, one-to-one observation, physical and chemical restraints, control of "sharps," cheeked pills, hoarded pills, vomiting, heavier overdosing, deeper cutting, fire setting, suicide pacts, elopement, breaking windows, starting fights, interfering with other patients, hitting nurses, refusing to eat, refusing to get up, refusing to go to bed, provocative sexual behavior, and more.

Gunderson (2001) and Paris (2002) suggest partial hospitalization as a successful alternative to hospital (Piper, Rosier, Azim, & Joyce, 1993). However, for this to work, a patient must be organized and motivated enough to get themselves to the day hospital every day, on time, and to remain there for the duration of the program—day after day, week after week. In Piper's study, there was a 42% drop-out rate. Thus, mobile crisis home treatment may have a role to play, but research studies show mixed results.

Links (1998) states that assertive community treatment (ACT), which, as we have seen, shares many features with MCHT, has been applied to patients with personality disorders. The effectiveness with this group parallels that of patients with chronic psychotic disorders; i.e., declines in hospitalization, increased reports of satisfaction with the program, and better overall compliance. The effects of ACT on symptom improvement is less clear, particularly the effect on the affective, cognitive, and behavioral symptoms of personality disorders.

Studies of home-based treatment for personality disorder patients are scanty. They suggest that patients with personality disorders don't do as well as those with Axis I diagnoses. Unfortunately, none of the studies distinguish between the various personality disorders; they are all lumped together. For example, Tyrer and Merson (1994) compare the home-based treatment and hospital-oriented treatment of emergency patients—with, and without personality disorders. Home-based treatment was superior and resulted in lower use of beds, but only for patients without personality disorder. Those with personality disorder showed greater improvement in depressive symptoms and social functioning when referred to the hospital-oriented service, a finding that does not support the principle of avoiding hospital. However, it is impossible to draw conclusions about the implications for treatment of BPD; of the 50 personality disorder patients studied, only 8 had BPD (emotionally labile in ICD 10 classification).

In a study of the St. Albans (U.K.) Community Treatment Team (profiled in Chapter 3), patients with personality disorder also fared less well than those with other diagnoses (Brimblecombe & O'Sullivan, 1999). They were much less likely to be accepted by the team—37.5% (about 70% for schizophrenia and 70% mood disorders), and more likely to be admitted at assessment—25% (18.5% schizophrenia and 7% mood disorder), and during treatment—22% (15.7% schizophrenia and 18.9% mood disorders). However, what proportion of these patients had BPD is not known.

Brimblecombe (2001c) states that increased admissions of personality disorder patients may relate to impulsiveness and the difficulty with which such individuals often have in negotiating in a meaningful way. The initial forming of rapport and development of a relationship is of tremendous importance in working with suicidal patients. Part of the relationship building involves the worker being honest with the patient about the risk of suicide and, in turn, the patient being honest with them. The worker offers help to the patient, who in turn offers to stay alive long enough to give the worker an opportunity to help them. It is a negotiation. Patients with personality disorder have less ability to negotiate and form supportive relationships with others, a prerequisite to working with suicidal patients in the community. Or is it? Perhaps, with borderline patients, the clinician has to negotiate differently. Dawson and MacMillan (1993) point out that in the case of borderline patients, the *process* level of communication is paramount; there is more important meaning to be found in the *interpersonal negotiations* than in the events the patient says brought about his state, and in his presentation of distress. Clues that the process of communication may be paramount in the interaction with a patient include incongruity between situation and affect, exaggeration, vagueness, an immediate sense of failure in the clinician, and the effect on the clinician, causing him to feel a sense of urgency, resentment, and strong and immediate sense of responsibility. The assumption of the usual role of helper and comforter is not useful here. Instead, they suggest such techniques as responding with empathic neutrality, using paradoxical statements, and assuming a position contrary to assigned attributes, such as saying that you don't know what should be done about the patient's situation instead of reassuring him that you can handle the crisis. If successful, these techniques can lead the borderline patient to switch to a more positive and competent mode of being, and therefore better able to negotiate their care in a home treatment setting.

SIDEBAR

Practical Tips

- They are less likely to run away from their own home or destroy their own stuff
- There will be increased expectation to control behavior—from self and family
- There is diffuse transference with team of staff, not one worker
- A discharge date is set, which at admission, which limits intensity of attachment and dependency
- It is short-term
- Limits and boundaries are set from the start
- Splitting is anticipated and addressed
- A high level of support is provided ad lib whenever the patient wants (within limits set)
- Goals are limited, past issues are not addressed, do not open patient up
- It is in the here and now; emphasize the positive
- Patients are given responsibility for their actions, autonomy is fostered, patients are provided with choices
- Dialectical behavior therapy techniques are to cope with crises and affect

If workers could be less anxious about litigation and more mindful of the negative effects of hospitalization and it's unproven efficacy in preventing suicide, maybe less patients would be admitted by home treatment teams. Not all staff's anxiety is about litigation though. In the U.K., community mental health services have received a lot of negative press, following some widely publicized incidents in which psychiatric patients injured someone, or committed suicide; enough to make admission—the "path of least resistance," attractive.

One mobile home crisis service that has developed comfort, and competence in treating patients with borderline personality disorder is the acute adult home support team in Edmonton, Alberta (described in Chapter 3).

Their approach is described in the sidebar, Table 7.7.

Case Histories from Adult Acute Home Support Team, Edmonton, Alberta

Bernice, aged 53

Bernice has been referred to the home support team 13 times since 1993. The majority of contacts took place between 1994 and 1995. A number of diagnoses (once, eight were given concurrently) were assigned over the years, but borderline personality disorder is the primary diagnosis overall. She has had contacts with psychiatric professionals since at least 1975 for mood disorder and alcoholism.

An alcoholic father and emotionally cool mother influenced Bernice's early years. She had a child at age 15 that was adopted, and later at 18 had another pregnancy, which required she marry the father. The marriage was never a good one, as Bernice's drinking and extramarital affairs caused strain and her husband was physically abusive. She frequently felt suicidal and self-mutilated as a result. She required frequent hospitalizations in the mid-1990s due to an increasing risk of self-harm following her divorce. The home support team prevented many hospitalizations after it was started in 1993; frequent support in the home or by telephone was enough to contain her. She always settled quickly from various personal issues she faced. She rarely had more than four or five visits per three-week stay with the team, and a half hour or less could contain her. She also began working and attending support groups, which she valued for the social contact, but also for the attention. The use of dialectical behavioral therapy (DBT) techniques were implemented, which reduced self-mutilation: distraction techniques were helpful with tolerating unpleasant feelings. Our last contact was four years ago.

Darlene, aged 57

Darlene is well known to the home support team, having been referred 12 times between 1996 and 2001. Eight of these contacts occurred in 1998. Borderline personality disorder is the most prominent diagnosis and the most influential in her need for support. Self-destructive behavior and mutilation are the usual reason for referral. Stress and disappointment are generally also cited as precipitants. She is employed in a managerial position, divorced, and is estranged from her children. Her mother was an alcoholic.

Adult relationships with men were mentally abusive; abandonment was a common theme. She is very well known to crisis services and the ambulance service due to frequent attempts at suicide.

Visits are generally lengthy (one hour) and reassurance is the most frequent technique used. DBT is used to decrease the impact of negative feelings, with some success. Feelings about medications and symptoms of anxiety/depression are reviewed repeatedly. Due to psychotherapy, insight is present, but coping techniques are not. DBT and relaxation techniques augment her intellectual gains. Referrals to the home support team are sometimes used as a reminder to use DBT skills. Hospitalization has not been needed since 1999. Phone calls in between referrals have been an added source of support that substituted for visits to emergency departments or self-harm.

Chapter Eight

Mobile Crisis Home Treatment of Mental Disorders: Part II

"Manic patients are not usually a problem—they usually have something you can help them with—want the window fixed—we give them some leeway with medication—let them know it's not just about medication."

Marcellino Smyth, consultant psychiatrist

"We used to be bad at manics—we have learned to be liberal with diazepam and hold our anxieties—have more faith in the team—and have a lower threshold for admission."

Sue Smith, RN, manager

TREATMENT OF MANIC DISORDER

When one asks MCHT clinicians which patients are difficult to treat in their service, manic patients are often mentioned. However, some report success, and our experience is that MCHT treatment can divert some of these patients from the hospital and shorten the length of admission for many others. Indeed, treatment in the home may have certain advantages for manic patients, whose behavior presents specific challenges to an in-patient milieu. Manic patients are often irritable, self-centered, grandiose, and demanding—characteristics that can quickly bring them into conflict with the rules and restrictions that are part of life on an in-patient ward. Busy nurses are not able to give these patients the leeway and control they need. Their over-activity, irritability, increased social and sexual drive, and lack of empathy for others causes concern for how they will affect other patients, many of whom are very vulnerable.

Table 8.1

Manic Disorder: Indications for Hospital Admission

- Patient lacks capacity to cooperate with treatment, cannot care for themselves adequately, or provide reliable feedback to clinician
- Patient at risk of suicide or harm to others; rapid mood fluctuation, especially if combined with substance abuse make risk assessment particularly difficult
- Patient lacks psychosocial supports; recovery from mania is helped by an environment that encourages safety, constructive activity, positive interaction, and compliance with treatment. If home environment lacks these features and exposes patient to undesirable activities, such as alcohol and drug abuse, hospitalization may be considered
- Other factors: complicating psychiatric or general medical conditions, engaging in bizarre or imprudent behavior that may endanger important relationships, severe psychotic features, ultra-rapid cycling

---

Of course, these features of manic patients can make it impossible for caregivers and the community to tolerate them also, but some of these patients do manage to stay within the limits of their environment's tolerance, and home treatment may be the best option. As with other disorders, the American Psychiatric Association "Practice Guidelines for the Treatment of Patients with Bipolar Disorder" (1994) recommends the least restrictive setting that is likely to allow for safe and effective treatment. This description of treatment of manic patients is based on the above guidelines and the revised practice guidelines (American Psychiatric Association 2002); Frances, Docherty, and Kahn's, "The Expert Consensus Guideline Series, Treatment of Bipolar Disorder" (1996) is also used.

Frances, et al. (1996) provide the following guidelines for level of care.

Almost always admit for one of the following:

- High risk for suicide, violence, or severe deterioration in self-care
- Severe psychosis (e.g., delusions influence behavior)

Usually admit for one of the following:

- Unlikely to cooperate with out-patient treatment
- Less severe psychotic symptoms
- Poor judgment about spending, business, or sexual behavior
- Poor psychosocial supports, or behavior that is alienating family

Sometimes admit for the following problems, depending on their number and severity:

- Poor general medical health
- Rapid cycling
- First episode of mania
- Mixed episode or dysphoric mania
- Has failed 1 or 2 out-patient trials of mood stabilizers
- Clinician has never treated this patient before

Frances, Dochert, and Kahn (1996), state "The experts set a low threshold for hospitalizing manic patients." On the other hand, manic patients themselves set a high threshold for hospitalization; the denial of their illness (anosognosia) is a frequent component of the disorder itself. Although home treatment of manic patients can be tricky, it may have a special role in this disorder because, in many jurisdictions, the laws governing involuntary admission often don't address manic patients' situations: the criteria are confined to threat of serious physical harm to self or others. It may be difficult to involuntarily admit the manic patient with grandiose delusions, over-activity, excessive spending, and reckless, irresponsible behavior if they are not an immediate danger to themselves or others. Or, one can admit them for a short while, but within a few days they sign out against medical advice or manage to improve enough, or "behave themselves" sufficiently, such that they no longer meet the criteria for involuntary admission. For these reasons, mobile crisis home treatment sometimes can be the only option, even if hospital treatment is the clinician's number one choice.

"Unlikely to cooperate with out-patient treatment" is one of the most common reasons for hospital admission. This lack of cooperation usually takes the form of refusing to attend, or missing appointments, poor adherence to medication regimes, giving inaccurate feedback to the clinician, and indulging in behavior guaranteed to make their illness worse and get them into trouble. Home treatment can sometimes engage the uncooperative manic patient because of its proactive, flexible approach and its capacity to tolerate their capricious behaviors. The more formal, structured, rulebound, typical in-patient unit or out-patient clinic can seem more like a challenge to a manic patient, rather than a place of healing and recovery.

Apart from high risk of suicide and violence and severe psychosis, the other clinical situations that can lead to admission, such as psychotic symptoms, poor judgment, and poor psychosocial supports, can often be addressed by such features of home treatment as close monitoring two or even three times a day, enlisting the family's aid, and 24-hour emergency coverage.

In the American Psychiatric Association "Practice Guidelines" (1994), specific goals of psychiatric management are

1. Establishing and maintaining a therapeutic alliance
2. Monitoring the patient's psychiatric status
3. Providing education about bipolar disorder
4. Enhancing treatment compliance
5. Promoting regular patterns of activity and wakefulness
6. Promoting understanding of and adaptation to the psychosocial effects of bipolar disorder.
7. Identifying new episodes early
8. Reducing the morbidity and sequelae of bipolar disorder

These goals will now be addressed in the context of the key components and daily operations of home treatment outlined in Chapters 4 and 6.

Approach to the Patient

At the end of the day, in spite of MCHT's greater capacity to adjust to a manic patient's behavior, the clinician sometimes just has to accept it is not working and admit the patient voluntarily, or involuntarily. As in other serious psychiatric disorders, much depends on the patient's attitude to the home treatment team, the family's relationship with the patient and their capacity to deal with the illness, and the specifics of their symptoms and behavior and consequent risk. There are many manic patients who cannot be treated at home, especially bipolar I manics with psychosis.

Sometimes MCHT can work after a brief initial hospital admission, even after one or two days—enough to get some sleep and start on medication.

A good place to start in engaging these patients is to implicitly acknowledge to oneself and to the patient that they have the power and control in the therapeutic relationship. Furthermore, at first blush, the patient cannot see anything that the clinicians have that he wants; he has no need of their services. A humble, tolerant approach, using humor and giving the patient control, can help diminish his irritability and antagonism. Sometimes this entails humoring the patient, and smacks of manipulation. Being willing to apologize when they take offence, acknowledging their claims to knowing better than you, and engaging with their intelligence and narcissism can soften the resistance and open up negotiation. Usually, one can find something they need; for example, help with a conflictual relationship—"I'll help keep your father off your back"—or help with an employment or social assistance issue. Or, one can point out possible consequences of their behavior—in a neutral, non-threatening, and non-judgmental way; e.g., "If you continue to drive recklessly, your license might get taken away—maybe you should give the car keys to your wife for the next week." Or, you can present them with your own dilemmas: "Your family is upset, what should we do? If this carries on, we'll be in trouble. Dr. X is worried, he wants me to admit you to the hospital, but maybe we can handle this situation at home." You can help the family to negotiate with them—usually they want something, such as money, that can be bargained for, say, taking medicine. A "motivational interviewing" approach, as is used in addiction counseling, can be helpful—listening to them and pointing out when they acknowledge indirectly that they are having difficulties that can be attributed to a mental health problem. It is important to avoid the appearance of being controlling. Often, concurrent with the elevated mood, one can identify and target, in the patient's own words, such dysphoric symptoms as feeling hyper, out of control, edgy, or cranky, that one can offer to relieve with medicine, thereby providing them with a rationale for taking it.

Assessment

The approach to assessment will depend on whether this is the patient's first diagnosed manic episode or whether they have a known previous history. If it is the first, the initial assessment will have to be accompanied by a great deal of education for the family and the patient, who may have difficulty conceptualizing the disturbed behavior as an illness; for example, in adolescents and young adults, manic illness can appear as misbehavior. One advantage of hospital treatment is that it is a powerful reminder that the person is "sick"—"if I am in the hospital—I guess I must be sick."

It is important to quickly identify four things: what has made the situation a crisis, what symptoms and behavior present what degree of risk—to the patient and their family—what is the capacity of the MCHT team and the family to exert sufficient influence on the patient, and what is the family's capacity to tolerate the patient remaining at home. To carry out home treatment of a manic patient, it is essential that the team are able to engage the patient, to find "a hook"—a sense that they begin to look to you for help—with something (even though it may not be a conventional clinical need). It is important that the relationship with the family is workable; if there is a lot of antagonism, pushing and shoving, with the patient trampling on the rights of others in the house, it is not going to work.

If the patient is psychotic, with delusions and hallucinations, the degree to which they influence the patient's behavior is important to assess—and what behavior the delusions may lead to. Writing "a great novel," or "talking to God" at home is less of a worry than harassing strangers in the street because of paranoia. Frequent areas of concern that need risk assessment are spending, driving, alcohol and substance abuse, aggressiveness, comorbid medical conditions, behavior towards the neighbors, and insisting on going to work or school; any of these issues can lead to demands for admission if not adequately dealt with. A patient who insists on driving around recklessly at night, snorting cocaine, and pressing his attentions on women in bars is not a candidate for home treatment. However, such a patient can present a clinical and ethical dilemma: it may be impossible to admit them to hospital because they don't meet the local criteria for involuntary admission, and yet their behavior and lack of treatment adherence make one uncomfortable at the prospect of assuming clinical responsibility for their care and being seen as accountable for harmful actions.

Medication

Rapid control of over-activity, irritability, and insomnia is very important; it is likely that most caregivers could not stand more than two or three days of round-the-clock manic behavior. This requires liberal use of benzodiazepine, anti-anxiety medication such as lorazepam, and the use of atypical anti-psychotic medications such as olanzapine. Having said this, it is important to not appear as an agent of chemical control, and when approaching the subject of medication to give patients some leeway, some sense that they have control. This can be achieved by giving them and their caregivers a range of dosages—some room to move—and adopting an attitude of inviting them to try out these medicines and go at their own pace. Reminding them of the effect of their behavior on the family may be productive: "How would you feel as a parent if your kid had not slept for four days? Sometimes, by listening carefully, one can elicit admissions of dysphoric symptoms or negative aspects of their behavior accompanying the high mood, and medicine can be offered as a solution; for example, "It will make you less likely to fly off the handle, feel more in control." It is often necessary for staff to observe the patient to make sure they actually take their medicine, once or twice a day; sometimes the caregivers can do this under staff supervision. It is not unusual for these patients to chafe at being at home for twice-daily visits; they have busy lives and may be out when you call—we have had to do treatment by voice mail for a few days. If adherence is poor, and the situation urgent, a short-acting depot injection of zupenthixol acetate is very helpful, as long as one can monitor the patient frequently.

Mood stabilizers are required, of course, and can be prescribed in the same spirit—"try it for the next week." Lithium and valproate require monitoring blood tests, and the patient will have to be taken to the laboratory by staff or family; some services will take blood at home.

Working with the Family and Social Networks

Education is especially important in treating mania at home. The family need to know what behavior and symptoms to expect—what they may be in for, and how to respond. Teach and model how to approach the patient, how to avoid getting into arguments, or at least pick their battles wisely. Establishing a normal, regular, 24-hour cycle of sleeping and eating is important, and creating a low-key atmosphere, with decreased stimulation. Write out a schedule of activities, with the aim of decreasing, channeling, and structuring over-activity. Identifying a space that can be the patient's own for their over-active, untidy behavior, can help make life tolerable for everyone in the house.

The family may need to be firm, however, especially in regard to driving and spending. They need to be alerted to the financial aspects of mania, and the importance of restricting access to credit cards, chequebooks, and bank accounts, and how to approach the bank and make the necessary legal arrangements regarding power of attorney, etc. Get them to enlist the help of other family members to spread the burden. Caregivers need to be reassured that they can bring the patient to the hospital for admission at any time—that this would not be a failure; or, they may need to be coached to call the police if the situation becomes too risky.

Education

Because of the nature of mania, caregivers will play a role in all phases of the illness; patients don't disclose their foolish, excessive, or risky behavior to others and can present surprisingly normal to the clinician for a half hour interview, deliberately "holding it together." Families frequently say that they have understood the patient's illness for the first time during an episode of home treatment; recurrent crisis treatments in hospital don't always lend themselves to family involvement with care and education. In home treatment, they "live" the illness, and education given in the context of their assisting with treatment is powerfully effective. The autonomous, cyclical, self-limiting nature of the illness needs to be explained, as well as the need to identify new episodes early; sometimes an MCHT team will meet the patient for the first time in hospital for early discharge, but can avoid hospital the next time, by encouraging early referral. A life chart provides a valuable display of the course of the illness and episode frequency, polarity, severity, frequency, and relationship, if any, to environmental stressors, as well as response to treatment.

Monitoring the Patient's Psychiatric Status

Careful, regular monitoring of mood and behavior is vital to successful drug treatment. Both the family and the patient need to keep mood charts, chronicling daily highs and lows and behavior such as hours of sleep. They need to be alerted to the possibility of rapid switches to depression, depending on the previous course of the illness and its natural cycle. Suicide risk needs to be established and discussed; mixed affective states or dysphoric mania can present a high risk.

Case Histories of Mania

Hannah, aged 50

Hannah is a 50-year-old arts administrator, married with two sons. She was referred by her family doctor at the request of her husband, who became concerned about the sudden onset of strange behavior the night before.

She had been under some stress at work, being heavily involved in some political infighting around the selection of a new executive director of the organization she worked for. Apart from some sleepless nights, she had remained well until the night before. After a stressful committee meeting, she had gone out with some friends for dinner, when she started to behave strangely. She had danced to music on the sidewalk, appeared to be listening to music in her head, waved her arms around, and talked incessantly using rhymes and puns.

Fifteen years previously, she had an episode of severe psychosis and spent ten weeks in a psychiatric ward. It had been a traumatic experience—once she was held down and given an injection and was locked in a seclusion room.

June 19, initial assessment at home by case manager

She sat cross-legged on the floor, mute at first, later talking in a whisper, saying she was getting messages coming at her from all directions. She gestured bizarrely and spoke nonsensically. Her husband James said she had slept little and ate little in the previous 24 hours. She said, "I want to work this out by myself," and did not want James or the case manager to interfere. James was very patient and supportive and appeared confident in his ability to handle things. They were both very keen to avoid hospital admission, because of the experience 15 years before. Toward the end of the interview, she became a bit aggressive, barring the case manager's exit at the door, saying she had not been given enough time, even though the interview had lasted over an hour.

June 19, later; psychiatrist's visit

She greeted the psychiatrist with a dreamy smile, stood, or wandered from room to room for most of the interview. She would not answer questions appropriately, talked about difficulties with her thinking, and said, "Mine is an old language." She came close to the psychiatrist, smiled intensely and seductively, putting her hand on his knee. She was difficult to engage and seemed uncomfortable with clinical questions; it would be easy to frighten her off, and therefore the interview was curtailed.

When told that she was likely ill, similar to 15 years previously, she was surprisingly acquiescent and agreed to take some medicine. She was prescribed trifluoroperazine, an anti-psychotic (this was before atypical anti-psychotics were available), to be supervised by her husband.

June 20, home visit

Slept 10 hours, took medicine. Sometimes answered questions in French, asked "where are all the little children," seemed confused and forgetful.

June 21, home visit

Slept well, speech still tangential, smiling inappropriately.

June 22, home visit

Slept well, visited neighbor.

June 23, phone contact at weekend

Some confusion at times; talked of "spinning" and being unable to settle at bedtime.

June 26, home visit

Feeling "euphoric," avoids questions about medication, James reports that she is more reluctant to take them, and missed this morning's dose. She complained of being sedated and dulled mentally and insisted on going to work today. Affect is giddy, talks in rhymes and puns. Case manager attempted a lot of negotiation, cajoling, to continue to take medicine, and find a substitute person for work.

June 27–July 6, phone contact only, refused visits

July 6, home visit, psychiatrist

Improving, behavior more normal.

July 13, home visit, psychiatrist

Appears back to normal, still taking medicine. After this time, she declined most visits, but the case manager kept in touch by phone. She refused to take a mood stabilizer, and the trifluoperazine was gradually discontinued. She allowed two more home visits by the psychiatrist, on August 3 and 27. The role of stress became clearer. She was very grateful for the help, and offered to write a supportive letter to the provincial health minister about our service.

Points Illustrated

This patient was quite resistant to psychiatric intervention—not surprising, given her previous experience which eventually may have been repeated were it not for home treatment. The role of a confident, tolerant, insightful caregiver, was paramount, and their relationship was good enough to enable him to exert influence on her.

   The team adopted a soft-pedaling approach; anything firmer, and this very bright, opinionated woman would have slammed the door shut. The team negotiated and allowed her to set the pace, to decline needed visits, and communicate by phone, relying on her husband to monitor her mental state. With early administration of anti-psychotic medication and daily home visits, she was able to get sufficient sleep, and symptoms were rapidly controlled.

Megan, aged 19

Megan is a teacher's aide taking an enforced break from university studies in another town, which had to be terminated last year due to an episode of severe depression. She lives with her parents in a large house; her father is a dentist and her mother is a homemaker.

   A family friend, Jane, with whom she had been staying overnight, brought her to the hospital 24-hour walk-in crisis clinic very early today. Jane said Megan was "manic"; what prompted the emergency visit was "a convulsion"—some kind of a spell in which Megan's eyes rolled back, she was "not with it," breathed hard, and moaned. They had tried to get her admitted to a hospital during the night in a nearby town, but they did not provide an emergency service.

   Megan behaved inappropriately from the beginning, greeting the psychiatrist carrying a large Snoopy doll, saying, "Do you like Snoopy, can he come in with me, although he does not talk much?" At times, her eyes would roll back and she would appear to lose consciousness and hyperventilate; if one did nothing, she would ask the psychiatrist to make a response, saying "I can't keep this up."

She told her life history, with much emphasis on sexual abuse from an uncle, and talked dramatically about how her kisses thrilled him, she wanted to marry him, and her great disappointment that he had recently married.

She gave a history of depression and cyclical mood swings, when she would become very active, spending a lot of money, including her university tuition money. She had been going to bars alone, drinking heavily, and acting promiscuously.

Her mother had tried to get her admitted two or three months previously, but she had refused. Jane was very concerned at her "self-destructive and risky behavior," going out alone to bars drinking; she had been emotionally labile, and holding on to the doll in a childlike fashion.

There was a strong family history of affective disorder, mainly depression; her mother and cousin had been diagnosed with bipolar affective disorder. Her father was described as very distant, always working, and had a drinking problem. Her parents had severe marital difficulties.

A diagnosis of bipolar affective disorder, manic phase, and likely histrionic personality traits was made.

Megan was adamant about not wanting admission and wanted to keep working at the school. She accepted referral to the mobile crisis treatment service for treatment of mania. Clonazepam (an anti-anxiety drug used in treatment of mania) was prescribed.

April 20 and 21, visit by case manager

Assessment carried out, home treatment explained. Pressured speech, flight of ideas, labile affect.

4 p.m.

Mother called: Megan out of control, running in the rain, and has been dancing on the stage at the school where she works and had been asked to leave. It was impossible to keep her at home, and admission was requested. This time, Megan agreed, saying she could not tolerate home because of extreme frustration with her family; admission was arranged on the hospital psychiatric unit.

April 26

Case manager informed that Megan had self-discharged the night before and had refused to take the lithium (a mood stabilizer) prescribed for her.

April 27

Mother had great difficulty disciplining Megan, was very anxious and frightened of her. Megan was all over the house, intrusive, interfering with everyone, including her two brothers, who also lived at home. She was rude and inappropriate with visitors. She was claiming to "write a novel" and her crafts were all over the house; she was using the phone a lot. The case manager helped the parents gain control. Megan was limited to her bedroom, from which many stimulating articles, such as the phone, were removed. She had to earn privileges by adhering to treatment recommendations and avoiding over stimulation.

Everybody's role in the family was outlined in a written treatment plan, a copy of which was given to everyone, including Megan. The emphasis was on setting boundaries and limits. Megan agreed to this plan.

April 28

Megan continues to be inappropriate and at times bizarre. Mother was over-involving friends, neighbors, and family in her care and asking their opinions about her diagnosis. Megan finally agreed to take lithium and also haloperidol (an anti-psychotic drug), as well as the clonazepam.

8 p.m.

Megan called the on-call worker, asking for admission "to get away from the house"; this was discouraged—there were no beds available anyway. Extra clonazepam was suggested.

April 29

Megan more settled—some extra-pyramidal side effects—stiffness and tremor. Discussed with psychiatrist on phone, haloperidol dose reduced.

May 1, 11 a.m.

Mother called the on-call worker: overwhelmed with Megan and also with husband—thinks he is drinking excessively. Advised to contact self-help group for families of alcoholics—Al-Anon; promised to call back at 4 p.m.

4 p.m.

On-call worker called mother back, as promised; mother more settled—not focusing on husband's drinking—was going to an Al-Anon meeting; feelings validated.

May 3

Mother talked at length about her own problems, with Megan, Megan's boyfriend Jack, her husband's drinking, and her two sons. Megan still has side effects; trihexyphenidyl (anti-Parkinson drug) prescribed. Case manager decided that all members of this disturbed family need help, and will help them obtain it.

May 4, 1:30 a.m.

Megan called the on-call worker; could not sleep, wanted to talk to someone. Had not taken her haloperidol—wanting to stop taking it.

May 4

Meeting with Megan, her mother and Jane. All acknowledged progress.

May 5

Megan improving; one of her brothers had been physically abusive to her—apologized, but declined professional help for himself.

May 7

Meeting with Megan and boyfriend to help with relationship problems.

May 10

Case manager and team social worker meet with Megan and her parents to discuss problems in family as a whole; encouraged parents and brothers to seek counseling.

May 11

Meeeting with Megan and her school principal to discuss her wishes to return to work. He was concerned that it was too soon. Wants Megan to be fully recovered; her mood is still high and she is anxious. Haloperidol discontinued.

May 12

Met Megan at restaurant. Still grandiose—she wants to rent a local theatre for $10,000; insists on applying for jobs.

May 13

Mother phoned on-call; Megan had locked herself in closet after argument with her father. Megan sobbing on phone—wants to kill herself. Case manage met her and mother at the hospital—settled after meeting.

May 15

Discussed over-activity, many inappropriate grandiose ideas. Megan responded to structure and gentle firm direction. Plans to go to Florida for vacation with Jack—discouraged.

May 18

Meeting with boyfriend Jack. Megan prescribed another anti-psychotic drug—perphenazine.

May 20

Phoned on-call worker. Megan "feels rejected by life," rejected after failed job applications. Has suicidal thoughts—of taking all her pills or slashing her wrists. Settled; used closet in her bedroom to calm self. Megan continued to improve, but with many ups and downs on the way. The case manager met with her and a sexual abuse counselor to start working on the childhood sexual abuse issues regarding the uncle. Megan was able to resume her university studies in her home town. Followup was also arranged with the program psychiatrist in his private office.

Length of stay: 90 days
Number of visits: 27
Number of phone calls during office hours: 9
Number of after hours calls to on-call worker: 12

Points Illustrated

The hospital was unable to treat this patient; the family had made two unsuccessful attempts to have her admitted but she refused. When she did agree, she only stayed four days before discharging herself against medical advice and did not take her medicine in hospital. She was not certifiable under Ontario's Mental Health Act.

The case manager was able to manage her by engaging her in a trusting relationship, negotiating with her about every step, and teaching her family how to deal with her behaviors very specifically, with written instructions for everyone.

The family was educated about bipolar disorder. Hospital management was "mimicked," by using her bedroom as a "seclusion room" (in a non-coercive fashion, mainly to decrease stimulation and create some boundaries that the family could live with), and by the use of "privileges."

The case manager met with everybody involved with this patient: family, family friend, boyfriend, and employer. Home treatment deals with not only the patient's immediate family group, but also the wider social context such as work; the aim is to deal with any problems relating to the illness in these various outside groups, with an emphasis on preserving the patient's role functioning.

The family, particularly the mother, was somewhat disturbed; but this was exacerbated by Megan's manic behavior. The case manager dealt not only with the patient but also with the family's pathology, arranging or encouraging help for them.

Telephone support, including after hours, was frequent. Case manager stayed on until patient stable; adequate follow-up was arranged. Even though this patient was quite ill, she had sufficient insight, was very bright, and had a positive attitude to home treatment. Also, although ill, her symptoms and behavior did not cause her or others to be at much risk, apart from some mild fleeting thoughts of suicide.

TREATMENT OF FIRST EPISODE PSYCHOSIS

"The experience of first-time admission to a psychiatric hospital is often seen as traumatic and has been compared to that of a disaster experience."

Paul Fitzgerald—psychiatrist

It can be argued that home treatment offers particular advantages over inpatient treatment in the treatment of first episode psychosis—more so than in any other condition, except perhaps acute postpartum disorders. Many patients with first episode psychosis who present acutely have a traumatic and negative introduction to the mental health system. Usually young, and treatment naïve, they often have to be involuntarily admitted, sometimes with use of police, physical restraints, forced injections, and seclusion. McGorry, et al., (1991) have found evidence of post-traumatic stress disorder symptoms in such patients. This alienating experience can lead to a high rate of service disengagement with consequent further crises and development of a vicious cycle. Birchwood (2002) reported that, in over 50% of first episode patients, the first experience of treatment was after involuntary admission; there was a high rate of disengagement (50% in 18 months) and over-representation in these figures by young Black males in Birminham U.K.

Clinical experience and research has shown that home treatment can replace hospital admission in a large proportion of these patients. Fitzgerald and Kulkarni (1998), in Victoria, Australia, successfully treated 22/37 first episode psychotic patients entirely at home; Malla (2002) reported 47% of patients treated without hospital admission in the Prevention & Early

Intervention Psychosis Program (PEPP) service in London, Ontario, Canada. Because these were not randomized controlled studies, it is unknown to what degree hospitalization was avoided by the use of home treatment. In the Australian study (Fitzgerald & Kulkarni, 1998), the initial measures of psychopathology were statistically equivalent in the successful and the unsuccessful home treatment patients; i.e., more severe psychopathology scores did not predict subsequent hospital admission. The unsuccessful patients had less social support and a longer duration of untreated psychosis.

Home treatment can also help to decrease the time it takes for the first episode patient to get treatment. The outcome of first episode psychosis is thought to be improved by shortening the length of time the patient's psychotic symptoms go untreated—the so-called DUP (duration of untreated psychosis; Malla & Norman, 2002) and best practice is to shorten the DUP as much as possible. As the early psychotic illness progresses untreated, there is more and more opportunity for serious physical, social, and legal harm to occur. Twenty to thirty percent of these patients have suicidal ideas and some have made suicide attempts before receiving effective treatment. Ten to fifteen percent of individuals with psychosis eventually commit suicide—two thirds in the first five years. Patients who become disabled usually do so in the first three years of their illness. Unemployment, loss of friends, and loss of self-esteem can develop and become entrenched. Giving anti-psychotic medicine early improves outcome, and with sustained treatment over 80% achieve remission of symptoms within the first six months. Relapse in the early phase of psychosis increases the chance of further relapse and persistent symptoms. Abnormal biological features usually seen in individuals with established schizophrenia can also be seen in a subgroup of patients during their first episode. Cognitive problems associated with schizophrenia can emerge at the onset of psychosis and quickly become established. All these observations give rise to the concept of early psychosis, being a psychosocially and biologically critical period.

Why the delay in treatment? Malla (2002) lists the seven milestones to appropriate treatment:

1. Recognizing that something is wrong—not quite right
2. Acknowledging it may be a mental illness
3. Seeking professional help
4. Accessing help
5. Appropriate diagnosis
6. Offer of appropriate treatment
7. Acceptance and continuation of appropriate treatment

It is in steps 3, 4, and 7 that home treatment can shine; the way services are delivered increases the chance of successful engagement in treatment. Young people may doubt the usefulness of professional help and their negative stereotype of mental illness and fear of mental health services can create a barrier to seeking medical attention. A flexible and informal service that does not require them to attend out-patient appointments in a clinic, that can meet them in their homes, their schools, in a coffee shop, or even on the street, and has the expressed intention of avoiding hospital admission, is more likely to engage them in a therapeutic alliance. Engagement is a crucial first stage—without this, treatment efforts are likely to fail; it is an independent predictor of treatment retention rates and good symptom and functional outcomes in psychosis (Spencer, Birchwood, & McGovern, 2001). Short waiting lists and frequent contact with a single worker are also thought to encourage the development of a therapeutic alliance (IRIS, 2002). These authors go on to espouse the "assertive outreach model," which shares many characteristics of mobile crisis home treatment, such as low case loads, allowing the time for development of a therapeutic relationship and home visiting for persistent followup of individuals in danger of being lost to service. The aims of an assertive outreach approach in first episode psychosis are twofold: 1) to engage the individual and their family in a collaborative relationship, which will provide a foundation for treatment and support, and 2) to maintain continuity of contact throughout the critical early phase. The web site www.iris.org (IRIS, 2002) lists the key elements of this treatment model, and they are almost exactly the same as those of MCHT outlined in Chapters 4, 5, and 6.

Of course, an acute home treatment service cannot provide all the services required in a team dedicated to the care of first episode patients. Prototypes of these services, such as Birmingam Early Intervention Service (Spencer, et al., 2001) and the Prevention and Early Intervention Program for Psychosis (PEPP) in London, Ontario, Canada, (Malla, 2002), treat patients for an extended period of time (three years) and address many issues, such as education, employment, and quality of life. However, these services use MCHT to deal with crises in the least restrictive setting (as well as using alternative accommodation such as respite beds and hostels). The importance of extended support for first episode psychosis is sadly highlighted by the case of David (see below). Although home treatment was highly successful in treating the acute episode in this man, who would have been very difficult to engage otherwise, he made a serious suicide attempt by jumping off a building within a year of discharge from our program. He eventually recovered after extensive surgery and rehabilitation, and is now psychiatrically stable, attending an out-patient clinic. The Birmingam Early Intervention Service was the first early intervention service in the U.K. and was granted NHS Beacon Service status. The National Service Framework (Department of Health, 1999) has plans for 50 such services to be developed throughout Britain. From Spencer, Birchwood, and McGovern, (2001) and Mental Health Policy Implementation Guide (Department of Health, 2001), IRIS (2002) and Fitzgerald and Kulkarni (1998), the following principles and clinical guidelines relevant to Mobile Crisis Home Treatment of first episode psychosis are described.

Engagement of Service Users

In addition to the previously mentioned service features, Spencer also recommend "low stigma treatment settings," to the degree of avoiding out-patient care and day care altogether. Patients who do not adhere to treatment are not discharged; the frequency of visits is stepped up.

Comprehensive Assessment

Comorbidity with problems such as substance misuse, depression, suicidal thinking, social avoidance, and PTSD symptoms is common, and needs assessment and treatment, not least because they can lead to crises and relapse.

It is also important to get a sense of patients' sense of stigma, their own explanatory model of the illness, and their views of the future. Avoid a premature confrontation of their beliefs about their problems if they don't accept that they are ill. Instead, search for common ground with the patient and offer practical assistance with a problem of importance to the individual; home treatment, which brings the clinician face to face with the patient's environment and social problems, makes it relatively easy to find something you can help them with.

Embrace Diagnostic Uncertainty

An acute first episode of psychosis is often difficult to diagnose with certainty: substance misuse often clouds the picture, symptoms and signs change frequently, and mania and schizophrenia can appear similar in cross section. A premature diagnosis, for example, of schizophrenia, can be harmful, engendering pessimism in the patient, staff and, family. Therefore, a symptom-based approach to treatment is advocated. This might mean prescribing a mood stabilizer for manic symptoms.

Medication

> *"The principle underlying the use of neuroleptic medication in the early stages of schizophrenia is simple; it is to ensure that the experience of medication is as positive as possible and should occur in the context of building a trusting relationship with the patient and providing information about their illness."*

Paul Bebbington, (IRIS, 2002)

Spencer recommends an anti-psychotic free observation period, during which the diagnosis of psychosis can be confirmed and organic causes excluded. Benzodiazepines can be used for tranquillization. This is not always possible; in the need to gain rapid control of psychotic symptoms and agitation in order to attain credibility with family and caregivers and prevent early demands for hospital, admission has to take precedence.

Low doses of anti-psychotics are recommended and the team should aim for complete remission of symptoms, which can be achieved in 70–80% of cases. The remission rate of positive and negative symptoms reaches a plateau after three to six months of treatment. Failure of symptoms to remit after six months of adequate treatment with two anti-psychotic drugs should prompt a review of diagnosis and treatment adherence, and clinicians should consider cognitive behavior therapy and/or clozapine. Great care needs to be taken to minimize side effects. Patients should be given time to decide whether to take medicine or not, and it should be offered in a low-key fashion. In the PEPP service (Malla, 2002), 17.5% start medication after one month, 4.2% after three months, and 2.3% never take it.

Spencer says patients should not be discharged if they refuse medication; however, there are limits to the degree to which a home treatment service can allow persistent non-adherence to treatment: in times of scarce resources, the patient may be taking up a space that somebody could benefit from. Can the team continue to accept responsibility for someone whose behavior is out of control and yet may not fit criteria for involuntary admission?

Focus on the Entire Family

The degree of family support is crucial to the success of Mobile Crisis Home Treatment. In Fitzgerald and Kulkarni's (1998) study, patients who were successfully treated at home had a higher degree of family support than those that did not. They found that it was important to introduce some structure for both the patient and the family and to adopt a clear, pragmatic, and optimistic approach. An early period of sedation for the patient allowed the family to regroup. Spencer says the traditional concept of expressed emotion that forms the rationale for family intervention in schizophrenia may be of less relevance in a family experiencing psychosis for the first time; issues of trauma and loss are usually uppermost. Families have a wide range of emotional reactions that need to be dealt with: feelings of loss—of the person they knew; disbelief regarding the teams assessment; and anger and frustration at the health services and the tortuous route they have taken to get help. Dealing with these issues early on may help prevent the development of a critical family atmosphere later.

They will need help in addressing the day-to-day difficulties of living with the patient and learning how to talk about and solve problems without rancor. They are provided with information about psychosis, including the rationale for embracing diagnostic uncertainty and the importance of time in clarifying the clinical picture. We find "small plant" analogy helpful: when you find a small plant in your garden, you don't know what kind of a weed or flower it will become—only time will tell.

The Birmingham early intervention team provide a clinical vignette of family work with such patients, which illustrates many of these points very well and is here quoted in full (IRIS, 2002)

> Tom had been experiencing difficulties since his early teens, and was referred by his GP to the mental health services when he stopped attending school at 16, complaining that he was being picked on by his peers. Initial meetings with him and his parents revealed that the difficulties were more widespread, with Tom keeping the family awake at night, talking to voices and becoming extremely angry and shouting when his parents and brother refused to say that they could hear them as well. The atmosphere was tense in the house, with the father being very critical of Tom's laziness, reflected as he saw it in his staying in bed until the afternoon. His mother's main concern was that he never wanted to wash, and was not eating properly. His brother resented the fact that Tom was getting all the attention in the family, and was spending more and more time outside the house.
>
> Tom started to take medication, which resulted in him feeling calmer and sleeping better at night. He also reported that the voices were not as loud as they previously had been. All family members were involved right from the start. Each was given time on their own to talk about their views of what was happening. Family sessions were held to provide information on psychosis to the family, and to help them look at the way they communicated with each other. Particular emphasis was placed on them noticing the good things that were going on, and in developing ways of asking each other for what they wanted without being critical and angry.

Good progress was made, but the father continued to be very negative towards Tom and the things he did. He was offered an individual session where he became extremely upset and talked about his sadness about what was happening with Tom. He always had very high hopes for him, as this was his "true son" (the other boy was adopted). Mostly he felt sad that he saw a very bleak future for Tom.

After the father's individual session, the family sessions became more productive, and they were all able to focus on more realistic things to work towards. All were very pleased when Tom got a part-time job in a local shop, as they saw this as the first step towards him leading a better quality of life.

Case history of first episode psychosis, David, aged 24

July 5

David is a 24-year-old single man, who plays in a band. He referred himself, at the urging of his friend Scott, with whom he had been living for 2 weeks, after being asked to leave his father's house. David had been continuously ill for well over a year, and so far, had been very difficult to engage. He had had one visit with a psychiatrist a year previously, and had been diagnosed with schizophrenia. He soon stopped the anti-psychotic prescribed due to side effects, and never returned. Scott was concerned about David's suicidal ideas and odd behavior. David was averse to psychiatric treatment and refused to be admitted to hospital; he had been seen briefly in June by the Hazelglen service but denied problems, and just wanted help with housing and finances. He left the service after two weeks.

July, 6 home visit by case manager

David appeared unkempt, stooped, and thin, with long greasy hair. Initially denying any problems, he opened up after his friend left the room. He described auditory hallucinations in which he could hear "the whole city talking to him." He described special powers, which enabled him to change TV programs by inserting himself invisibly into the TV and claimed to be an emissary from God, sent to protect people on earth. He was upset at TV news about wars; it meant that he had not fulfilled his role.

Scott described his friend as always introverted and quiet, a good drummer, whose mental state had deteriorated in the last month—he would go into a "trance" for a long time, just sitting and staring.

July 6, office visit with psychiatrist

Unable to give coherent history, little spontaneous speech, questions have to be repeated two or three times; mentioned command hallucinations—nature unclear.

Flupenthixol (an anti-psychotic) 3 mg at night, and benztropine (for extra-pyramidal side effects) prescribed. Diagnosis of paranoid schizophrenia reconfirmed. Global assessment of functioning (GAF) score 35.

July 8, phone call from hospital crisis clinic:

David had a severe extra-pyramidal reaction, given intramuscular injection in the emergency room.

July 11, home visit by case manager

Told her he had taken 14 flupenthixol tablets at once; hence, the severe side effects. Education about medication; arrangements made for Scott's mother to control his medication and give it to him daily. Housing problem addressed by involving mental health housing agency.

July 15, phone contact

Tolerating medication.

July 20, home visit

Case manager accompanied David to group home for psychiatric patients to see if it would be suitable—not so; would have to mix with others and join in to do household duties and cooking. Arrangements made to see a social worker about apartments. Scott's mother phoned; David had found an apartment.

July 25, home visit by case manager

David had stopped taking his medication, due to side effects—slurred speech and thick tongue.

July 26, office visit, accompanied by case manager

Depot intramuscular anti-psychotic started—pipotiazine palmitate.

August 2, home visit by case manager

Injection given. Apartment filthy, smelly, with old, half-eaten food and dirty dishes piling up—assistance and education about activities of daily living arranged. Calmer, fewer hallucinations.

August 17, office visit

Injection given. Has moved back with father temporarily. Hallucinations decreasing, clearer thoughts, calmer, functioning better in band.

August 24, office visit with psychiatrist

Little spontaneous speech, denies hearing voices, and having special powers—still withdrawn, tense.

August 31, office visit with father

Education provided about David's illness, given information to read.

September 6, office visit to case manager

Hair cut and clean, pleasant, more spontaneous, fewer hallucinations.

September to November 15

Discharge planning; referred to mental health association case manager and family doctor.

Home visits: 7
Office visits: 7
Phone contact: 2
Length of treatment: 3½ months

Postscript

Within one year of discharge, David made a serious suicide attempt by jumping off a building. His father had once again been unable to cope with him and asked him to leave; David could not cope living alone, and this was thought to be a major precipitant of the suicide attempt. He sustained multiple fractures, but was able to make a recovery. He became psychiatrically stable and attended an out-patient clinic for schizophrenic patients.

Points Illustrated

Home treatment was able to engage an unwilling patient who, if he were hospitalized, would likely have self-discharged. Treatment was achieved by home visits, working with his friend and the friend's mother, and by the relationship with the case manager.

David's friend Scott provided support, temporary housing, and Scott's mother administered the medication. Practical help with housing and activities of daily living was provided. The patient had very unstable life style, moving from one unsatisfactory place to another; case manager had to "follow him around." His stay was lengthy, partly due to housing problems. His condition deteriorated after intensive level of care ceased, even though a competent community case manager cared for him. A relatively small number of visits were accomplished due to David's reluctance to see staff often.

Case history of first episode psychosis, Helen, aged, 23

Helen is divorced and lives on social assistance in a townhouse with her two children, a girl aged three and a boy, four. After she refused admission to hospital, she was referred for Mobile Crisis Home Treatment by her primary care physician because of the sudden onset of strange behavior 11 days prior.

July 21, morning

Initial assessment by case manager, carried out at mother's home where Helen had been living for the past two weeks. She could not give a history, was unable to answer the case manager's questions, and was emotionally labile—crying one minute and laughing the next. Mother reports that she is unable to care for the children, has hardly eaten in two weeks, and spends many hours in the bathroom for no apparent reason. She has a long history of severe social anxiety and concerns that people were talking about her, such that she was unable to complete high school or keep a job. She had been married to an abusive man and separated 2½ years previously. She spends a lot of time at her mother's house.

July 21, afternoon

Home visit to mother's house by psychiatrist and case manager (patient unlikely to be able to attend at office). She had been having a bath when we arrived and came downstairs inappropriately dressed just in a towel; agreed to dress when mother asked her to. Her two children were unusually rambunctious and it was with some difficulty that the patient's sister kept them away from their mother, outside in a wading pool.

Helen was almost mute, looked baffled, perplexed, and very anxious. She seemed to understand who we were and why we were there; most of the history was from mother.

Eleven days previously, Helen spent 6 hours in the bathroom instead of watching TV with her mother as usual in the evening. She said cameras were watching her all the time (the bathroom seemed to be a place where she thought she could avoid the scrutiny of "people watching her"). She heard voices of "famous people," thought the radio and TV were talking about her. She thought she was a special religious person and had told mother a complicated story about the Pope, "Our Lady of Fatima," and a letter she thought was meant for her.

She wanted to die, had considered overdosing but wouldn't because of the children. She had eaten little for two weeks, slept poorly, but could help care for her children bathing and changing their clothes, but no cooking.

A diagnosis of schizophreniform psychosis and social anxiety disorder was made. She likely had a long prodromal phase with long-standing worries about people talking about her and severe dysfunction, not completing school or being able to sustain employment.

Helen and her parents did not want hospital admission. Her parents had not left her alone for the past two weeks. Although they both worked, they staggered their shifts and used up some vacation time to stay with her.

Risperidone (an anti-psychotic drug) and lorazepam (an anti-anxiety drug) were started; she was given some samples that had been brought to the home visit. Parents were asked to take her for a physical assessment from her primary care physician. Basis 32 score was 88 overall, 93 on psychosis scale.

July 21, after hours phone call by case manager

Helen had taken her medicine, and was doing "excellent" and slept one hour. Mother discussed diagnosis; case manager will bring booklet on first episode psychosis.

July 22, home visit

Helen is more active, had slept 12 hours, and was able to discipline her son. Her goals were to sleep better, stop hearing voices, and be less fearful when she goes out. Case manager will visit daily.

July 23, home visit

Appears brighter and well groomed. Health teaching about proper nutrition and excessive smoking, and stress of motherhood. Still has delusions.

July 28, office visit with psychiatrist

Having daily home visits with case manager. Has inappropriate affect—giggling, talks about voices, thought disordered. Medication adjusted.

July 31, phone call

Mother called: Helen had not eaten for two days, talking "nonsense," going from room to room to avoid her mother, not interacting with children, talking to herself, and laughs suddenly. Psychiatrist adjusts medication.

August 6, office visit with psychiatrist

Having frequent visits. Getting worse. Giggling openly and is suspicious, accusing psychiatrist of "not being a real doctor"and the case manage of "not being a real nurse." Medication increased. Psychiatrist explained her diagnosis of schizophrenia.

August 7, home visit

Improved; given booklet and video about schizophrenia.

August 11, home visit

Using large amounts of shampoo and bubble bath, spending many hours in bathroom; continues to be plagued with auditory hallucinations, delusional mood, delusions, and depressed. Medication switched to olanzopine (different anti-psychotic drug).

August 12, office visit with psychiatrist

Improving; less anxious, affect more appropriate, still delusional.

August 13, home visit

Able to stay alone overnight at her own house and go shopping with mother.

August 18, office visit with psychiatrist

Considerable improvement. Had opened up to mother about her delusions, including the thought that movie star Brad Pitt had been at the door. Discussed her gradual move back to her own home with the children; mother works close by in case needed urgently.

August 25, office visit with psychiatrist

Still delusional and frustrated that people that don't believe her. Thinks ex-husband put porno movie about her on the Internet Medication increased.

August 29, office visit with psychiatrist

Looks very ill: pale, haggard, weepy, frustrated, and frightened. Hearing voices accusing her of molesting her children and giving her grandfather AIDS. Offered admission to hospital for more support and break from child care; said she would think about it. Olanzopine ineffective, therefore switched gradually to perphenazine (older anti-psychotic).

September 1, mother telephoned on-call number

Helen had just taken an overdose of perphenazine. Advised to go to emergency room; case manager advised ER staff.

September 2, office visit with psychiatrist
Kept overnight in hospital, then discharged. She took 24 four-mg tablets of perphenazine—not to harm herself, but she just "wanted to sleep and get rid of the voices" Looks better!

After this episode, Helen continued to improve, and the auditory hallucinations finally became much less and she was much less delusional. Case manager started to meet her in coffee shop, for two reasons: to help her overcome social anxiety, and to talk to her away from her mother. Mother has been indispensable to home treatment and very supportive. However, she clearly has difficulty loosening up her involvement with Helen when she functions better, and seems to resent case manager's attempts to deal separately with Helen; for example, she looked displeased at the plan to meet in coffee shop, and did not give Helen any money (the case manager paid).

At this point, discharge from Mobile Crisis Home Treatment is being planned. A family meeting is planned to discuss diplomatically the need to separate from Helen a bit and not to make premature plans "to all live together in a bigger house."

Home visits: 27
Phone contacts: 30
Hours of direct care: 22

Points Illustrated

This patient was very ill. She had very poor premorbid functioning, with severe social anxiety, probably mild paranoia, and a lengthy prodromal period before the acute psychosis started.

She did not respond to two anti-psychotic medicines, thereby lengthening her stay in MCHT.

Her parents were extremely supportive, but will need help with being over-involved and learning how and when to allow their daughter more autonomy.

Her clinical course was very uneven and unpredictable, such that with conventional in-patient treatment and out-patient followup it would have been very difficult to adjust the intensity of treatment quickly enough.

Family burden was high; however, it would likely have been greater with hospital treatment. Helen could contribute a great deal to the care of her two unusually rambunctious children most of the time. Fortunately, none of Helen's psychotic thinking ever presented a safety concern, to her, her children, or her parents.

The case manager had to continually assess Helen's parenting ability as well as her self-care, because she was constantly wanting to "try it on my own with the children." A fine line was trodden in respecting her wishes for independence and her perception that in some ways it would be easier to care for her children away from doting, inconsistent grandparents vs. the danger of putting herself in a position of high stress and risking further demoralization.

TREATMENT OF SEVERE POSTPARTUM DISORDER

Hospital admission for severe postpartum disorder is likely viewed as especially devastating for patients and their families. To wrench a new mother, who may have had little exposure to psychiatry before, away from her newborn baby, her husband, and her other children, puts a blight on what is supposed to be a joyful occasion; it is hard to think of a more paramount indication for non-hospital treatment. Prolonged separation of mothers from their infants is potentially damaging to the mother/infant relationship. Even in the nineteenth century, thoughtful clinicians urged that postpartum psychosis be treated at home. There, the patient can maintain her role as wife, homemaker, and mother of her other children and can maintain her relationship with her newborn. This discussion is based on the work of Brockington (1996) and Oates (1988).

Clouston, in 1896 (Brockington, 1996), described the treatment of a patient who was sleepless and restless, uncooperative and deluded, and absolutely refused food. He sent a "first-rate attendant from the asylum" in addition to an ordinary nurse and servants. She was fed, controlled, taken out, and nursed through her attack in six weeks. Connolly (Brockington, 1996), in an 1846 article in the *Lancet,* describes the precautions that must be taken against suicide and filicide while treating these patients at home. Brockington states that "it is still preferable to treat this disorder at home wherever possible. If hospital admission is necessary, there are great advantages in joint mother and baby admission."

However, there were several disadvantages to joint admissions of mother and baby:

- Risk of injury to baby from other patients exists
- Many profoundly ill women and their families were reluctant to accept admission. This seemed to be particularly common among women who had other children and did not want to be separated from them.

- Another group of women, initially admitted, made constant pleas for discharge, seriously interfering with their treatment and progress, while on the ward and dominating all therapeutic interaction.
- In 1992, the cost of care was 50% higher than admitting the mother alone.

These drawbacks to joint admission, and the wish to keep mothers at home with their babies, led Oates (1988), in Nottingham, U.K., to develop a team to provide home treatment for patients with severe postpartum disorders—mainly bipolar and schizophrenic disorders. The team consisted of Dr. Oates, 2 residents, a psychologist (all half time), plus 2 community nurses and a social worker. Volunteers from the Homestart organization helped them. This is a national voluntary organization consisting of mothers who offer support and practical help to families with young children; the basic idea is to establish a bond of friendship between an experienced mother and a younger mother who is finding it difficult to cope. The volunteers receive a six-week intensive training and regular supervision from a social worker. A group of six volunteers received extra training from the home treatment team and had close contact with the community nurses, receiving supervision with the clinical team.

Oates studied 31 patients treated at home, all suffering from bipolar disorder or schizophrenia; all, save one, were psychotic at the start of home treatment. There were two groups of women: The first group (n = 20), the majority of whom were initially seen on the postnatal ward, were admitted to a psychiatric Mother and Baby Unit but were discharged home early, at a stage when their psychiatric state would normally have required a continuing stay in hospital. The second group (n = 11) were seen initially on a home visit and managed completely at home, thus avoiding admission. Patients in which the psychotic process involved the baby or who were engaged in potentially hazardous behavior towards the baby were not treated at home; nor were actively suicidal or infanticidal patients. The patients had to live within a 20-minute car journey from the hospital.

Three levels of MCHT were used:

- **Level 1.** The nurse spent 8 hours a day in the patient's home, leaving only when a reliable family member took over the care. A psychiatrist visited the home on alternate days.

    Case example: A 26-year-old woman, married to a miner, with two children. This was her fourth illness: she had been admitted

twice with mania before having children, and had had a manic illness starting on the fifth day after the birth of her first child, which
necessitated an in-patient stay. She had recovered from all her illnesses within four weeks and was known to be a caring and competent mother of her first child. She was admitted on the sixth day
postpartum in a state hallmarked by insomnia, motor over-activity, flight of ideas, and pressure of speech. She was noisy, restless,
angry, and argumentative towards staff and refused to move from
the nursery or be separated from her baby for even a few minutes.
Despite her disturbed mental state, she was affectionate and caring towards her baby. She was continuously demanding to go
home and refused all medication. Her husband felt she would settle at home and would be more amenable to treatment in that environment. However, he did not feel he could manage her on his
own and there were no other family members available for help.
The patient's mental state continued unchanged for four days before she was sent home for MCHT.

From 7 a.m. to 8 p.m. there was continuous nursing presence in
the home for seven days. The psychiatrist and midwife visited
daily. She immediately cooperated with medication, her behavior
settled, and she assumed responsibility for the baby, although caring for it always in the presence of another person.

On the eighth day, the nursing presence was reduced to two visits
for two hours each day, from 7 a.m. to 9 a.m., when her husband
left for work, and from 4 p.m. until 6 p.m., when her husband returned from work. By week three the visits were reduced to alternate days, and by week four they were reduced to weekly, with the
patient attending the hospital out-patient clinic. Negotiations with
her husband's employer resulted in his being allowed to work regular shifts during this period.

- **Level 2.** The nurse visited at least twice daily, each visit lasting at
  least two hours. During her absence from the house, either a family member, another health professional (health visitor, midwife,
  or Homestart volunteer) was present. A psychiatrist visited twice
  a week.

Case example: A 21-year-old woman, married to a miner, having her
first illness. She was re-admitted to the Maternity Hospital on the
12th postpartum day after the birth of her first child because she was

weepy and not coping. After three days she was referred for MCHT and was found to be suffering from a mixed affective disorder. She was restless, could not sleep, had pressure of speech and flight of ideas, but also experienced depressive ideation and was very tearful. Both she and her husband were distressed at the prospect of a psychiatric admission. She had a supportive mother living close by.

During week 1, The nurse visited twice a day from 7 a.m. to 9 a.m. and from 4 p.m. until 6 p.m., coinciding with her husband leaving for and returning from work. The patient's mother relieved the nurse.

During week 2, The patient's mental state changed. She became profoundly depressed with marked psychomotor retardation. ECT was started, the nurse transporting her to hospital twice weekly and returning with her, where she stayed for the rest of the day. During weeks 3 and 4 she steadily improved, receiving six ECT treatments and, after a brief hypomanic period lasting 48 hours made a recovery by the end of the fourth week. She was then seen on alternate days for a further two weeks (Level 3) before transfer to "orthodox community psychiatric nursing support and the out-patient clinic.

- **Level 3.** The nurse visits the home on alternate days, alternating her care with either family members or other health professionals. The psychiatrist visits weekly.

The maximum capacity of the service was one patient at Level 1, three at Level 2, and six at Level 3. At all levels, a medical team member could be summoned to the house immediately. A bed was available for the nurse to admit the patient immediately on her own authority and all forms of physical treatment could be provided. A nurse was available by phone 24 hours a day/seven days a week.

The patients with mania and schizophrenia received the most intensive nursing care, had the youngest babies, and were the most disturbed women. Over half of the patients managed at Level 3 had not been admitted at all. They had older babies and the choice of Level 3 nursing was indicated by the continuous presence of a family member and a clinical state that was stable and predictable over a 24-hour period. The majority of patients in Levels 1 and 2 moved on to a lower level of nursing, and only three were re-admitted. The majority of Level 3 patients moved on to conventional out-patient care and community nursing with only two admissions and one-day hospital admission. None of the manic patients required re-admission. All three re-admissions were patients suffering from depressive psychosis.

Table 8.2 Diagnoses and Level of Nursing Care

Diagnosis of study patients	No.	Highest Level of Nursing		
		1	2	3
Schizophrenia-like conditions	3	1	2	0
Mania	10	4	2	2
Depressive psychosis	18	2	2	14
Total	31	7	8	16

The patients included in this study represented 66% of all the post-partum patients referred to the psychiatric services with a new episode of psychotic illness and 76% of all those admitted.

MCHT was considered to be a workable alternative to hospital. This seemed to be particularly effective with manic conditions as well as in severe depressive illness. Women with older children and those who have had a previous episode of postpartum psychosis appear to have welcomed this treatment. Anxieties about the patient's welfare only led to admission on three occasions. All three of these patients were depressed, but only one was admitted because of suicidal behavior (she took an overdose of her antidepressants). None of the manic or schizophrenic patients required admission because their behavior was hazardous to themselves or their babies. None of the mothers injured their babies, nor did any on them engage in behavior that was neglectful of the infant's emotional or physical well-being that could not be easily and quickly overcome by the support and assistance of the nurse and the patient's family. MCHT minimized disruption to the family and facilitates an early resumption of maternal autonomy and self-esteem. The clinical recovery of those 17 patients in the study who had been admitted for a previous episode of postpartum psychosis was the same with MCHT: most of these patients thought that they had recovered more quickly when they were managed at home with their second episode.

In 1988, Brockington developed a similar team to Oates, but they have never been able to achieve Level 1 care, nor did they develop a liaison with voluntary agencies like Homestart. The number of patients receiving daily visits of at least a week has never been more than 10 per year. He lists what he perceives as "difficulties" in treating these patients at home:

- It is hard to maintain the standards of caretaking that are the norm in hospital-based psychiatry. There are logistical difficulties in developing an effective records system for patients who never come to the hospital. It is essential to have a coordinator whose office is in the in-patient unit.

- There is risk that medical examination and treatment is neglected.
- There is an "ever-present" risk that the patients or their babies come to harm. The first patient treated at home, who was mute and deluded, climbed onto the roof, while husband was asleep in bed beside her. "We instruct the family that the mother must never be left alone, and must not leave the house. We review any points of danger such as window latches and the storage of medication."

The first two of these difficulties are hard to understand; they are not seen as problems with MCHT in general and would appear to be easily overcome. The third difficulty, that of risk, would appear to be one of adequate risk assessment, apparently achieved in Oates' study.

In spite of these caveats, Brockington states "From this more limited experience, we can confirm that this form of care is feasible, and is appreciated by mothers and their families"; he lists home treatment as one of the elements of "the ideal service."

Case history of postpartum depression, Heidi, aged 29

June 20

This patient came to the hospital 24-hour walk-in crisis clinic in the morning having been told to do so by a friend. She is married and has three children, a nine-year-old, three-year-old, and a baby, three months, whom she is still breast feeding.

She complained of numerous severe symptoms of depression, some borderline psychotic symptoms, and decreased inability to function for the past four weeks. She was restless and pacing at night, had nightmares of snakes and worms coming out of her body, and a "shivering sensation" in her vagina, as though she were being penetrated. She had flashbacks of sexual abuse. She was extremely weepy and disheveled and feeling she is not worthy to be a mother.

She wishes she would die, and not have to deal with the pain, although thinking of her children prevents her from harming herself. She was afraid to pick up the baby but seemed evasive as to why. She ate poorly and had lost weight.

Her son had been born three weeks prematurely, he had been jaundiced, and she needed to use a breast pump, all causing increased stress.

She had been depressed after the 3-year-old's birth, also; at that time she had separated temporarily from her husband.

She was born and raised in Germany, an only child, raised by her mother. She had a diploma in social work.

Her mother, had been visiting from Europe for seven months, and recently she had asked her to leave because of confrontations over what she perceived as mother controlling the children and the home, and also because of issues concerning childhood sexual abuse.

Mother had a history of depression. Identified sexual abuse by neighbor when 5 years old. The psychiatrist recommended admission to hospital but she refused; she was therefore referred to Mobile Crisis Home Treatment. She was diagnosed as having major depressive disorder in the postpartum period with some borderline psychotic features present. Scored 76 on the Basis-32, in the severe range of psychopathology.

June 21

Called by case manager; message left for her to call back.

June 21

Called emergency pager at 11 p.m.; unable to sleep.

June 22

Called case manager crying, distressed. Home visit made. Having panic attacks with flashbacks of sexual abuse. Thinking of "taking a knife to her head." Feeling ashamed of wanting to do this—not worthy as a mother. Discussed at length idea of being admitted to hospital, and of having extra support at home during weekend. Called her husband at work to discuss admission to hospital. Unable to guarantee her safety. Asking for medication for anxiety; agreed to get support from her friends to help with the children. Call placed to psychiatrist—will prescribe alprazolam (an anti-anxiety drug). Reviewed use of pager and crisis clinic if needed over weekend.

June 25

Pacing floor during interview; continues to have flashbacks of sexual abuse—upset stomach, shaky legs, feels weak. The week before, when case manager came close to her for a few seconds she thought she might hurt her. Today, when case manager held the baby, her comment was, "you won't hurt her." Health teaching re: depression and medication, reassured that she will feel "normal again."

June 26

Interview with psychiatrist. She had vague, disjointed, wandering speech; seemed "on the borderline of psychosis." Quetiapine (anti-psychotic) added at bedtime. Started on venlafaxine (anti-depressant).

June 27

Called case manager: "waves of heat" since starting Venlafaxine; cannot stand it—wanted to take cold shower but couldn't because she had to take care of children. A few times, after "waves of heat" had thoughts "of hurting someone or myself. I would never hurt my children—I would hurt myself first." Took alprazolam—alleviated these feelings.

After this, she continued to improve. Was discharged three months later. She had a series of home visits, telephone calls, interviews with psychiatrist. Emphasis was on support, encouragement, education, and practical help, particularly with obtaining social services financial assistance. Followup arranged with counselor she had seen off and on over the years. Referred to cognitive therapy group starting in November.

Total interviews: 13
Total direct hours: 29.3
Total indirect hours: 1 (numerous brief phone calls)

Points Illustrated

Factors contributing to success included rapid control of insomnia, anxiety, and quasi-psychotic thoughts with medicine; ready availability of phone support including after hours; supportive husband and friends; practical help.

Sandra, aged 35

December 27

Sandra' primary care physician referred her to the 24-hour walk-in crisis clinic at the hospital. She was a dental hygienist, married for the second time, living with her husband and a blended family of four teenagers.

She had given birth to twins 3 weeks premature 4 weeks previously. For the past 2 weeks she had not been sleeping and the family thought she had the blues. She had become worse in the previous 24 hours and had come to the clinic the previous night, where she had been given lorazepam (an anti-anxiety medicine) to calm her down. When she visited her primary care physician that morning she was very agitated. She was continuously crying, pacing, and having racing thoughts.

When she tries to be with the babies she just cries. She worries a great deal about whether they are getting enough milk when she breastfeeds. She denied any thoughts of harming herself or the babies. She felt a great pressure to do everything for the babies, and guilty that she needed help from the family. She had no previous psychiatric history. She had low energy, insomnia, anhedonia. Her mental status examination showed a woman who was tearful, exhausted, overwhelmed, and markedly anxious, with depressed affect. She was admitted to the psychiatric ward, and started on olanzapine (an antipsychotic medicine also used for severe agitation), citalopram (an anti-depressant), and lorazepam.

December 31

Discharged herself from hospital against medical advice after five days. Referred to Mobile Crisis Home Treatment service. Basis 32 score 73, in severe range.

January 3

First assessment by case manager. Still extremely anxious and irritable. Thoughts race, she can't turn them off, has a lot of guilt. Requires much help with day-to-day activities from her family. Sleeping better. Short-term memory and concentration poor; eats with encouragement. Husband is very supportive and has taken paternity leave to care for her and children. Her mother and mother-in-law are taking turns to stay with her at night to care for the babies. Sandra is negative about her experience on the psychiatric ward and upset at the doctors and nurses. Her medication is citalopram (an anti-depressant), temazepam (a hypnotic), and risperidone (an anti-psychotic medicine also used for severe agitation). It was clear that Sandra's premorbid personality was perfectionist, with rigid rules for herself, very independent, with difficulty depending on others. Her mental state was one of extreme anxiety, with frequent questions, and seeking of reassurance, but, at the same time, challenging the treatment plan and the medications. She wants information, thinks in black-and-white, wants control of the conversation, and does not take kindly to interruptions from the family, talking non-stop.

January 4

Several phone contacts to monitor and assess mental state. Still very anxious, wanting concrete details about exactly what day she will get better, and black and white answers about how the medicines will work. Struggling with obsessional thinking. Education and reassurance given; psychiatrist called; risperidone increased.

Case manager phones Sandra numerous times over the weekend. Sandra called the on-call worker on Sunday about not sleeping and racing thoughts. On-call worker made a follow-up call later—more settled.

January 7

Encouraged to walk daily, gradually increase workload, and use relaxation techniques. Starting to settle down, but unable to admit progress. Family report progress in areas of confusion, sleep, and worry.

January 8, 9

Daily phone contact—settling down.

January 10

Interview with home treatment psychiatrist (hospital psychiatrist had been medically responsible up to this time). Medications adjusted.

January 14, phone contact

January 15

Improving; mother continues to sleep overnight to care for the babies.

January 21

Phone contact. Had been doing well, enjoying increased activities, but yesterday had increased symptoms of irritability and anxiety. She had called the on-call worker yesterday (Sunday).

January 22, phone contact

Less anxious.

January 23, home visit

More settled but still frustrated with not being 100%. Very poor insight into the role of stress: blended family, twins. Unable to accept help. Husband said he was annoyed at his wife's impatience.

Sandra had met another mother with postpartum depression in the waiting room at the office. The case manager arranged for the two women to get together for mutual support.

January 28, phone contact

Not as well, upset and guilty at the thought of wishing she did not have children; crying a lot. Caring for twins alone at night now—finding it stressful.

9 p.m.

Phoned on-call worker.

January 29, inteview with psychiatrist

He concludes that she has an obsessional personality, examines and analyses every detail of her life, never had any hobbies or interests outside the home. Even when she leaves the house for a short walk, she has to telephone home to see if the babies are OK and that her husband is doing the job right.

More attempts will be made to get her out of the house; the case manager will take her for walks and bring her to the office.

February 11

Doing better. Able to discuss problems with 18-year-old stepson, who resents her and the twins—refers to her as "psycho bitch."

February 27

Discharge to care of primary care physician and a therapist in the out-patient clinic.

Total number of interviews: 9
Total direct hours of care: 16.7
Total phone contac indirect hours of care: 2.21

Points Illustrated

As mentioned above, women with severe postpartum disorders are often difficult to keep in hospital. This patient signed herself out of hospital after five days, and found the hospital experience negative.

Home treatment was helped a great deal by having a very supportive family who could stay with her all the time. Much use was made of phone support, both during office hours and after hours. She was a difficult patient to engage; very irritable, questioning and challenging everything in her attempt to be in control. Her functioning was very poor; had difficulty leaving the home, needing family to care for the babies. Practical help was given such as case manager going for walks with her.

Home treatment was very flexible. This patient's symptoms and dysfunction waxed and waned; at times, she would not need much support for a few days, but then would suddenly get worse and need much more contact, this would have been difficult to respond to in a conventional out-patient clinic.

SIDEBAR

Practical Tips (Oates, 1988)

- Nurse's assessment of patient's behavior in the home, her social situation, and her supports in the home is paramount.
- A great deal of nursing effort is devoted to the task of increasing the mother's self-confidence and her feelings of mastery and pleasure in her relationship with her baby. She works alongside the mother, ensuring that all the baby's needs are met and relieves her of tasks she is unable to do.
- As far as possible, all nursing involvement with the baby takes place in the presence of the mother and with her permission.
- As she improves, mother is encouraged to do more, but preventing her from becoming agitated and flustered.
- Support husband and other relatives; this often means advising them not to take over care of baby.
- Help mother to create own style of mothering; may bear little resemblance to her preconceived ideas and expectations.
- Help mother understand that negative emotions are common.
- Help mother have more realistic expectations of herself and motherhood.

Appendix

EVALUATION TOOLS

This is simply a list of tools commonly used in the evaluation of MCHT services. No opinion about them is implied by their inclusion here.

Measures of Acuity, Symptoms, and Functioning

Brief Psychiatric Rating Scale, BPRS

This is the most commonly used scale; use of this enables one to compare the acuity of one's patients to those of patients in numerous studies. It is a brief, clinician-rated scale used to assess the global severity of a range of psychiatric symptoms. Scores range from 24 (not present) to 168 (extremely severe impairment). Hoult, Rosen, and Reynolds (1984), used this scale in his study.

> Overall, J.E.R. & Gorham, D.R. (1962). The brief psychiatric rating scale. *Psychological Reports, 10,* 799–812.

Short Clinical Rating Scale (1978)

This scale was used by Stein and Test.

> French, M. H., & Henninger, G. R. (1970). A short clinical rating scale for use by nursing personnel 1. Development and design. *Archives of General Psychiatry, 23,* 233–240.

Health Sickness Rating Scale

This scale measures functioning and was used by Hoult, et. al., (1984).

> Luborsky, L. (1962). Clinical judgement of mental health. *Archives of General Psychiatry, 7,* 407–417

Present State Examination PSE

This scale measures symptoms and is more suitable for research evaluation, as opposed to program evaluation for on-going management. It is a clinician-rated scale measuring mental status. Syndrome and sub-syndrome scores are derived by rating and combining 142 sympton items. Higher scores indicate greater clinical impairment. This was used in Hoult, Rosen, & Reynolds (1984) and Muijen (1992).

Wing, J. K., Cooper, J. E., & Sartorious, N. (1974). *Measurement and classification of psychiatric symptoms: An instruction manual for PSE and Catego program.* Cambridge: Cambridge University Press

Morningside Rehabilitation Scale

This scale measures social function, with four subscales measuring dependency, activity levels, social integration, and current symptoms or behaviour. Dean, et al., (1993) used this scale in Birmingham.

Affleck, J. W., & McGuire E. J. (1984). The measurement of psychiatric rehabilitation status. A review of the needs and a new scale. *British Journal of Psychiatry, 145,* 517–525.

Comprehensive Psychiatric Rating Scale, CPRS

This scale was used by Merson, et al., (1992).

Asberg, M., Montgomery, S. A., Perris, C., Schally, D., & Sedvall G. (1978). A comprehensive psychopathological rating scale. *Acta Psychiatrica Scandinavica, 271* (Suppl. 5–27).

Montgomery and Asberg Depression Rating Scale, MADRS

This provides subscale of above—measures depression CPRS and used by Merson, et al.

Montgomery, S. A., & Asberg, M. (1979). A new depression scale designed to be sensitive to change. *British Journal of Psychiatry, 134,* 382–389

Brief Scale for Anxiety BAS

This also provides subscale of CPRS and was used by Merson, et al., (1992).

Tyrer, P., Owen, R. T., & Cicchetti, D. (1984). The brief scale for anxiety: A subdivision of the comprehensive psychopathological rating scale. *Journal of Neurology, Neurosurgery, Psychiatry, 47,* 970–975.

Global Assessment Scale

The Global Assessment Scale is a clinician-rated assessment of overall functioning on a scale of 1 to 100. Lower scores indicate poorer functioning. This scale was used in the study by Marks, (Marks, I. & Connely, et al., 1994).

Endicott, J., Spitzer, R. L., Fleiss, J. L., & Cohen, J. (1976). The global assessment scale. A procedure for measuring overall severity of psychiatric disturbance. *Archives of General Psychiatry, 33,* 766–771.

Psychiatric Evaluation Form, PEF

This scale measures psychological state and role functioning. It is a clinician-rated scale used to assess psychological functioning during the week prior to interview. Consists of 24 individual and 8 summary scales. Scoring on each scale ranges from 1 to 5 with higher scores indicating greater impairment. It was used by Fenton, et al., 1982.

Endicott, J., & Spitzer, R. L. (1972). What! Another rating scale: The psychiatric evaluation form. *Journal of Nervous and Mental Diseases, 154,* 88–104.

Social Adjustment Scale

This scale measures social functioning in a number of life domains (work, social, extended family, marital, parental, family unit and economic adequacy) on a scale of 1 to 7, with lower scores indicating poorer functioning. It was used by Marks, (Marks, Connelly, et al., (1994).

Weissman, M. M., Klerman, G. L., Paykel, E. S., Prusoff, B., & Hanson, B. (1974). Treatment effects on the social adjustment of depressed patients. *Archives of General Psychiatry, 30,* 771–778.

Social Functioning Schedule, SFS

This scale measures social functioning in 12 areas. It was used by Burns, et al., 1993).

Remington, M., & Tyrer, P. (1979). The social functioning schedule—A brief semi-structured interview. *Social Psychiatry, 14,* 151–157.

Social Functioning Questionnaire, SFQ

The Social Functioning Questionaire is a self-rated 8 items that correlate and is highly with Social Functioning Questionnaire, an observer, rated instrument. It was used in the study by Merson, et al., (1992).

Tyrer, P. (1990). Personality disorder and social functioning. In D. F. Peck, & C. M. Shapiro (Eds.), *Measuring human problems: A practical guide* (pp. 119–142). Chichester: John Wiley.

Behavior and Symptom Identification Scale, BASIS 32

The BASIS 32 has been a widely used behavioural health outcome assessment tool since 1985.

Developed by Susan V. Eisen, Ph.D., at McLean Hospital, Belmont, Massachusetts, it is used by the following mental health agencies for population profiling and outcomes measurement: California, Michigan, Nevada, and South Carolina. It is used by the Hazelglen home treatment service (see Chapter 3).

The McLean BASIS 32 plus system includes: a Perceptions of Care Survey, an 18-item, self-report rating scale incorporating patient/client perspectives on the quality of (in-patient and out-patient) behavioural health services received.

Information can be obtained at http://www.basis-32.org/new/b32.html or by phone at 617-855-2424.

Eisen, S.V. (2000). *Behavior and symptom identification scale. Basis-32 application guide: Community norms and clinical benchmarks.* The McLean Hospital Corporation.

Measures of Family Burden

Social Behaviour Assessment Schedule, SBAS

The SBAS assesses objective burden and distress of relatives. It was used in the study by Dean, et al., (1993).

Platt, S., Weyman, A. Hirsch, S., & Hewett, S. (1980). The social behavioural asessessment schedule (SBAS). Rationale, contents, scoring, and reliability of a new interview schedule. *Social Psychology, 15,* 43–55.

Family Burden Scale

This scale includes 31 items measuring objective and subjective burden and subjective stress. It was used in the study by Burns, Beadsmoore, et al. (1993).

Paykel, E. S., Morgen, S. P., & Griffiths, J. H. (1982). Community psychiatric nursing for neurotic patients—A controlled trial. *British Journal of Psychiatry, 140,* 573–581.

Family Evaluation Form—Adapted FEF

Fenton, et al., (1982), used a 61-item instrument developed from the FEF, which reflects different aspects of the psychological, social, and economic burden caused by the patient's illness.

Spitzer, R. L. Gibbon, M., & Endicott, J. (1971). *Family evaluation form.* New York State Psychiatric Institute.

CBS-R

Bergman, K., & Wistedt, R. (1985). CBS-R: *A new scale for burden on relatives of schizophrenic patients and effects of education.* Unpublished report, Dandevyd Sweden, Karolinska Institute.

Measures of Satisfaction—patients and families

Client Satisfaction Questionaire, CSQ

The CSW is an 8-item, patient-rated scale measuring patients' satisfaction with different aspects of their care (quality of service, amount of support received, needs and preferences). Each item is measured on a scale of 1 to 4. Higher scores indicate greater satisfaction. It has been widely used; e.g., by Minghella, et al. (1998), and Muijen, et al. (1992).

Larsen, D. L., Atkinson, C. C., Hargreaves, W. A., & Nguyen, T. D. (1979). Assessment of client/patient satisfaction: Development of a general scale. *Evaluation and Program Planning, 2,* 197–207.

Consumer Satisfaction Scale

The Consumer Satisfaction Scale contains 37 items eliciting assessments of quality, appropriateness and accessibility of care.

Paykel, E. S. &Griffiths, J. H. (1983) Satisfaction with treatment. In E. S. Paykel, & J. H. Griffiths (Eds.), *Community psychiatric nursing for neurotic patients* (pp. 46–53). London: Royal College of Nursing.

Treatment Comparison Questionnaire

This questionaire elicits patient and family members' opinions of home treatment compared to hospital treatment and was used in a study by Wasylenki, et al. (1997).

Wasylenki, D., Gehrs, M., Goering, P., & Toner, B. (1997). A home based program of treatment of acute psychosis. *Community Mental Health Journal, 33,* 151–162.

Measuring Costs

Client Services Receipt Inventory

The Client Services Receipt Inventory records retrospective information on community supports. It was used in the study by Connolly, Knapp, Beecham, et al. (1994).

Beecham, J. C., Knapp, M. R. J. (1992). Costing psychiatric options. In G. Thornicroft, C. Brewin, & J. Wing (Eds.), *Measuring mental health needs,* (pp. 170–190). Oxford: Oxford University Press.

Bibliography

Agus, D. (1991). *Proposed crisis system*. Baltimore Mental Health System.

Alexander, C., & Zealberg, J. J. (1999). Mobile crisis: moving emergency psychiatry out of the hospital setting. *New Directions for Mental Health Services, No. 82, summer 1999*, 93–96.

Allen, M. H., Forster, P., Zealberg, J., & Currier, G. (2002). American Psychiatric Association Task Force on Psychiatric Emergency Services: Report and recommendations regarding psychiatric emergency and crisis services. Retrieved website: http:// www.psych.org/downloads/EmergencyServicesFinal.pdf

Allen, M. (1999). Level 1 psychiatric emergency services: The tools of the crisis sector. *The Psychiatric Clinics of North America, 22*, 713–734.

Allness, D. J., & Knoedler, W. H. (1998). *The PACT model of community-based treatment for persons with severe and persistent mental illnesses: A manual for PACT start-up*. Arlington, VA: National Alliance for the Mentally Ill.

American Psychiatric Association. (1994). Practice guidelines for the treatment of patients with bipolar disorder. *American Journal of Psychiatry, 151* (Suppl. 12).

American Psychiatric Association. (1997). Practice guidelines for the treatment of patients with schizophrenia. *American Journal of Psychiatry, 154* (Suppl. 4).

American Psychiatric Association. (2000). Practice guidelines for the treatment of patients with major depressive disorder (revision). *American Journal of Psychiatry, 157* (Suppl. 4).

American Psychiatric Association. (2001). Practice guideline for the treatment of patients with borderline personality disorder. *American Journal of Psychiatry, 158* (Suppl. 10).

American Psychiatric Association (2002). Practice guidelines for the treatment of patients with bipolar disorder (revision). *American Journal of Psychiatry, 159* (Suppl. 4).

Arce, A. A., & Vergare, M. (1985). An overview of community residences as alternatives to hospitalization. *Psychiatric Clinics of North America, 8*, 423–437.

Audini, B., Marks, I. M., Lawrence, R. E., Connolly, J., & Watts, V. (1994). Home based versus out-patient/in-patient care for people with serious mental illnesses. Phase II of a controlled study. *British Journal of Psychiatry, 165*, 204–210.

Baron, S. T., Agus, D., Osher, F., & Brown, D. (1998). The city of Baltimore, USA: The Baltimore experience. In D. Goldberg, & G. Thornicroft (Eds.) *mental health in our future cities.* (pp. 57–76). Psychology Press Hove, East Sussex, U.K.

Barrow, S. M., Hellman, F., Lovell, A. M., Plapinger, J. D., & Struening, E. L. (1991). Evaluating outreach services: Lessons from a study of five programs. *New Directions for Mental Health Services*, No. 52, pp. 29–44.

Bazelon Center for Mental Health Law. Olmstead v. L.C. Retrieved March 23, 2003, from http://www.bazelon.org/issues/communitybased/olmstead/index.htm

Bengelsdorf, H., & Alden, D. C. (1987). A mobile crisis unit in the psychiatric emergency room. *Hospital and Community Psychiatry, 38,* 662–665.

Bengelsdorf, H., Levy, L. E., Emerson, R. L., & Barile, F. A. (1984). A crisis triage rating scale: Brief dispositional assessment of patients at risk of hospitalization. *The Journal of Nervous and Mental Diseases, 172,* 424–430.

Bennet, R. (1995). Family placement schemes as an alternative to short term hospitalization. In M. Phelan, G. Strathdee, & G. Thornicroft (Eds.), *Emergency mental health services in the community* (pp. 259–275). Cambrige University Press.

Birchwood, M. (2002). *Strategies for early intervention in psychosis.* Paper presented at Facing the challenges of early intervention in psychosis conference Prevention & Early Intervention Psychosis Program, University of Western Ontario, London.

Braun, P., Kochansky, G., Shapiro, R., Greenberg, S., Gudeman, J., Johnson, S., et al. (1981). Overview: Deinstitutionalization of psychiatric patients, a critical review of outcome studies. *American Journal of Psychiatry, 138,* 738–749.

Breakey, W. R. (1996). Inpatient services. In W. R. Breakey (Ed.), *Integrated mental health services* (pp. 264–275) New York: Oxford University Press.

Brent, D. A. (2001). Achieving better outcomes in early onset depression. In M. Weissman (Ed). *Treatment of depression.* (pp. 175–196). Washington, DC: American Psychiatric Press.

Breslow, R. (2001). Emergency psychiatric services. In G. Thornicroft, G., & Szmukler (Eds). *Textbook of community psychiatry.* (pp. 265–276). Oxford University Press.

Brimblecombe, N. (2001a). Assessment in crisis/home treatment services. In N. Brimblecombe, (Ed.), *Acute mental health care in the community: Intensive home treatment* (pp. 78–101) London: Whurr Publishers.

Brimblecombe, N. (2001b). Developing intensive home treatment services: Problems and issues. In N. Brimblecombe (Ed.), *Acute mental health care in the community: Intensive home treatment* (pp. 187–210). London: Whurr Publishers, and personal communication April 21, 2002.

Brimblecombe, N., & O'Sullivan, G. H. (1999). Diagnosis, assessments, and admissions from a community treatment team. *Psychiatric Bulletin, 23,* 72–74.

Brockington, I. F. (1996). *Motherhood and mental health.* Oxford University Press

Brook, B. D. (1973). Crisis hostel: An alternative to psychiatric hospitalization for emergency patients. *Hospital and Community Psychiatry, 24,* 621–623.

Burns, T. (1990). The evaluation of a home-based treatment approach in acute psychiatry. In D. Goldberg & D. Tantum (Ed.), *The public health impact of mental disorder.* (pp. 197–205). Lewiston, NY and personal communication, August 24, 1998: Hogrefe & Huber.

Burns, T., Beadsmoore, A., Bhat, A. V., Oliver, A., & Mathers, C. (1993). A controlled trial of home-based acute psychiatric services 1: Clinical and social outcome. *British Journal of Psychiatry, 163,* 49–54.

Burns, T., Knapp, M., Catty, J., Healey, A., Henderson, J., Watt, H., et al. (2001). Home treatment for mental health problems: A systemic review. *Health Technology Assessment, 5,* 15.

Burns, T., Raftery, J., Beadsmoore, A., McGuigan, S. & Dickson, M. (1993). A controlled trial of home-based acute psychiatric services. II: Treatment patterns and costs. *British Journal of Psychiatry, 163,* 55–61.

Burti, L. (2001). Italian psychiatric reform 20 plus years after. *Acta Psychiatrica Scandinavica, 104* (Suppl. 410), 41–45.

Canadian Psychiatric Association (1998). Canadian clinical practice guidelines for the treatment of schizophrenia (revised). *Canadian Journal of Psychiatry, 43* (Suppl. 2).

Canadian Psychiatric Association and the Canadian Network for Mood and Anxiety Treatments. (2001). Clinical guidelines for the treatment of depressive disorders. *Canadian Journal of Psychiatry, 46* (Suppl. 1).

Carse, J., Panton, N. E., & Watt, A. A. (1958). A district mental health service. The Worthing experiment. *Lancet, 174,* 39–41.

Catty, J., Burns, T., & Knapp, M. (2001). Evaluating innovative mental health services: Lessons from a systematic review of home treatment. *Eurohealth, 8,* 34–36.

Chiu, T. L., & Primeau, C. (1991). A psychiatric mobile crisis unit in New York City: Description and assessment, with implications for mental health care in the 1990's. *The International Journal of Social Psychiatry, 37,* 251–258.

Christie, W. R. (1985). The moment of admission. *Psychiatric Clinics of North America, 8,* 411–421.

Coates, D. B. (1982) [Review of the book *Home and hospital psychiatric treatment*] *Canadian Journal of Psychiatry, 27,* 436–437.

Coates, D. B., Kendell, L. M., & MacCurdy, M. A. (1976). Evaluating hospital and home treatment for psychiatric patients. *Canada's Mental Health, 24,* 28–33.

Collins English dictionary. (1991). HarperCollins Publishers. Glasgow. U.K.

Commonwealth of Australia. (1992). *National Mental Health Policy.* Retrieved January 18, 2004, from http://www.mmha.org.au/Policy/NationalMental HealthPolicy

Connolly, J., Marks Il, Lawrence, R., McNamee, G., & Muijen, M. (1996). Observations from community care for serious mental illness during a controlled study. *Psychiatric Bulletin, 20,* 3–7.

Creed, F. (1995) Acute day hospital care. In G. Strathdee & M. Phelan (Ed.), *Emergency mental health services in the community.* (pp. 298–319) Cambridge University Press.

Creed, F., Black, D., & Anthony, P. (1990). Randomized controlled trial of day patient versus in-patient psychiatric treatment. *British Medical Journal, 300,* 1033–1037.

Dawson, D. & MacMillan, H. L. (1993). *Relationship management of the borderline patient.* New York: Brunner-Mazel.

Dean, C. (1993). The development of a local service in Birmingham. In C. Dean, & H. Freeman (Eds.), *Community mental health care: international perspectives on making it happen.* Washington, DC: Gaskell.

Dean, C., & Gadd, E. M. (1990). Home treatment for acute psychiatric illness. *British Medical Journal, 301,* 1021–1023.

Dean, C., Phillips, J., Gadd, E. M., Joseph, M., & England, S. (1993). Comparison of community based service with hospital based service for people with acute severe psychiatric illness. *British Medical Journal, 307,* 473–476.

Department of Health. (1999). *A national service framework for mental health.* Retrieved January 12, 2003, from http://www.nelh.nhs.uk/nsf/mental health/default.htm

Department of Health. (2000). *The NHS plan.* Retrieved January 12, 2003, from http://www.nhs.uk/nationalplan

Department of Health. (2001). *Mental health policy implementation guide.* Retrieved January 12, 2003, from http://www.doh.gov.uk/mentalhealth/implementationguide.htm

Department of Health, NSW. (1987). *Guidelines for psychiatric crisis teams and extended hours services.* State Health Publication No. (RIU) 87–1074 ISBN 0-7305-3250-X, Sydney, Australia.

Driver, D. (2001). Sask. mental patients' hospital stays too long. *Medical Post.*

Dunn, L. M. (2001). Mental Health Act assessments: Does a home treatment team make a difference? In N. Brimblecombe (Ed.), *Acute mental health care in the community: Intensive home treatment* (pp. 102–121). London. Whurr Publishers.

Fassler, D., Hanson-Myer, G. & Brenner, D.G.(1997). Home-based care. In L. I. Sederer, & A. J. Rothschild (Eds.), *Acute care psychiatry: diagnosis and treatment.* (pp. 391–414). Baltimore: Williams & Wilkins.

Fenton, F. R., Tessier, L., & Struening, E. L. (1982). *Home and hospital psychiatric treatment.* University of Pittsburgh Press.

Fink, M., Abrams, R., Bailine, S., & Jaffe, R. (1996). Ambulatory electroconvulsive therapy: Report of a task force of the association for convulsive therapy. *Convulsive Therapy, 12,* 42–55.

Fisher, W. E., Geller, J. L., & Wirth-Cauchon, J. (1990). Empirically assessing the impact of mobile crisis capacity on state hospital admissions. *Community Mental Health Journal, 26,* 245–252.

Fitzgerald, P., & Kulkarni, J., (1998). Home-oriented management programme for people with early psychosis. *British Journal of Psychiatry, 172* (Suppl. 33), 39–44.

Ford, R., Minghella, E., Chalmers, C., Hoult, J., Raftery, J., & Muijen, M. (2001). Cost consequences of home-based and in-patient-based acute psychiatric treatment: Results of an implementation study. *Journal of Mental Health, 10,* 467–476.

Forster P., & King, J. (1994). Definitive treatment of patients with serious mental disorders in an emergency service, part 1. *Hospital and Community Psychiatry, 45,* 867–869.

Frances, A., Docherty, J. P., & Kahn, D.A. (1996). The expert consensus guideline series: Treatment of bipolar disorder. *The Journal of Clinical Psychiatry, 57*

(Suppl. 12A).

Geller, J. L., Fisher, W. H., & McDermeit, M. (1995). A national survey of mobile crisis services and their evaluation. *Psychiatric Services, 46,* 893–897.

Friedman, T. T., Becke, A., & Weiner, L. (1964). The psychiatric home treatment service: Preliminary report of five years of clinical experience. *American Journal of Psychiatry,* 120, 782–788.

Gillig, P. M. (1995). The spectrum of mobile outreach and it's role in the emergency service. *New directions for mental health services,67.*

Godfrey, M., & Townsend, J. (1995). *Intensive home treatment team: Users' and carers' experiences of the service and the outcomes of care. Working Paper 1.* University of Leeds.

Goodacre, R. H., Coles, E. M. & MacCurdy, E. A., Coates, D. B., & Kendall, L. M. (1975). Hospitalization and hospital bed replacement. *Canadian Journal of Psychiatry, 20,* 7–14.

Grad, J., & Sainsbury, P. (1966). Evaluating the community psychiatric service in Chichester: Results. In E. M. Gruenberg (Ed.), *Evaluating the effectiveness of community mental health services.* (pp. 246–278). New York: Milbank Memorial Fund.

Grad, J., & Sainsbury, P. (1968). The effects that patients have on their families in community care and a control psychiatric service: A two year follow up. *British Journal of Psychiatry, 114,* 265–278.

Greenberger, D. & Padesky, C. A. (1995). *Mind over mood: Change how you feel by changing the way you think.* New York: The Guildford Press.

Gunderson, J. G. (2001). *Borderline personality disorder: a clinical guide.* Washington DC: American Psychiatric Press.

Guo, S., Biegel, D. E., Johnsen, J. A. & Dyches, H. (2001). Assessing the impact of community-based mobile crisis services on preventing hospitalization. *Psychiatric Services, 52,* 223–228.

Harrison, J., Alam, N., & Marshall, J. (2001). Home or away: Which patients are suitable for a psychiatric home treatment service? *Psychiatric Bulletin, 25,* 310–313.

Harrison, J., Poynton, A., Marshall, J., Gater, R., & Creed, F. (1999). Open all hours: Extending the role of the psychiatric day hospital. *Psychiatric Bulletin, 23,* 400–404.

Hibbard, R., Bahrey, F., Guinhawa, D., & Stevenson, D. (1998). *Intensive Home Treatment of the Acutely Mentally Ill: Experience of a General Hospital Based team.* Paper presented at the meeting of the Canadian Psychiatric Association, Halifax, Nova Scotia.

Hoge, M., Davidson, L., Hill, W. L., Turner, V. E., & Ameli, R. (1992). The promise of partial hospitalization: A reassessment. *Hospital and Community Psychiatry, 43,* 345–354.

Hoult, J. (1986). Community care of the acutely mentally ill. *British Journal of Psychiatry, 149,* 137–144.

Hoult, J. (1999 September). How to Set Up a Home Treatment Service. Paper presented at the Good Practices in Home Treatment conference. University of Wolverhampton, U.K. and personal communication, April 23, 2003.

Hoult, J., & Reynolds, I., (1984). Schizophrenia: a comparitive trial of community oriented and hospital oriented care. *Acta Psychiatrica Scandinavica, 69,* 359–372.

Hoult, J., Rosen, A., & Reynolds, I. (1984). Community oriented treatment compared to psychiatric hospital oriented treatment. *Social Science and Medicine, 18,* 1005–1010.

IRIS. *The initiative to reduce the impact of schizophrenia.* Retrieved May 20, 2002, from http://iris-initiative.org.uk

Johnson, S., Hoult, J., Nolan, F., Sandor, A., Pilling, S., Bebbington, P. et al. (2001). Evaluation of the South Islington crisis resolution team. Unpublished manuscript.

Joy, C. B., Adams, C. E. & Rice, K. (2001). Crisis intervention for people with severe mental illnesses (Cochrane Review). *The Cochrane Library.*

Kennedy, P. (2003). CHRT for rural areas: The Monaghan story. In *More than the sum of all the parts: Improving the whole system with crisis resolution and home treatment* (pp. 21–23). Northern Centre for Mental Health Publications. Retrieved March 14, 2004, from http://www.scmh.org.uk/wbm23.ns4/weblaunch/launchme

Kennedy, P., & Smyth, M. (2003). CHRT really works—What's stopping you? In *More than the sum of all the parts: Improving the whole system with crisis resolution and home treatment* (pp. 24–28). Northern Centre for Mental Health Publications. Retrieved March 14, 2004, from http://www.scmh.org.uk/wbm23.ns4/weblaunch/launchme

Kessler, K. A. (1994). R. K. Schreter, (Ed.), *Allies and adversaries: The impact of managed care on mental health services* (pp. 31–41). Washington DC: American Psychiatric Press.

Kluiter, H. (1997). Inpatient treatment and care arrangements to replace or avoid it—Searching for an evidence-based balance. *Current Opinion in Psychiatry, 10,* 160–167.

Knapp, M., Beecham, J., Koutsogeorgopoulo, V., Hallam, A., Fenyo, A., Marks, I. M., et al. (1994). Service use and costs of home-based versus hospital-based care for people with serious mental illness. *British Journal of Psychiatry, 165,* 195–203.

Knapp, M., Marks, I. M., Wolstenholme, J., Beecham, J., Aston. J., Audini, B., Connolly, J. & Watts, V. (1998). Home-based versus hopital-based care for serious mental illness. Controlled cost-effectiveness study over four years. *British Journal of Psychiatry, 172,* 506–512.

Kwakwa, J. (1995). Alternatives to hospital based mental health care. *Nursing Times, 23,* 38–39.

Langsley, D. G., Flomenhaft, K., & Machotka, P. (1969). Follow-up evaluation of family crisis therapy. *American Journal of Orthopsychiatry, 39,* 753–759.

Langsley, D. G., Machotka, P., & Flomenhaft,K.(1971). Avoiding mental hospital admission: A follow-up study. *American Journal of Psychiatry, 127,* 1391–1394.

Langsley, D. G., Pittman, F. S., & Machotka, P. (1968). Family crisis therapy, results and implications. *Family Process, 7,* 145–158.

Leaman, K. (1987). A hospital alternative for patients in crisis. *Hospital and Community Psychiaty, 38*, 1221–1223.

Linehan, M. M., (1993). *Skills training manual for treating borderline personality disorder.* New York: The Guilford Press.

Links, P. S. (1998). Developing effective services for patients with personality disorders. *Canadian Journal of Psychiatry, 43*, 251–259.

Lipton, L. (2001). Few safeguards govern elimination of psychiatric beds. *Psychiatric News.*

Malla, A. K. (2002). *An Overview of Early Intervention in Psychosis: The PEPP Project.* Paper presented at "Facing the challenges of early intervention in psychosis conference" University of Western Ontario, London.

Malla, A. K., & Norman, R. M. G. (2002). Early intervention in schizophrenia and related disorders: advantages and pitfalls. *Current Opinion in Psychiatry, 15*, 17–23.

Marks, I. M., Connolly, J., Audini, B., & Muijen, M. (1994). Service use and costs of home-based versus hospital-based care for people with serious mental illness. *British Journal of Psychiatry, 165*, 195–203.

Marks, I. M., Connolly, J., Muijen, M., Audini, B., McNamee, G., & Lawrence, R. E. (1994). Home-based versus hospital-based care for people with serious mental illness. *British Journal of Psychiatry, 165*, 179–194.

Marshall, J., & Harrison, J. (1998). Opting to stay home. *Mental Health Care, 11*, 344–346.

McEvoy, J. P., Schleifler, P. L., & Frances, A. (1999). The expert consensus guidelines series: Treatment of schizophrenia. *The Journal of Clinical Psychiatry, 60*, (Suppl. 11).

McGlynn, P., & Smyth, M. (1998). The home treatment team: Making it happen. The Sainsbury Centre for Mental Health/North Birmingham Mental Health Trust, London.

McGorry, P. D., Chanen, A., & McCarthy, E. (1991). Post-traumatic stress disorder following recent-onset psychosis—An unrecognized syndrome. *Journal of Mental and Nervous Disease, 197*, 253–258.

Melton, G. B. (1997). Why don't the knuckleheads use common sense? In S. W. Henggeler, & A. B. Santos (Eds.) *Innovative approaches to difficult-to-treat populations.* (pp. 351–370). Washington DC: American Psychiatric Press Inc.

Mendel, W. M., & Rapport, S. (1969). Determinants of the decision for psychiatric hospitalisation. *Archives of General Psychiatry, 20*, 321–325.

Menninger, W. W. (1995). Role of the psychiatric hospital in the treatment of mental illness. In H. I. Kaplan, & B. J. Sadock (Eds.), *Comprehensive textbook of psychiatry* (pp. 2690–2696). Philadelphia: Williams & Wilkins.

Merson, S., Tyrer, P., Onyett, S., Lack, S., Birkett, P., Lynch, S., et al. (1992). Early intervention in psychiatric emergencies: A controlled clinical trial. *The Lancet, 339*, 1311–1314.

Minghella, E., Ford, R., Freeman, T., Hoult, J., McGlynn, P., & O'Halloran, P. (1998). *Open all hours: 24-hour response for people with mental health emergencies.* London: The Sainsbury Centre for Mental Health.

Moy, S., & Pigott, H. E. (1998). Home based services. In R. K. Schreter, S. S. Scharfstein, & C.A. Schreter (Eds.), *Managing care, not dollars—The contin-*

uum of mental health services (pp. 27–41). Washington, DC: American Psychiatric Press.

Muijen, M., Marks, I. M., Connolly, J., & Audini, B. (1992). Home based care and standard hospital care for patients with severe mental illness: A randomised controlled trial. *British Medical Journal, 304,* 749–754.

Niemiec, S. Personal Communication, May 3, 2003.

Oates, M. (1988). The development of an integrated community—oriented service for severe postnatal mental illness. In R. Kumar, & I. F. Brockington (Eds.), *Motherhood and mental illness: causes and consequences* (pp. 133–158). London: Wright.

Ontario Ministry of Health. (1988). *Building community support for people: A plan for mental health in Ontario.* Ontario: Queen's Printer.

Ontario Ministry of Health. (1993). *Putting people first.* Ontario: Queen's Printer.

Orme, S. (2001). Intensive home treatment services: The current position. In N. Brimblecombe (Ed.), *Acute mental health care in the community: Intensive home treatment.* (pp. 29–53). London: Whurr Publishers.

Pai, S., & Kapur, R. L. (1982). Impact of treatment intervention on the relationship between dimensions of clinical psychopathology, social dysfunction and burden on the family of psychiatric patients. *Psychological Medicine, 12,* 651–658.

Paris, J. (2002). Chronic suicidality among patients with borderline personality disorder. *Psychiatric Services,53,* 738–742.

Pasamanick, B., Scarpitti, F., & Dinitz, S. (1967). *Schizophrenics in the community. An experimental study in the prevention of hospitalization.* New York: Appleton-Century-Crofts.

Perry. S., Frances, A., & Clarkin, J. (1990). *A DSM-III-R casebook of treatment selection.* New York: Brunner/Mazel.

Pigott, H. E., & Trott, L. (1993). Translating research into practice: the implementation of an in-home crisis intervention triage and treatment service in the private sector. *American Journal of Medical Quality, 8,* 138–144.

Piper, W. E., Rosie, J. S., Azim, H. F. A., & Joyce, A. S. (1993). A randomized trial of psychiatric day treatment for patients with affective and personality disorders, *Hospital and Community Psychiatry, 44,* 757–763.

Polak, P. R., & Kirby, M. W. (1976). A model to replace psychiatric hospitals. *The Journal of Nervous and Mental Disease, 162,* 13–22.

Polak, P. R., Kirby, M. W., & Deitchman, W.S. (1995). Treating acutely psychotic patients in private homes. In R. Warner (Ed.), *Alternatives to the hospital for acute psychiatric treatment.* (pp. 213–233). Washington, DC: American Psychiatric Press.

Reding, G. R., & Raphelson, M. (1995). Around-the-clock mobile psychiatric crisis intervention: Another effective alternative to psychiatric hospitalization. *Community Mental Health Journal, 31,* 179–190.

Romanow, R. (2002*). Building on values: The future of health care in Canada.* Retrieved October 4, 2003, from http://cbc.ca/healthcare/final_report.pdf

Rush, A. J. (2001). Practice guidelines and algorithms. In M. Weissman (Ed.), *Treatment of Depression* (pp. 213–242) Washington, DC: American Psychiatric Press.

Sainsbury Centre for Mental Health. (2001). *Mental Health Topics: Crisis Resolution.* Retrieved May 1, 2002, from http://www.scmh.org.uk/wbm.23.ns4/weblaunch/launchme

Santos, A. B. (1997). Guest editor's introduction—ACT now! *Administration and Policy in Mental Health, 25,* 101–104.

Schene, A. (2001). Partial hospitalization. In G. Thornicroft, & G. Szmukler (Eds.), *Textbook of Community Psychiatry* (pp. 283–294). Oxford University Press.

Schreter, R. K. (1997). Psychiatric care for the 21st century. *Psychiatric Services, 48,* 1245–1246.

Segal, S. P., Egley, L. & Watson, M. A., (1995). Factors in the quality of patient evaluations in general hospital psychiatric emergency services. *Psychiatric Services, 46,* 1144–1148.

Segal, S. P., Watson, M. A., & Akutsu, P. D., (1996). Quality of care and use of less restrictive alternatives in the psychiatric emergency service. *Psychiatric Services, 47,* 623–627.

Sledge, W. H., Tebes, J., Rakfeldt, J., Davidson, L., Lyons, L., & Druss, B. (1996). Day hospital/crisis respite care versus inpatient care, part I: Clinical outcomes. *American Journal of Psychiatry, 153,* 1065–1072.

Sledge, W. H., Tebes, J., Wolff, N. & Helminiak (1996). Day hospital/crisis respite care, part II: Service utilization and costs. *American Journal of Psychiatry, 153,* 1074–1083.

Smyth, M. G. (1999 September). Welcome address presented at Good Practices in Home Treatment Conference. University of Wolverhampton,U.K.

Smyth, M. G., & Hoult, J. (2000). The home treatment enigma. *British Medical Journal, 320,* 305–309.

Spencer, E., Birchwood, M., & McGovern (2001). Management of first-episode psychosis. *Advances in Psychiatric Treatment, 7,* 133–142.

Stein, L. I., & Santos, A. B. (1998). *Assertive community treatment of persons with severe mental illness.* New York, W. W. Norton.

Stein, L. I., & Test, M. A. (1978). An alternative to mental hospital treatment. In L. I. Stein, & M.A. Test (Eds.), *Alternatives to mental hospital treatment* (pp. 43–55). New York: Plenum Press.

Stein, L. I. & Test, M. A. (1980). Alternatives to mental hospital treatment.I. Conceptual model, treatment program and clinical evaluation. *Archives of General Psychiatry, 37,* 392–397.

Strauss, J. S., & Carpenter, W, T. (1974). Prediction of outcome in schizophrenia. Part II. *Archives of General Psychiatry, 37,* 37–42.

Stroul, B. A. (1988). Residential crisis services: a review. *Hospital and Community Psychiatry, 39,* 1095–1099.

Surgeon General. (1999). Mental health: A report of the surgeon general. Retrieved October 4, 2003, from http://www.surgeongeneral.gov/library/mentalhealth

Szmukler, G., & Holloway, F. (2001). In-patient treatment. In G. Thornicroft, & Szmukler (Eds.), *Textbook of community psychiatry.* (pp. 265–276). Oxford University Press, Oxford.

Test, M. A., & Stein, L. I. (1980). Alternative to mental hospital treatment III. Social cost. *Archives of General Psychiatry, 37,* 409–412.

Thornicroft, G. H., & Bebbington, P. (1989). Deinstitutionalisation—from hospital closure to service development. *British Journal of Psychiatry, 155,* 739–753.

Thornicroft, G., & Tansella, M. (1999). *The mental health matrix: A manual to improve services.* Cambridge University Press.

Thornicroft, G., & Tansella, M. (2001). The planning process for mental health services. In G. Thornicroft, & G. Szmukler (Eds.), *Textbook of community psychiatry.* (pp. 179–192). Oxford University Press.

Torrey, W. C., Drake R. E., Dixon, L., Burns, B. J., Flynn, L., & Rush, A. J. (2001) Implementing evidence-based practices for persons with severe mental illnesses. *Psychiatric Services, 52,* 45–50.

Tufnell, G., Bouras, N., Watson, J. P., & Brough, D. I. (1985). Home assessment and treatment in a community psychaiatric service. *Acta Psychiatrica Scandinavica, 72,* 20–28.

Tyrer, P., (1995). Maintaining an emergency service. In M. Phelan, G. Strathdee, & G. Thornicroft (Eds.), *Emergency mental health services in the community* (pp. 197–212). Cambridge University Press.

Tyrer, P., & Merson, S. (1994). The effect of personality disorder on clinical outcome, social networks, and adjustment: a controlled clinical trial of psychiatric emergencies. *Psychological Medicine, 24,* 731–740.

Warner, R. (1995). *Alternatives to the hospital for acute psychiatric treatment.* Washington, DC: American Psychiatric Press.

Wasylenki, D, Gehrs, M., Goering, P., & Toner, B. (1997). A home-based program for the treatment of acute psychosis. *Community Mental Health Journal, 33,* 151–162.

Weisbrod, B. A., Test, M. A., & Stein, L. I. (1980). Alternative to mental hospital treatment II. Economic benefit-cost analysis. *Archives of General Psychiatry, 37,* 400–405.

Weisman, G. K. (1985). Crisis oriented residential treatment as an alternative to hospitalization. *Hospital and Community Psychiatry, 36,* 1302–1305.

Williams, L. (1998). A "classic" case of borderline personality disorder. *Psychiatric Services, 49,* 173–174.

Wood, H., & Carr, S. (1998). Designing local mental health services. In H. Wood, & S. Carr (Eds.) *Locality services in mental health.* The Sainsbury Centre for Mental Health.

Wynne, L. C. (1978). *The nature of schizophrenia: New approach to research and treatment.* New York: John Wiley.

Zealberg, J. J., Christie, S. D., Puckett, J. A., McAlhany & Durban, M. (1992). A mobile crisis program: Collaboration between emergency psychiatric services and police. *Hospital Community Psychiatry, 43,* 612–615.

Zealberg, J. J. & Santos, A. B. (1996). *Comprehensive emergency mental health care.* New York: W. W. Norton.

Zealberg, J. J., Santos, A. B., & Fisher, R. K. (1993). Benefits of mobile crisis programs. *Hospital and Community Psychiatry, 44,* 16–17.

Zwerling, I., & Wilder, J. F. (1964). An evaluation of the applicability of the day hospital in treatment of acutely disturbed patients. *Israel Journal of Psychiatry and Related Disciplines, 2,* 162–185.

Index

287